Get FIT Stay FIT

WILLIAM E. PRENTICE, PH.D., P.T., A.T.C.

Professor, Coordinator of the Sports Medicine Specialization,
Department of Exercise, and Sports Science
The University of North Carolina
Chapel Hill, North Carolina

Fourth Edition

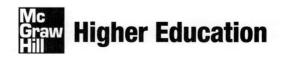

Mc Graw Hill Higher Education

Boston   Burr Ridge, IL   Dubuque, IA   Madison, WI   New York
San Francisco   St. Louis   Bangkok   Bogotá   Caracas   Kuala Lumpur
Lisbon   London   Madrid   Mexico City   Milan   Montreal   New Delhi
Santiago   Seoul   Singapore   Sydney   Taipei   Toronto

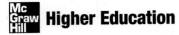

Higher Education

GET FIT, STAY FIT, FOURTH EDITION

Published by McGraw-Hill, a business unit of The McGraw-Hill Companies, Inc., 1221 Avenue of the Americas, New York, NY, 10020. Copyright © 2007, 2004, 2001, 1996 by The McGraw-Hill Companies, Inc. All rights reserved. No part of this publication may be reproduced or distributed in any form or by any means, or stored in a database or retrieval system, without the prior written consent of The McGraw-Hill Companies, Inc., including, but not limited to, in any network or other electronic storage or transmission, or broadcast for distance learning.

Some ancillaries, including electronic and print components, may not be available to customers outside the United States.

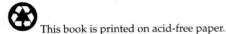 This book is printed on acid-free paper.

1 2 3 4 5 6 7 8 9 0 DOC/DOC 0 9 8 7 6

ISBN-13: 978-0-07-304685-3
ISBN-10: 0-07-304685-X

Vice President and Editor-in-Chief: *Emily Barrosse*
Publisher: *William R. Glass*
Senior Sponsoring Editor: *Christopher C. Johnson*
Director of Development: *Kathleen Engelberg*
Developmental Editor: *Gary O'Brien, Van Brien & Associates*
Executive Marketing Manager: *Pamela S. Cooper*
Managing Editor: *Jean Dal Porto*
Project Manager: *Meghan Durko*
Art Director: *Jeanne Schreiber*
Lead Designer: *Gino Cieslik*
Photo Research Coordinator: *Natalia C. Peschiera*
Cover Designer: *Gino Cieslik*
Cover Credit: *© James R. Wvinner/Workbook Stock/Getty Images*
Media Producer: *Michele Borrelli*
Production Supervisor: *Janean A. Utley*
Composition: *10/12 Palatino, by GTS, New Delhi, India Campus*
Printing: *#45 New Era Matte Plus., R.R. Donnelley & Sons*

Photo Credits: **Page 7:** (top right) © Chris Falkenstein/Getty Images; **9:** (right) © Royalty-Free/CORBIS; **76:** (left to right) © Getty Images, © Ryan McVay/Getty Images; **78:** © Karl Weatherly/Getty Images; **79:** (both) © Royalty-Free/CORBIS.

Library of Congress Cataloging-in-Publication Data

Prentice, William E.
    Get fit, stay fit/William E. Prentice.—4th ed.
        p. cm.
    Includes bibliographical references and index.
    ISBN-13: 978-0-07-304685-3 (pbk. : alk. paper)
    ISBN-10: 0-07-304685-X (pbk. : alk. paper)
        1. Physical fitness. 2. Exercise. 3. Health. I. Title.
RA781.P67 2007
613.7—dc22   2005054124

The Internet addresses listed in the text were accurate at the time of publication. The inclusion of a Web site does not indicate an endorsement by the authors or McGraw-Hill, and McGraw-Hill does not guarantee the accuracy of the information presented at these sites.

www.mhhe.com

BRIEF CONTENTS

CONTENTS

PREFACE

If you believe what you hear, see, and read in the media, you would think that every person in America has become a "fitness junkie." It is true that millions of people exercise in some way, shape, or form on a somewhat consistent basis. But the fact is, that for the vast majority of Americans the thought of going out and "exercising" never even crosses their minds. Through TV and videos, on the Internet, in magazines or newspapers, our society is constantly bombarded by images that suggest the importance of being physically fit and healthy. It seems that people in your generation, in contrast to all the previous ones, are finally starting to realize that there really is a reason for living a healthy lifestyle and for incorporating regular exercise into that lifestyle.

Get Fit, Stay Fit is a text designed to tell you not only how you can go about getting yourself fit, but also why it is to your advantage to make fitness and exercise a regular part of your lifestyle. It begins by discussing the basic principles of fitness that apply to any type of exercise program, and then explains how being fit relates to a healthy lifestyle. Specific techniques and guidelines for developing cardiorespiratory endurance, for improving muscular strength and endurance, for increasing flexibility, and for maintaining appropriate body weight and composition are described in detail so that you can put together a personalized fitness program based on your individual needs. This book also provides recommendations and suggestions on selecting and using the exercise equipment available to help you get fit, as well as tips for making your exercise program as safe and free of injury as possible.

FEATURES

- *Practical application chapters are dedicated to starting your own fitness program (3), practicing safe fitness (9), and becoming a wise consumer (10). These chapters cut through the confusion and provide essential information on how to start up, equip yourself, and safely execute an individual fitness program.*
- *Special boxes—Fit Lists, Health Links, and Safe Tips—highlight, summarize, and provide quick reference to important information.*
- *Lab Activities assist in evaluating a number of personal measures of fitness as well as providing guidelines for increased health.*
- *Key terms are in color and are defined in boxes to help build a working vocabulary of concepts, terms, and principles necessary for understanding, beginning, and maintaining any fitness program.*
- *Chapter pedagogy also includes chapter objectives, key terms, definition boxes, bulleted summaries, and suggested readings to enhance the learning process.*
- *All exercise safety information and illustrations have been updated to provide proper fitness techniques for a safe and effective fitness program.*

- *Each chapter contains an expanded list of reviewed Web sites relevant to the chapter topic. Using the power of the World Wide Web as a resource, students will be able to obtain further information to take their studies beyond the classroom.*
- *An updated and expanded list of references provides a significant resource for students as well as instructors for further study of key issues and topics.*
- *The Appendix includes an extensive Food Composition Table that provides the nutritive value of commonly used foods.*

NEW TO THIS EDITION

CHAPTER 1

- *Added statistics on participation in physical activity in the United States*
- *Expanded information on the physical benefits on various physiological systems of being physically active*
- *Expanded information on the psychological benefits of being physically active*
- *Added new Healthlink on the Healthy People 2010 objectives to improve health, fitness, and quality of life through daily physical activity*

CHAPTER 2

- *Added new information on hypertension*
- *Added new Healthlink on Stress and specific physical disorders*
- *Added new Fit List on suggestions for managing and coping with stress*

CHAPTER 3

- *Added diminishing returns and reversibility to the basic principles of a fitness program*
- *Introduced the concept of the FITT principle*
- *Added information to the Activity Pyramid*

CHAPTER 4

- *Expanded information comparing aerobic and anaerobic activities*
- *Added information on heart rate monitors*
- *Discussed the FITT principle as it applies to improving cardiorespiratory endurance*
- *Added new information on calculating working heart rate*
- *Added new information on hiking and backpacking*
- *Added The Rockport Fitness Walking Test as a new Lab Activity*

CHAPTER 5

- *Emphasized that the FITT principle can be applied to strength training*
- *Clarified information on one repetition maximum*
- *Added new strength training worksheet for the lower extremity*
- *Added new information on functional strength training*
- *Expanded coverage of core stability training*
- *Increased the number of photos demonstrating a variety of strength training exercises*

CHAPTER 6

- *Expanded information on dynamic or ballistic stretching*
- *Added information on the controversy over whether stretching prevents injury or improves performance*

CHAPTER 7

- *Updated information on the 2005 U.S. Dietary Guidelines*
- *Added new Healthlink which details the new 2005 U.S. Dietary Guidelines*
- *Added information to MyPyramid which has replaced the old food pyramid*
- *Updated information on the nutritional label*
- *Added new nutritional information to the fast foods table*
- *Added new information on vegetarianism*

CHAPTER 8

- *Changed emphasis from controlling body weight to controlling body fat*
- *Emphasized the importance of body mass index*
- *Redefined lean body mass*
- *Added measurement of waist circumference as an estimate of overweight and obesity*
- *Added information on incorporating the FITT principle in burning body fat*
- *Updated the overview of diet plans table*
- *Added female athlete triad syndrome to eating disorders*

CHAPTER 9

- *Moved old Chapter 10 (Practicing Safe Fitness) to make it Chapter 9*
- *Added discussion of exercises for treating low back pain*

CHAPTER 10

- *Added new information and guidelines for selecting fitness shoes*

ANCILLARIES

COMPUTERIZED TEST BANK CD-ROM

Brownstone's Computerized Testing is the most flexible, powerful, easy-to-use electronic testing program available in higher education. The Diploma system (for Windows users) allows the test maker to create a print version, an online version (to be delivered to a computer lab), or an Internet version of each test. Diploma includes a built-in instructor gradebook, into which student rosters and files can be imported. The CD-ROM includes a separate testing program, Exam VI, for Macintosh users. The Computerized Test Bank for *Get Fit, Stay Fit* contains more than 300 multiple choice, true-false, fill-in, and short essay test questions for convenience in preparing examinations.

FITSOLVE II SOFTWARE

The Fitsolve software package enhances learning of health concepts by personalizing information and explaining the meaning of the results, rather than just grading students. It begins with a heart-disease risk questionnaire, followed by input of fitness test scores. Features include a score summary, heart-attack risk categorization, and assessment of health-related fitness. This product is available on diskette for Windows users.

HEALTHQUEST CD

The HealthQuest CD helps students explore their personal wellness behaviors using state-of-the-art interactive technology. Students will be able to assess their current health status, determine their risks, and explore options for positive lifestyle change. Tailored feedback gives a meaningful and individualized learning experience. Modules include the Wellboard (a health self-assessment); Stress Management; Fitness; Nutrition; Communicable Diseases; Cardiovascular Health; Cancer; Tobacco; Alcohol; and other Drugs.

LAB ACTIVITIES

ACKNOWLEDGMENTS

In revising *Get Fit, Stay Fit,* my editor Gary O'Brien has been instrumental in the development of the fourth edition, and has provided a great deal of help and support. The reviewers provided many constructive recommendations about content and organization. Their input and suggestions have been greatly appreciated and are reflected throughout the text. They include the following:

Megan D. Franks
North Harris College (TX)

Serena Reese
East Tennesse State University

Diana Mozen
Virginia State University

And finally, as always, this is for my wife Tena and our boys, Brian and Zach, who each day make my life more worthwhile.

By writing this book, I have tried to provide you with all the details you need to know about getting yourself fit and to stress the importance of developing a healthy lifestyle. But the bottom line is that, to get fit, you need to stop reading about it and start doing it. There is no better time than now!

William E. Prentice

CHAPTER 1

Getting Fit Why Should You Care?

Objectives

After completing this chapter, you should be able to do the following:

- Give several reasons why being fit should be important to you.
- Discuss the physical, social, and psychological benefits of being fit.
- List the component parts of physical fitness.
- Determine your reasons for wanting to become physically fit.

So, you've finally decided it's time to get fit. Why is that? People have many different reasons and motivations for beginning a physical activity program. Are you interested in improving your overall health and well-being? Are you concerned about the way you look to your friends? Are you tired of being a couch potato? Are you interested in fitness primarily because you are required to take this fitness class? Whatever your motivation happens to be, consistently engaging in physical activities can make you physically fit, and can have many positive benefits on your style of living.

WHY SHOULD YOU CARE ABOUT BEING PHYSICALLY ACTIVE?

Have you noticed that it is virtually impossible to go through a day without being exposed to something involving **physical fitness** or wellness? We eat, sleep, go to class, and some of us even try to include some form of exercise in our busy schedules. Fitness information comes from many sources. "Experts" give advice on television or radio and in magazines, books, and newspapers. Even our friends and classmates are willing to give opinions on the best

KEY TERMS

physical fitness	caloric intake
wellness	caloric expenditure
health-related components	skill-related components
cardiorespiratory endurance	speed
muscular strength	power
muscular endurance	neuromuscular coordination
flexibility	balance
body composition	agility
atherosclerosis	reaction time

1

ways to work out or on how to lose weight. Furthermore, the image of the attractive, healthy, physically active person is used to market everything—clothing, food, cosmetics, health care products, sports equipment, weight loss programs—the list goes on.

Our society is characterized by a fast-paced lifestyle, with obligations and stresses that affect our physical and emotional fitness. A common misconception is that daily living incorporates enough exercise to maintain an adequate level of fitness. Surveys indicate that virtually all adults believe that exercise is important to health and wellness and that regular physical activity is essential for themselves and for their children. Still, despite this increased interest in fitness and wellness, the U.S. Department of Health and Human Services reports that only 24 percent of adults participate in a minimum of 30 minutes of light-to-moderate exercise at least five times per week and only 12 percent are active seven times per week. Approximately 60 percent of the population is somewhat active but fails to achieve exercise intensity levels necessary for improving cardiorespiratory endurance.

Unfortunately, approximately 25 percent of American adults are essentially sedentary and do not engage in any type of leisure-time physical activity. Technological advances, such as the automobile, television, elevators, escalators, and moving sidewalks, eliminate the need for physical exertion and contribute to a sedentary lifestyle. The 1996 *Surgeon General's Report of Physical Activity and Health* reviewed mounting evidence that relates physical activity to reduced risks of a variety of health problems. This lack of regular physical activity has resulted in an epidemic of overweight and obesity.

Physical fitness is not entirely dependent on exercise. Choosing a healthy lifestyle also plays an important role. Physical fitness affects the total person, including intellect, emotional stability, physical conditioning, and stress levels. The road to achieving a healthy lifestyle includes proper medical care, eating the right foods in the right amounts, appropriate physical activity that is adapted to individual needs and physical limitations, satisfying work, healthy play and recreation, and proper amounts of rest and relaxation.

Engaging in physical activity to get yourself fit allows you to satisfy your needs regarding mental and emotional stability, social consciousness and adaptability, spirituality and morality, and physical health consistent with your heredity. This is the definition of the term **wellness.** Being fit means that the various systems of your body are healthy and function efficiently to enable you to engage in activities of daily living, as well as recreational pursuits and leisure activities, without unreasonable fatigue.

HEALTHY PEOPLE 2010 OBJECTIVES

Healthy People 2010 is a set of health objectives for the nation to achieve over the first decade of the new century. It can be used by many different people, states, communities, professional organizations, and others to help them develop programs to improve health. Healthy People

physical fitness: the various systems of your body are healthy and function efficiently to enable you to engage in activities of daily living, as well as recreational pursuits and leisure activities, without unreasonable fatigue

wellness: Satisfying your needs regarding mental and emotional stability, social consciousness and adaptability, spiritual and moral fiber, and physical health consistent with your heredity

2010 builds on initiatives pursued over the past 2 decades. The 1979 surgeon general's report, *Healthy People,* and *Healthy People 2000: National Health Promotion and Disease Prevention Objectives* both established national health objectives and served as the basis for the development of state and community plans. Like its predecessors, Healthy People 2010 was developed through a broad consultation process, built on the best scientific knowledge and designed to measure programs over time. The 28 focus areas of Healthy People 2010 were developed by leading federal agencies with the most relevant scientific expertise. Additionally, through a series of regional and national meetings and an interactive Web site, more than 11,000 public comments on the draft objectives were received. The Secretary's Council on National Health Promotion and Disease Prevention Objectives for 2010 also provided leadership and advice in the development of national health objectives.

The leading health indicators will be used to measure the health of the nation over the next 10 years. Each of the 10 leading health indicators has one or more objectives from Healthy People 2010 associated with it. As a group, the leading health indicators reflect the major health concerns in the United States at the beginning of the 21st century. The leading health indicators were selected on the basis of their ability to motivate action, the availability of data to measure progress, and their importance as public health issues. The leading health indicators are:

- Physical activity
- Overweight and obesity
- Tobacco use
- Substance abuse
- Responsible sexual behavior
- Mental health
- Injury and violence
- Environmental quality
- Immunization
- Access to health care

Healthy People 2010 offers a simple but powerful idea: Provide health objectives in a format that enables diverse groups to combine their efforts and work as a team. It is a road map to better health for all. The initiative has partners from all sectors. Health Link Box 1-1 lists the Healthy People 2010 objectives for improving health, fitness, and quality of life through physical activity.

THE PHYSICAL BENEFITS OF BEING PHYSICALLY ACTIVE

Human beings are designed to be active creatures. Although changes in civilization have resulted in a decrease in the amount of activity needed to accomplish the basic tasks associated with living, the human body has not changed. Therefore, it is important to be aware of the requirements for good health and recognize the importance of vigorous physical activity in your life. If you do not, your health, productivity, and effectiveness are likely to suffer. Health Link Box 1-2 summarizes 10 physical benefits associated with physical activity.

THE SOCIAL REWARDS OF BEING PHYSICALLY ACTIVE

If you are willing to participate in physical activities that help keep you fit, you create outlets, companionship, and feelings of belonging inherent in such activities. Physical activity can provide a great mechanism for exploring strategies to resolve conflicts, act fairly, comply with rules and fair play, and to generally develop a moral and ethical code of behavior. Participation in physical activity provides an opportunity for socializing. Physical fitness affects the entire person, and rich dividends come to the person who concentrates on the development of the body as well as the mind.

HEALTH LINK 1-1

Healthy People 2010 Objectives to Improve Health, Fitness, and Quality of Life Through Daily Physical Activity

- Reduce the proportion of adults who engage in no leisure-time physical activity.
- Increase the proportion of adults who engage regularly, preferably daily, in moderate physical activity for at least 30 minutes per day.
- Increase the proportion of adults who engage in vigorous physical activity that promotes the development and maintenance of cardiorespiratory fitness 3 or more days per week for 20 or more minutes per occasion.
- Increase the proportion of adults who perform physical activities that enhance and maintain muscular strength and endurance.
- Increase the proportion of adults who perform physical activities that enhance and maintain flexibility.
- Increase the proportion of adolescents who engage in moderate physical activity for at least 30 minutes on 5 or more of the previous 7 days.
- Increase the proportion of adolescents who engage in vigorous physical activity that promotes cardiorespiratory fitness 3 or more days per week for 20 or more minutes per occasion.
- Increase the proportion of the nation's public and private schools that require daily physical education for all students.
- Increase the proportion of adolescents who participate in daily school physical education.
- Increase the proportion of adolescents who spend at least 50 percent of school physical education class time being physically active.
- Increase the proportion of adolescents who view television 2 or fewer hours on a school day.
- Increase the proportion of the nation's public and private schools that provide access to their physical activity spaces and facilities for all persons outside of normal school hours (that is, before and after the school day, on weekends, and during summer and other vacations).
- Increase the proportion of worksites offering employer-sponsored physical activity and fitness programs.
- Increase the proportion of trips made by walking.
- Increase the proportion of trips made by bicycling.

THE PSYCHOLOGICAL BENEFITS OF BEING PHYSICALLY ACTIVE

Physical activity generally has a positive influence on a person's psychological health throughout a lifetime cycle by improving health and enhancing function and quality of life. Some of the psychological benefits include enhanced motivation, increased self-perception and esteem, improved mood states, emotional well-being, reduction of stress and anxiety, and creation of a realistic body image. Physical activity has a positive impact on mental health and appears to alleviate the symptoms of depression, anxiety, and, to a lesser extent, panic disorder.

Many people use regular exercise, especially of a recreational nature, as a means of mental relaxation. Exercise can play a significant role in reducing stress. It diverts attention from

HEALTH LINK 1-2

Physical Benefits of Being Physically Active

1. Regular, vigorous activity increases muscle size, strength, and power and develops endurance for sustaining work and resisting fatigue.
2. Exercise strengthens the heart muscle and improves the efficiency of the vascular system in delivering oxygenated blood to the working tissues and in using it, thereby improving cardiorespiratory endurance.
3. Exercise improves the functioning of the lungs by deepening the respiration process.
4. Exercise helps to keep the digestive and excretory organs in good condition.
5. Muscular exercise enhances nerve-muscle coordination.
6. Exercise helps a person to maintain a healthy body weight by reducing the percentage of total body weight that is made up of fat tissue.
7. Exercise contributes to improved posture and appearance through the development of proper muscle tone, greater joint flexibility, and a feeling of well-being.
8. Physical activity generates more energy and thus contributes to greater individual productivity for both physical and mental tasks.
9. The person who is fit has more strength, energy, and stamina; an improved sense of well-being; better protection from injury (because strong, well-developed muscles safeguard bones, internal organs, and joints and keep moving parts limber); and improved cardiorespiratory function.
10. It is often the case that people who become physically active will pay more attention to such things as proper nutrition, rest, and relaxation and may also drink less alcohol and stop smoking because they do not want to undo the benefits gained through physical activity. They are likely to be committed to engaging in health-promoting, rather than health-harming, behavior.

www.health.gov/healthypeople/

---

stress-producing thoughts to a more relaxing and positive focus. Exercise may also help us to feel better about ourselves and to feel that we are more capable of handling potential stress-producing situations. Some people say that engaging in physical activity gives them an "exercise high." It is true that exercise causes the release of chemicals called endorphins in the brain that can positively affect your attitude and outlook.

It has also been shown that regular exercise and increased physical fitness increase *serotonin* levels in the brain which lead to improved mood and feelings of well-being.

Serotonin is an important neurotransmitter (brain chemical) that contributes to a range of functions, including sleep and wake cycles, libido, appetite, and mood. Lack of serotonin has also been linked to depression.

THE BENEFITS OF EXERCISE IN THE AGING PROCESS

For the traditional student, at this point in your life it is likely that your physical health is fine. However, a fact that we wish we could change, but unfortunately cannot, is that aging begins immediately at birth and involves a lifelong series of changes in physiological and performance capabilities. These capabilities increase as a function of the growth process throughout adolescence, peak sometime between the ages of 18 and 30 years, then steadily decline with increasing age. Interestingly, this decline may be caused by the sociological constraints of aging as much as by biological effects. It is possible for you to maintain a relatively high level of physical function if you maintain an active lifestyle.

In most cases, after age 30, qualities such as muscular endurance, coordination, and strength begin to decrease. Furthermore, as we age, recovery from vigorous exercise requires a longer amount of time. Regular physical activity, however, tends to delay and in some cases prevent the appearance of certain degenerative processes. If you were active as a child, became fit as a teenager, and continue to stay fit throughout your life, it is very likely that you will have greater strength, flexibility, and cardiorespiratory health and a lower percentage of body fat than if you chose a more sedentary lifestyle.

WHAT COMPONENTS OF FITNESS ARE IMPORTANT TO YOU?

Engaging in physical activities can have a positive effect on many different physical attributes. For the vast majority of people in our society, regardless of age, the focus should be on those components of fitness that are concerned with the development of qualities necessary to function efficiently physically and to maintain a healthy lifestyle. Those fitness components include cardiorespiratory endurance, muscular strength, muscular endurance, flexibility, and body composition. Collectively, they are referred to as **health-related components.** The Fit List Box 1-1 summarizes the fitness components.

FIT LIST 1-1

Fitness Components

Health-related components

- Cardiorespiratory endurance
- Flexibility
- Muscular strength
- Muscular endurance
- Body composition

Skill-related components

- Speed
- Power
- Agility
- Coordination
- Balance
- Reaction time

Cardiorespiratory endurance is the ability to persist in a physical activity requiring oxygen for physical exertion without experiencing undue fatigue (Figure 1-1). If you go out and run 2 miles or swim 2,000 yards, you are displaying cardiorespiratory endurance. The functioning of the heart, lungs, and blood vessels is essential for distribution of oxygen and nutrients and removal of wastes from the body. For performance of vigorous activities,

health-related components: components of a healthy lifestyle, including muscular strength, muscular endurance, cardiorespiratory endurance, flexibility, and body composition

cardiorespiratory endurance: the ability to persist in a physical activity requiring oxygen for physical exertion without experiencing undue fatigue

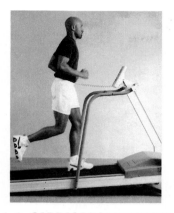

FIGURE 1-1. CARDIORESPIRATORY ENDURANCE.
Perhaps the most essential fitness component for both good health and skill-related performance.

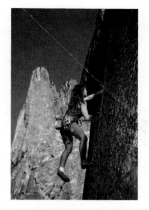

FIGURE 1-3. MUSCULAR ENDURANCE.
The ability to perform muscular contractions repeatedly over a period of time.

efficient functioning of the heart and lungs is necessary. The more efficiently they function, the easier it is to walk, run, work, and concentrate for longer periods. Exercise of this nature involves the heart, the vessels supplying blood to all parts of the body, and the oxygen-carrying capacity of the blood.

Muscular strength is the ability or capacity of a muscle or muscle group to exert force against resistance (Figure 1-2). It refers to a muscle's ability to exert maximal force in a single effort. Strength is needed in all kinds of work and in physical activity, and strong muscles provide better protection of body joints, resulting in fewer sprains, strains, and muscular difficulties. Furthermore, muscle strength helps in maintaining proper posture and provides greater endurance, power, and resistance to fatigue.

Muscular endurance is the ability of muscles to perform or sustain a muscle contraction repeatedly over a period of time (Figure 1-3). Muscular endurance is closely related to muscular strength. If you are strong, you will be more resistant to fatigue because relatively

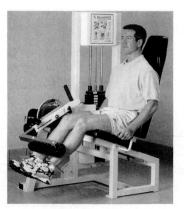

FIGURE 1-2. MUSCULAR STRENGTH.
The ability to generate force against resistance.

muscular strength: the ability or capacity of a muscle or muscle group to exert force against resistance

muscular endurance: the ability of muscles to perform or sustain a muscle contraction repeatedly over a period of time

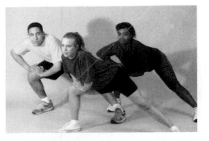

FIGURE 1-4. FLEXIBILITY.
The ability to move freely through a full range of motion.

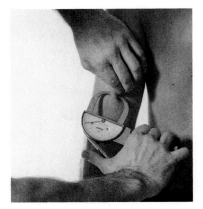

FIGURE 1-5. MEASURING BODY COMPOSITION.
Exercise can reduce the percentage of total body weight that is fat tissue.

less effort will be required to produce repeated muscular contraction.

Flexibility is the ability to move the joints in your arms, legs, and trunk freely throughout a full, nonrestricted, pain-free range of motion (Figure 1-4). It may be improved by engaging regularly in stretching. Flexibility is important for performance in most active sports; it is also important for maintaining good posture. Flexibility is also essential in carrying on many daily activities and can help to prevent muscle strain and muscular problems such as backaches.

Body composition refers to the different types of tissues that make up your body. These primarily include bones, muscles, tendons, ligaments, skin, and fat (Figure 1-5). Body composition particularly refers to the percentage of fat in the body relative to the percentage of all the other tissues. An excess of fat in the body is unhealthy because it causes the body to expend more energy for movement, and it may reflect a diet in which an individual is consuming more calories than he or she needs. The demand on the cardiorespiratory system is greater when the percent body fat is high. Furthermore, it is believed that obesity contributes to degenerative diseases such as high blood pressure and **atherosclerosis.** It has also been linked to diabetes and certain cancers. Obesity can also result in psychological maladjustments and may shorten life. A balance between caloric

intake and caloric expenditure is necessary to maintain proper body fat content. Adequate exercise, therefore, is effective in controlling body fat. **Caloric intake** is the total number of calories consumed in a 24-hour period regardless of the type of foods ingested. **Caloric expenditure** is the number of calories burned

flexibility: the ability to move your arms, legs, and trunk freely throughout a full, nonrestricted, pain-free range of motion

body composition: the percentage of fat in the body relative to the percentage of all the other tissues

atherosclerosis: a process by which fatty plaques are deposited along arterial walls

caloric intake: the number of calories consumed in the diet

caloric expenditure: the number of calories expended through basal metabolism and exercise

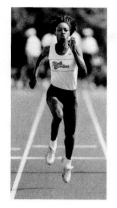

FIGURE 1-6. SPEED.
Speed is an important component in many competitive athletic situations.

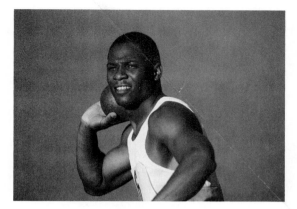

FIGURE 1-7. POWER.
The ability to generate large amounts of force rapidly.

off in a 24-hour period from basal metabolism and exercise.

Other components of fitness, called **skill-related components,** are also important for any physically active person. These components deal more with performance in sports and other physical activities than with basic physical health and include speed, power, coordination, balance, and agility.

Speed is the ability to perform a particular movement very rapidly. It is a function of distance and time (Figure 1-6). Speed is an important component for successful performance in many competitive athletic situations.

Power is the ability to generate great amounts of force against a certain resistance in a short period (Figure 1-7). Power is a function of both strength and speed. The ability to drive a golf ball, hit a softball, or kick a ball a long distance requires some element of power.

Neuromuscular coordination is the ability to integrate the senses—visual, auditory, and proprioceptive (knowing the position of your body in space)—with muscle function to produce smooth, accurate, and skilled movement (Figure 1-8).

Balance is the ability to maintain some degree of equilibrium while moving or standing still (Figure 1-9).

skill-related components: fitness components associated with athletic performance, including speed, power, coordination, balance, and agility

speed: the ability to perform a particular movement very rapidly. It is a function of distance and time

power: the ability to generate great amounts of force against a certain resistance in a short period of time

neuromuscular coordination: the ability to integrate the senses with muscle function to produce smooth, accurate, and skilled movement

balance: the ability to maintain some degree of equilibrium while moving or standing still

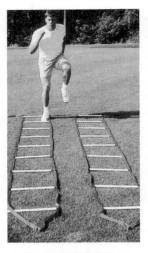

FIGURE 1-8. NEUROMUSCULAR COORDINATION.
The ability to integrate the senses with motor function to produce coordinated movement.

Agility is the ability to change or alter—quickly and accurately—the direction of body movement during activity. Agility to a large extent depends on coordination. Agility may be improved with increased flexibility and muscular strength (Figure 1-10).

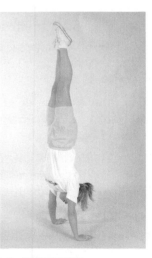

FIGURE 1-9. BALANCE.
The ability to maintain equilibrium when moving or stationary.

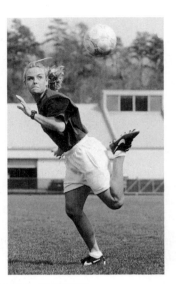

FIGURE 1-10. AGILITY.
The ability to change direction of movement quickly and accurately.

Reaction time is the time required to produce an appropriate and accurate physiological or mechanical response to some external stimulus.

DETERMINING YOUR REASONS FOR WANTING TO BE FIT

Perhaps the most important thing that you have learned by this point in your life is that people are different. These differences are evident in all aspects of our being. Certainly, each person has his or her individual reasons for choosing to engage in physical activity. Before you begin your personal fitness program, it may be helpful to

agility: the ability to change or alter—quickly and accurately—the direction of body movement during activity

reaction time: the length of time required to react to a stimulus

determine your personal reasons for wanting to get fit and your present level of activity.

Regardless of whether you are just starting an individualized fitness program or if you are already exercising, you should first consider exactly what it is that you are trying to accomplish. The exercise program you choose should be one that results in the development of the desired fitness component(s). This means that activities selected should be specific to goals. For example, if your goal is increasing stamina or endurance, this may be achieved effectively by engaging in activities such as running, swimming, skating, or cycling—all activities that maximize the use of the circulatory system. Lab Activity 1-1 will help you to determine your individual reasons for wanting to become physically fit.

DETERMINING HOW FREQUENTLY YOU ENGAGE IN PHYSICAL ACTIVITY

Before you begin any type of fitness program, it is essential for you to establish some baseline information relative to your existing exercise habits. It is important to appraise your daily schedule regularly to determine if you are devoting the proper amount of time to keeping yourself fit. Lab Activity 1-2 will help you determine your current levels of fitness activity. There is little question that incorporating consistent, regularly scheduled exercise into your lifestyle may be difficult, especially in light of existing demands on your time.

HOW LONG WILL IT TAKE YOU TO GET FIT?

There is no shortcut to fitness; it takes time. You should not expect results in a matter of hours or even days. After a month of appropriate activity on a regular basis, some improvement should be noted, depending on what your physical condition was when you started. After an extended period of gradual improvement, you may reach a plateau at which you experience no improvement but instead seem to stay at the same level of fitness. This is a natural phenomenon. In time, with regular workouts, improvement will occur; after several months, the desired results will be attained. Make a commitment to your fitness program and keep at it; you will feel better, and this will in turn motivate you to continue. Once you have attained a desirable physical fitness level, you will be strongly motivated to maintain this level through regular workouts.

Any physical fitness program requires effort to produce results. Too often, people look for the easy way to achieve their goals. Steam baths, sauna baths, fitness machines, massages, and gimmicks such as body wraps or fad diets may be relaxing or produce short-term effects, but it is necessary to exert effort to achieve the lasting benefits of physical fitness. The body must do the work. You can't sit and be fit!

The purpose of the chapters that follow is to provide you with knowledge about and understanding of the various aspects of fitness. They are designed to show the importance of its essential ingredients. They will explain how you can assess, develop, and maintain your fitness. Finally, they will show you how to plan, develop, and implement a personalized physical activity program based on your individual interests.

SUMMARY

- Being fit means that the various systems of your body are healthy and function efficiently to enable you to engage in activities of daily living, as well as recreational pursuits and leisure activities, without unreasonable fatigue.
- Being physically active produces various physiological, social, and psychological benefits.

- Engaging in regular exercise throughout your lifetime can delay many of the degenerative processes associated with aging.
- Most people should focus on those components of fitness that are concerned with maintaining a healthy lifestyle, including cardiorespiratory endurance, muscular strength, muscular endurance, flexibility, and body composition.
- Other components of fitness are more closely related to skill of performance in sports and other physical activities than to good health; such components include speed, power, coordination, balance, agility, and reaction time.
- Before starting a personal training program, it is helpful to examine your attitude toward physical fitness and your reasons for wanting to be physically fit, and your present level of activity.
- There is no short-cut to becoming physically fit. It requires time, hard work, and determination.

Suggested Readings

American College of Sports Medicine. 2003. *Fitness book.* Champaign, IL: Human Kinetics.

Baumann, A. E. 2004. Updating the evidence that physical activity is good for health: An epidemiological review 2000–2003. *Journal of Science and Medicine in Sport* 7(1 Supplement): 6–19.

Blair, S. N., Y. Cheng, and S. Holder. 2001. Is physical activity or physical fitness more important in defining health benefits? *Medicine and Science in Sports and Exercise* 33(6 Suppl.): S379–99.

Bouchard, C. 2000. *Physical activity and obesity.* Champaign, IL: Human Kinetics.

Brown, D. W. D. R. Brown, and G. W. Heath. 2004. Associations between physical activity dose and health-related quality of life. *Medicine and Science in Sports and Exercise* 36(5):890–96.

Buckworth, J., and R. K. Dishman. 2002. Interventions to change physical activity behavior. In *Exercise psychology,* edited by J. Buckworth. Champaign, IL: Human Kinetics.

Centers for Disease Control and Prevention. 1977. Guidelines for school and community programs: Promoting lifelong physical activity. *CAHPERD Journal/Times* 60(2):7–12.

Corbin, C. B. 2002. Physical activity for everyone: What every physical educator should know about promoting lifelong physical activity. *Journal of Teaching in Physical Education* 21(2): 128–44.

Corbin, C. B., R. P. Pangrazi, and G. C. Le Masurier. 2004. Physical activity for children: current patterns and guidelines. *President's Council on Physical Fitness and Sports Research Digest* 5(2):1–8.

Epstein, L. H., and J. N. Roemmich. 2001. Reducing sedentary behavior: Role in modifying physical activity. *Exercise and Sport Sciences Reviews* 29(3):103.

Erikssen, G. 2001. Physical fitness and changes in mortality: The survival of the fittest. *Sports Medicine* 31(8):571–76.

Fleck, S. J. and W. J. Kraemer. 2004. Integrating other fitness components. In Fleck, S. J. (ed.), *Designing Resistance Training Programs* edited by S. J. Fleck. 3rd ed. Champaign, IL: Human Kinetics.

Hawkins, S. A., M. G. Cockburn, A. S. Hamilton, and T. M. Mack. 2004. An estimate of physical activity prevalence in a large population-based cohort. *Medicine and Science in Sports and Exercise* 36(2):253–60.

Heyward, V. H., ed. 2002. *Advanced fitness assessment and exercise prescription.* 4th ed. Champaign, IL: Human Kinetics.

Jackson, A. W. 2003. *Physical activity for health and fitness.* Champaign, IL: Human Kinetics.

Krems, C., P. M. Luehrmann, and M. Neuhaeuser. 2004. Physical activity in young and elderly subjects. *Journal of Sports Medicine and Physical Fitness* 44(1):71–76.

McKormack-Brown, K., D. Thomas, and J. Kotecki. 2002. *Physical activity and health: An interactive approach.* Boston: Jones & Bartlett.

Melville, D. S., and B. J. Cardinal. 2002. Physical activity and fitness recommendations for physical activity professionals: Highlights of a position statement. *Strategies* 15(5):19.

Nieman, D. C. 1998. *The exercise-health connection.* Champaign, IL: Human Kinetics.

Pate, R. 1998. Physical activity for young people. *President's Council on Physical Fitness and Sports Research Digest* 3(3):1–6.

President's Council on Physical Fitness and Sports. 1998. Physical activity and aging: Implications for health and quality of life in older persons. *President's Council on Physical Fitness and Sports Research Digest* (3/4):1–6.

Seefeldt, V., R. M. Malina, and M. A. Clark. 2002. Factors affecting levels of physical activity in adults. *Sports Medicine* 32(3):143–68.

Sharkey, B. J., ed. *Fitness and health.* 5th ed. Champaign, IL: Human Kinetics. 2001.

Sparling, P. B., and T. K. Snow. 2002. Physical activity patterns in recent college alumni. *Research Quarterly for Exercise and Sport* 73(2):200–205.

Stone, W. J. and D. A. Klein. 2004. Long-term exercisers: What can we learn from them? *ACSM's Health & Fitness Journal* 8(2):11–14.

U.S. Department of Health and Human Services, Office of Disease Prevention and Health Promotion. 2000. *Healthy People 2010.* Washington, DC: U.S. Government Printing Office.

Zhang, K. and C. N. Boozer. 2004. Improving energy expenditure estimation for physical activity. *Medicine and Science in Sports and Exercise* 36(5):883–889.

SUGGESTED WEB SITES

American College of Sports Medicine

ACSM promotes and integrates scientific research, education, and practical applications of sports medicine and exercise science to maintain and enhance physical performance, fitness, health, and quality of life.
www.acsm.org

American Council on Exercise

The American Council on Exercise (ACE) is committed to promoting active, healthy lifestyles and their positive effects on the mind, body, and spirit.
www.acefitness.org

Canada's Physical Activity Guide Web site

Physical Activity Guide for older adults.
www.hc-sc.gc.ca/hppb/paguide

CDC's Nutrition and Physical Activity Program

This site provides science-based activities for children and adults that address the role of nutrition and physical activity in health promotion and the prevention and control of chronic diseases.
www.cdc.gov/nccdphp/dnpa

FitnessLink

FitnessLink is a fitness information resource for news, articles, and tips on health, fitness, sport, diet, and exercise, and it provides links to hundreds of quality fitness Web sites.
www.fitnessLink.com

FitnessWorld Homepage

This Web site features health and fitness information for both professionals and enthusiasts.
www.fitnessworld.com

Guide to Physical Activity

Talks about an increase in physical activity as an important part of a weight management program.
www.nhlbi.nih.gov/health

Healthy People 2010

Healthy People 2010 challenges individuals, communities, and professionals to take specific steps to ensure that good health, as well as long life, are enjoyed by all.
www.health.gov/healthypeople

International Society for Aging and Physical Activity

The ISAPA is an international not-for-profit society promoting research, clinical practice, and public policy initiatives in the area of aging and physical activity.
www.isapa.org

National Center on Physical Activity and Disability

This site provides references for articles, books, videos, Web sites, vendors for specialized products and services, recreational programs, and other information available on physical activity and disability.
www.ncpad.org

National Institute for Fitness and Sport

NIFS is a nonprofit organization committed to enhancing human health, physical fitness, and athletic performance through research, education, and service.
www.nifs.org

Nutrition and Fitness Software by NutriStrategy

This diet and exercise software helps you meet your nutrition and fitness goals. This site features nutrient information, weight training exercises, charts on calories burned during exercise, and facts about the health benefits of physical activity.
www.nutristrategy.com

Physical Activity Home Page

Discusses physical activity relative to the current World epidemiological transition that calls for higher levels of physical activity.
www.who.int/hpr/physactiv

1   2

○   ○

79

CHAPTE

Creating a **Healthy** Lifestyle

Objectives

After completing this chapter, you should be able to do the following:

- Discuss the importance of creating a healthy style of living and how fitness fits into this lifestyle.
- Recognize the impact of stress on the healthy lifestyle and identify stress management techniques.
- Identify risk factors present in your lifestyle that may predispose you to coronary artery disease.
- Explain how unhealthy lifestyle practices may contribute to the development of cancer.
- Explain why alcohol, drugs, and tobacco are considered deterrents to fitness.

WHY SHOULD YOU BE CONCERNED ABOUT YOUR LIFESTYLE?

Being physically active is critical to a healthful style of living but is perhaps no more important for total well-being than is your social, emotional, mental, or spiritual stability. Fitness can affect each of these components in either a positive or a negative manner.

Choosing a healthy lifestyle encourages you to prevent illness by improving your positive well-being in various ways, including (1) developing yourself physically, (2) expressing your emotions effectively, (3) having good relations with those persons around you, (4) being concerned about your decision-making abilities, and finally (5) paying attention to ethics, values, and spirituality. All these

KEY TERMS

stress management	hyperlipidemia
coronary artery disease	stress
	drug abuse
cancer	anabolic steroids
coping	alcoholism
relaxation techniques	tobacco use
lipoproteins	

of
rs,
est
e a
nce
ore
on

ing
ess-
ing
am,
and

reassessing your goals and plan.

Those who adhere to this approach believe it is the responsibility of the individual to work toward achieving a healthy lifestyle and thus realize an optimal sense of well-being. A healthy lifestyle should reflect the integration of such components as regular and appropriate physical activity, **stress management,** and elimination of controllable risk factors such as alcohol, smoking, and drug abuse. Many diseases, such as **coronary artery disease** or **cancer,** may ultimately be the result of an unhealthy lifestyle.

This chapter focuses on various lifestyle choices or practices that potentially interfere with or are deterrents to achieving a healthy lifestyle and, in particular, physical fitness.

WHAT IS THE EFFECT OF STRESS ON A HEALTHY LIFESTYLE?

It is important for the health-conscious, physically active individual to understand the potential effect of stress on the body. Stress has been linked to many diseases. It may also interfere with performance of daily tasks or the attainment of one's goals. Most importantly, poorly managed stress greatly reduces the quality of one's life.

The term *stress* comes from the Latin word *stringere,* meaning "to draw tight." The term refers to the responses that occur in the body as a result of what is called a stressor, or stimulus. Stress occurs when the internal balance or equilibrium of the body systems is disrupted.

Everyone experiences stress, and some stress is needed to perform the daily tasks of life and, more importantly, to stimulate growth and development. Stress can be beneficial. However, too much stress, especially when it exists for a prolonged period and is unrelieved, can result in physical and mental illness. Stress is caused or triggered by stressors that may be physical, social, or psychological and negative or positive in nature. Human reactions to positive stressors are called *eustress;* that is, stress that is beneficial. The term *distress* denotes detrimental responses or negative stressors. Often, only a fine line distinguishes whether a situation or action causes eustress or distress. For example, moderate physical training is a stressor that can make you stronger and more fit. However, if you do too much too soon, it can produce distress in the form of soreness or injury.

Sometimes the difference between eustress and distress is only a matter of interpretation; do you interpret the stressor as a threat or a challenge? Although we may habitually

stress management: involves techniques that attempt to reduce both the quantity and the quality of stress in your life

coronary artery disease: disease that results from the accumulation of fatty deposits (atherosclerotic plaque) within the coronary arteries

cancer: a collection of abnormal cells that tends to invade and ultimately take over normal tissue

respond in ways that seem automatic and beyond our control, we can choose to examine the way we think and then work on changing counterproductive thinking or beliefs. In many instances, the way we react to stressful situations is learned from our parents.

Stress should not, however, be considered solely a physiological phenomenon. Stress has also been viewed from a psychological or cognitive perspective. Current research suggests that the stress response is not a simple biological response. It is an interrelated process that includes the presence of a stressor, the circumstances in which the stressor occurs, the interpretation of the situation by the person, that person's typical reaction, and the resources the person has available to deal with the stressor.

For example, some people may find downhill skiing fun and exciting. They look forward to taking winter vacations to ski the slopes. Other people may have tried to ski, but their dislike of cold weather and fear of injury make skiing a distressing activity. Therefore the stress response in a given situation depends on the individual's perceptions. Individuals under stress usually exhibit certain warning signs and symptoms that may vary from person to person. Health Link 2-1 lists the potential signs of stress.

THE PSYCHOLOGICAL OR COGNITIVE RESPONSE TO STRESS

Once the stress process is initiated by the presence of a stressor, psychological or thought processes that determine how the stressor is perceived take over. An individual's perceptions of a particular situation can cause a response that may vary from arousal to anxiety. The degree to which a particular situation elicits an emotional response depends greatly on how the individual views the situation and how well prepared he or she feels to handle the situation.

HEALTH LINK 2-1

Signs of Stress

Irritability and depression
Heart palpitations
Dryness of throat and mouth
Impulsive behavior
Inability to concentrate
Feelings of weakness or dizziness
Crying
Anxiety
Emotional tension
Nervous tics
Vomiting
Easily startled by small sounds
Nervous laughter
Trembling hands
Stuttering or other speech problems
Insomnia

Breathlessness
Sweating
Frequent urination
Diarrhea and indigestion
Migraine headaches
Premenstrual tension or missed menstrual cycles
Pain in back
Increased smoking
Loss of appetite
Nightmares
Fatigue

www.futurehealth.org/stresscn.htm
www.cdc.gov/nasd/docs

THE PHYSIOLOGICAL RESPONSE TO STRESS

Every organ system in the body is affected by the stress response. The physiological response to stress follows a three-stage pattern of alarm, resistance, and exhaustion. There are two regulatory systems in the body that govern the stress response: the nervous system and the endocrine system. Differences between the nervous and endocrine systems are found in terms of how quickly they respond to a stressor and how long their responses are sustained. The endocrine system secretes hormones that prepare the body to deal with a stressful situation. These hormones may remain in the bloodstream for several weeks. The endocrine system's response to stress endures, whereas the nervous system's response is short-lived. This suggests that the endocrine system is more important to investigate for any connection between stress and disease.

During the alarm stage, the body undergoes physiological changes that are collectively referred to as the fight-or-flight syndrome (e.g., increased heart rate, blood pressure, respiratory rate). These physiological changes are primarily a nervous system response to prepare the body for vigorous muscular action. In the resistance stage, the body adjusts to stress and appears to return to its normal state of internal balance. If stress persists for a long time, exhaustion sets in. The person becomes less able to resist stress. Sustained stress can affect various body systems so that illness and even death may result. Health Link 2-2 summarizes specific physical disorders associated with stress.

HEALTH LINK 2-2

Stress and Specific Physical Disorders

Heart Disease Personality:	Having the characteristics of a Type A personality is a risk factor for coronary artery disease.
High Blood Pressure:	Individuals who are under stress are more likely to have high blood pressure. This may have some relationship to personality type.
Immune System:	Chemicals released during the stress response suppress the immune system, which involves a network of organs, tissues, and white blood cells that fight disease.
Digestive System:	Stress can cause heartburn, diarrhea, gastritis, and gas. Stress will not cause an ulcer but can make an ulcer feel worse.
Headaches:	Tension headaches and migraine headaches are both more likely to occur with increased stress.
Skin Problems:	Certain skin conditions such as acne, herpes simplex, psoriasis, hives, and eczema are likely to appear or worsen with increased stress.
Muscles:	Stress causes increased tension, particularly in the muscles of the neck and upper back, that can lead to the development of painful trigger points.
Respiratory Problems:	Stress can worsen asthma, especially the type of asthma that is exercise-induced.
Diabetes:	Stress can affect blood sugar levels, which is a potentially dangerous problem for a diabetic.

►Exercise and Stress Reduction

Engaging in physical activity is widely used as a means for reducing or alleviating stress. Many people who exercise report the feeling of a "high" both during and immediately following exercise. This euphoric feeling may be attributed to the release of opiate-like chemicals called endorphins in the brain. Consistent exercise also lowers both resting blood pressure and cholesterol, both of which can help to minimize the insidious damage caused by stress.

PERSONALITY AND STRESS

In identifying people who are at risk for developing cardiovascular disease, researchers believed that there was a connection between behavior pattern and risk of heart disease. People were classified as being either "type A" or "type B" personalities. The type A person is always "on the go," never satisfied with his or her level of achievement, appears tense, suffers from a sense of time urgency, and is competitive and impatient. In contrast, the type B person is more easy-going and relaxed, more patient, and satisfied with his or her level of achievement. The type A person was believed to have a higher risk of developing cardiovascular disease. However, recent research suggests that only those individuals who have hostile or angry behavior patterns are at risk. Therefore, identifying the sources of anger and hostility in these people and helping them with behavior modification may allow them to cope more effectively with stress.

COPING WITH STRESS AND STRESS MANAGEMENT

Life is filled with many challenges, some of which represent potential obstacles in the path of your career and life goals. **Coping** is an attempt to effectively manage or control stress

adequacy. For example, a commonly used defense mechanism is projecting blame for failure on someone or something else. Defense mechanisms are not necessarily the most effective way to deal with stress. They may bolster the ego, but they can also circumvent managing real problems.

Various methods of coping are beneficial because they allow people to achieve self-fulfillment. People learn to manage conflicts, sources of pressure, and frustration without experiencing harm to their bodies.

It is important for you to develop and incorporate into your lifestyle any techniques that will help you effectively reduce stress. Fit List 2-1 identifies some general guidelines for reducing stress. Lab Activity 2-1 will help you become more aware of your response to stress and how you cope with stress.

Stress management involves more than simply reducing the total quantity of stress in your life; it also means being able to change

coping: an attempt to effectively manage or control stress by using techniques that alter the physiological and psychological consequences of stress

... honest with yourself about all the things that are going on in your life, and then ... worries with someone you love, trust, or respect.

... you are feeling hassled and little things upset you that shouldn't, take a deep breath, count ..., and then put everything in perspective. Ask yourself, "Is this the worst thing that is ever ...oing to happen to me? Has anyone I love been hurt or affected? Will this still make me mad tomorrow?"

3. Become a better time manager. Keep a prioritized list of things to be done each day. Break down large, time-consuming projects into small chunks and reward yourself when you complete each part. Accept the fact that there is only so much time each day and that as long as you're working consistently, what you don't get done today you can finish tomorrow.

4. Work on developing healthy lifestyle habits that will enhance your resistance to stress (e.g., exercise), and avoid negative addictions such as smoking and drinking.

5. Keep a diary of things that seem to cause you stress so that over a period of time you can identify patterns or situations that cause problems. Then figure out how you can eliminate these stress-inducing situations.

6. Try to be positive and optimistic. If you constantly look for what's wrong with you or others around you, you will always find something, which often makes you feel even worse. Instead, focus on the positive aspects of all situations and try to find a little something that is good about each situation.

7. Laugh at yourself and try to maintain a sense of humor no matter what the situation.

8. Accept the fact that you can't control everything in your life and realize that your way is not always going to be the best way. Try to relax and accept other ways of doing things.

9. Develop a network of people—both family and friends—whom you love and trust, and put a degree of faith in their support when things get tough. Live your life for the good times that you share with these people, but make sure they will be there for your when things aren't so good.

10. Try to constantly focus on the pleasant aspects of your life and on the things that you can do to improve your situation.

11. Don't procrastinate. If you constantly put off things that you don't want to deal with or that are unpleasant, and you know that sooner or later you are going to have to address them, your level of frustration escalates and you feel more stressed. Deal with every situation as soon as you can.

the quality of stress in your life. Uncontrolled stress can result in physical and psychological disorders that pose a real threat to well-being. To manage stress effectively you must realize that you are responsible for your own emotional and physical well-being. Your perception of events (but not the events themselves) is under your control. You do not need to allow other people's behavior to affect your ability to maintain a relatively stable emotional and physical condition. Besides using physical activity, learning to control thought processes can be an effective method of managing stress. Collectively referred to as relaxation techniques, these methods have been demonstrated to be helpful.

▶ Relaxation Techniques

Relaxation is essentially a mental phenomenon concerned with the reduction of tensions that could originate from muscular activity but are more likely to result from psychological

FIT LIST 2-2

Relaxation Techniques

Muscle-to-mind techniques

- Progressive relaxation
- Massage
- Biofeedback

Mind-to-muscle techniques

- Yoga
- Meditation
- Imagery
- Autogenic training

responses to our hectic lifestyles. **Relaxation techniques** may be broadly classified as either muscle-to-mind techniques, which control the level of stimulation going to the brain from the muscles (progressive relaxation, massage, and biofeedback), or mind-to-muscle techniques, which control the level of stimulation along the nerve pathways coming from the brain to the muscles (yoga, meditation, imagery, and autogenic training). Fit List 2-2 summarizes these relaxation techniques.

Progressive Relaxation. Progressive relaxation involves alternately tensing (5 to 10 seconds) and relaxing (45 seconds) the muscles, moving through the body in a systematic fashion to tense and relax all major muscle groups. Concentrate first on the large muscle groups in the arms, legs, trunk, and neck. Then ease tension in the forehead, eyes, face, and even the throat through a program of progressive relaxation. The program teaches the person to relax his or her whole body to the point of negative exertion. The result is a release of tension, which is an antidote to fatigue; the result is also an inducement to sleep.

Massage. Massage can be useful as a stress-reducing technique, as it induces relaxation. You can massage your neck, face, head, and shoulders, or massage also can be done by another

person. To many, touch is a useful form of non-verbal communication and can be reassuring.

Biofeedback. Biofeedback is a common form of stress management and relaxation therapy. Its main goals are to teach concentration, relaxation, awareness, and self-control. A machine monitors various body functions and relays the information to the subject in the form of either sounds or lights. Biofeedback helps people to become aware of tensions they had not previously perceived and learn to reduce them, eventually without relying on the monitoring machines.

Yoga. Yoga uses several positions for the body through which the practitioner may progress, beginning with the simplest and moving to the more complex. The purpose of the various positions is to increase mobility and flexibility of the body. Slow, deep, diaphragmatic breathing can help in alleviating stress and also help to lower blood pressure and heart rate. Deep breathing has a calming effect on the body. It also increases production of endorphins, the body's own natural, morphinelike painkilling substances.

Meditation. Meditation uses mind-focusing exercises to control or concentrate one's attention. In most forms, meditation involves sitting quietly for a certain period, usually 15 to 20 minutes, and concentrating on a single word or image while breathing slowly and rhythmically to produce decreases in respiratory rate, heart rate, blood pressure, and muscle tension.

Imagery. Imagery can be used as a means of relaxation to cope with stressful situations. Images are pictures formed within the mind. The procedure is to sit relaxed, close your eyes,

relaxation techniques: techniques for reducing tensions that could originate from muscular activity but are more likely to result from psychological responses to hectic lifestyles

and concentrate on a particular image. With practice, you can learn to project your own body image into this picture and ultimately to perform various tasks within the mind, learning to cope with all possible variations of a situation that may be stress-producing before confronting the situation in real life.

Autogenic Training (Hypnosis). Autogenic training involves a series of specific exercises and autohypnosis that are designed to achieve a deep mental and physical state of relaxation.

HOW CAN YOU PREVENT CORONARY ARTERY DISEASE?

Half of all people who die in the United States each year die of coronary artery disease (CAD). The lifestyle you choose plays a major role in determining whether you develop CAD. Coronary artery disease results from the accumulation of fatty deposits (atherosclerotic plaque) within the coronary arteries (Figure 2-1). The coronary arteries supply blood to the heart muscle, which functions properly only when provided with a steady blood supply. The deposition of fatty plaque often begins early in life, and the continued, gradual deposition of plaque can lead to a significant narrowing of the coronary arteries, or *atherosclerosis*. The partial or complete blockage of one or more of the major coronary arteries can lead to a condition called *myocardial ischemia*, in which the heart muscle fails to receive an adequate supply of oxygen. This can produce symptoms such as chest pain (angina pectoris)

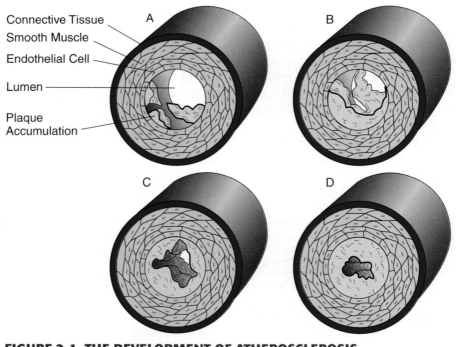

FIGURE 2-1. THE DEVELOPMENT OF ATHEROSCLEROSIS.
(A) Normal coronary artery. (B) Beginning stages of atherosclerosis; fatty plaque is deposited in vessel walls. (C) Advanced stage of atherosclerosis. (D) Completely blocked coronary artery.
Modified from Hahn D, Payne W: Focus on health, St Louis, 1991, Mosby.

and, if severe, can precipitate a heart attack. A heart attack can occur suddenly and without warning. The factors that ultimately lead to a cardiac arrest are present early in life but mostly go undetected until they manifest as a potentially life-threatening heart attack.

Among the cardiovascular diseases, coronary artery disease has the highest incidence of occurrence. Other cardiovascular diseases include hypertension, stroke, congenital heart disease, rheumatic heart disease, peripheral heart disease, and congestive heart failure.

RISK FACTORS

Coronary artery disease is related to personal lifestyle health habits known as *risk factors*. These risk factors cannot be labeled as causes but are instead characteristics that increase the probability of one's having CAD. The risk factors are summarized in Health Link 2-3.

Risk factors may be divided into those risk factors *that cannot be changed*, risk factors *that can be changed*, and *contributing risk factors* whose significance and prevalence have yet to be precisely determined. Some of them can be changed, treated, or modified, and some cannot. Each of these risk factors is related to CAD in an additive fashion; the greater the number of risk factors present, the greater the likelihood of developing CAD. Also, each of these factors is, at least in part, a function of individual lifestyles

o̶
mat̶
factors.̶
and heredi̶
altered throug̶

▶Risk Factors ̶ Changed

Family History. A histor̶ ily is considered a predisp̶ when parents or siblings experi̶ of the atherosclerotic disease pr̶ the age of 55 to 60 years.

Age. As age increases, so do the chanc̶ person's having some type of CAD.

Gender. More females than males die from̶ CAD each year, although males tend to develop CAD at a younger age.

Race. African Americans have a higher incidence of hypertension than caucasians.

▶Risk Factors That Can be Changed

Cigarette Smoking. Of all the risk factors listed, perhaps none is as great a risk factor as cigarette smoking. It should be noted that all cigarette smokers have a much higher risk than nonsmokers. Recently it has also been shown that individuals exposed to second-hand smoke (the smoke from a cigarette that enters the environment) are also at higher risk for coronary artery disease and lung cancer.

HEALTH LINK 2-3

Risk Factors for Coronary Artery Disease

Risk Factors That Cannot be Changed
Family History
Age
Gender
Race

Risk Factors That Can be Changed
Cigarette smoking
Hypertension

High blood-cholesterol level
Physical inactivity

Contributing Risk Factors
Obesity
Diabetes
Stressful living

American Heart Association, www.americanheart.org

and behavior patterns. This observation holds
out hope that it may be possible to prevent premature CAD through modification of the risk
...ly. With the exception of age, gender, race,
...y, each of the other risk factors can be
...ch lifestyle modification.

...That Cannot be

...y of CAD in the fam-
...osing risk factor
...enced evidence
...cess before
...es of a

rt disease when compared with
not exercise.

ing Risk Factors

sity is related to CAD only in that
are obese tend to have higher
res as well as **hyperlipidemia.**
individuals are more likely to de-
of diabetes. Obesity reduces the
gage in exercise, thus impacting on
factor—physical inactivity. All of
sk factors for CAD.

Type 2 (non-insulin-dependent di-
has an onset in adulthood produces
ies in lipoproteins, which seems to
atherosclerosis. Also, diabetics fre-
ave a weight problem which places
stress on the cardiovascular system.
l Living. **Stress** increases blood pres-
forcing the heart to work harder.

tributes to the deposition...
plaque. Thus serum cholesterol levels are directly related to the incidence of CAD. The
higher the serum cholesterol level, the greater
the risk of CAD. **Lipoproteins** are carriers
of cholesterol. Low-density lipoprotein (LDL)
deposits cholesterol into the arterial wall,
whereas high-density lipoprotein (HDL) seems
to be able to remove the cholesterol deposited
by LDL from the arterial walls. Thus the more
HDL present, the better off you are, because it
appears to be an anti-risk factor. It is recommended that total cholesterol be below 200 mg
per dl (milligrams per deciliter), LDL be less
than 100 mg per dl, HDL be greater than 60 mg
per dl. Research has shown that individuals
who engage in regular physical activity can increase HDL levels.

Physical Inactivity. Those individuals who
lead a relatively sedentary style of living are
more likely to suffer from CAD and are less
likely to survive a heart attack than are those
who maintain an active lifestyle. Recent evidence indicates that individuals who expend
a minimum of 2,000 calories of energy a week
in physical activity, significantly reduce death

EFFECTS OF EXERCISE AND DIET ON RISK FACTORS

As physical activity levels increase, the number
of deaths attributed to CAD decrease. These
findings are consistent for both men and
women. Even moderate levels of physical fitness that are attainable by most adults appear
to provide some protection against early death.

Like exercise, diet can affect many of the risk
factors identified. There is little doubt that
adopting a healthful style of living, which incorporates good exercise and dietary habits,

lipoproteins: a compound of fat and protein that carries cholesterol

hyperlipidemia: an excessively high level of fat in the blood

stress: the responses that occur in the body when the internal balance or equi-librium of the body systems is disrupted

has the greatest influence in reducing the incidence of CAD.

WHAT IS CANCER?

Cancer is the second leading cause of death in adults, falling behind coronary artery disease. Cancer is a condition in which cellular behavior becomes abnormal. The cells no longer perform their normal functions. In general, cancer cells do not multiply at an increased rate. Instead, whatever causes the cancer alters the cell's genetic makeup and changes the way the cell functions. This abnormal cell then divides, forming additional cancer cells, and over a period of time this tumor, or collection of abnormal cells, tends to invade and ultimately take over normal tissue.

Tumors are either benign or malignant. Benign tumors typically pose only a small threat to tissue and tend to remain confined in a limited space. Malignant tumors, however, are cancerous, grow out of control, and spread within a specific tissue. Unfortunately, malignancies can invade surrounding tissues and spread via the blood and lymphatic systems (metastasize) throughout the entire body, thus making it difficult to control the cancer.

Malignancies are classified according to the types of tissues in which they occur as well as according to the rate at which they affect the tissue. Although different types of cancer cells share similar characteristics, each is separate and distinct. Some types are relatively easy to cure, whereas others are difficult to cure and

even life threatening. Skin cancer is the most common type of cancer; fortunately, it is one of the easiest to detect and cure.

Males and females have a different incidence in other types of cancers. In the male, the highest incidence of cancer is in the prostate, followed closely by lung, colon/rectal, and urinary tract cancers and leukemias/lymphomas. In the female the highest incidence is found in the breast, followed by colon/rectal, lung, and uterine cancers and leukemias/lymphomas.

The precise causes of cancer are not easily identified. Researchers have identified more than 100 types of cancer with genetic origins. Certain cancers appear to occur along family lines. The onset of most cancer has also been attributed to certain environmental factors, including viruses, exposure to ultraviolet light, radiation, alcohol use, and certain chemicals, including tobacco. A fatty diet has also been linked to cancer. Probably a combination of heredity and environmental factors is responsible for the development of cancer.

The American Cancer Society has identified warning signs of cancer, which are listed in Health Link 2-4. Unquestionably, early detection and treatment of cancer markedly improve the patient's chances of beating the disease.

EFFECTS OF EXERCISE AND DIET ON CANCER

Physical activity has been associated with a reduced risk of certain types of cancer. Moderate

HEALTH LINK 2-4

American Cancer Society's Cancer Warning Signals

Change in bowel or bladder habits
A sore that does not heal
Unusual bleeding or discharge
Thickening or lump in breast or elsewhere
Indigestion or difficulty in swallowing

Obvious change in wart or mole
Nagging cough or hoarseness

Modified from the American Cancer Society, *Cancer facts and figures*, New York, 2002, The Society. www.cancer.org

exercise has been shown to produce certain enzymes that reduce the formation of free radicals formed with incomplete oxidation of nutrients. These free radicals enhance the risk of chronic illnesses including cancer. However, some researchers are concerned that excessive exercise may potentially reduce the body's ability to produce these enzymes, thus increasing the chances of free radical-based cellular changes, including cancer.

Eating a healthy diet also has the potential to reduce the risk of cancer. The American Cancer Society recommends the following dietary precautions:

- Reduce total fat intake
- Eat more high-fiber foods
- Eat foods rich in Vitamins A and C
- Include vegetables in your diet (broccoli, brussels sprouts)
- Avoid smoked, salt-cured, and charred foods
- Limit alcohol consumption
- Avoid obesity

WHAT LIFESTYLE HABITS ARE DETERRENTS TO FITNESS?

Physical fitness involves more than exercise. To be physically fit means that a person must develop lifestyle habits that exclude negative practices such as abusing drugs, drinking excessive amounts of alcohol, and smoking.

DRUG USE AND ABUSE

Drug abuse differs from drug use and drug misuse. Drug use refers to the taking of any

drug abuse: the use of drugs for non-medical reasons; that is, with the intent of getting "high"—altering mood or behavior

drug for medical purposes. Drug misuse refers to the irresponsibility that many individuals show in the use of drugs. People who ignore medical advice about proper use of a prescribed drug or lend prescriptions to others are displaying a misuse of drugs. Drug abuse may be defined as the use of drugs for nonmedical reasons; that is, with the intent of getting "high"—altering mood or behavior.

After time, the body builds a tolerance to the usual level of certain drugs. Therefore, after abusing one of these drugs for a certain period, a person no longer gets the same "high" unless the dosage is increased. This is one reason that chronic drug abusers continually need to increase their number of "fixes" or doses of a drug.

Habituation is defined as psychological dependence as a result of continued use. People can be habituated to the use of alcohol, cigarettes, or drugs. They can become habituated to almost anything if they feel that it is helping them. In other words, drug abuse can become a habit if the individual feels psychologically that it is helping him or her in some way.

The term *addiction* means physical dependence. An addicted individual's body (1) needs a drug to function, (2) builds a tolerance to that drug, and (3) in most cases suffers from withdrawal symptoms. Withdrawal symptoms are the unpleasant physical problems that occur when the drug is taken away.

Drugs are most commonly abused because of their effects on mood and behavior. For example, a drug may produce a feeling of euphoria, often called a "high." These drugs are often referred to as psychoactive or psychotropic drugs. However, certain drugs, when abused, can distort the personality to such a degree that the individual may become dangerous to self or society. Research has indicated that most individuals who abuse psychoactive drugs have the type of personality that is often impressionable, escapist, or fragile. Persons with stronger personalities may experiment with drugs but are less likely to become dependent on them because the drugs do not satisfy their needs.

Drug abuse can cause both personal and family problems such as domestic violence, crime, and relationship difficulties.

▶ Recreational Drugs

Obviously, there are many drugs of abuse in our society. Recreational drugs are not only a deterrent to a healthy lifestyle, but their use or possession is also illegal. Among the more common "recreational" drugs are marijuana and cocaine.

Marijuana. When used in small doses, marijuana produces a "high" feeling and sense of relaxation lasting for several hours after use. The immediate effects of use are relaxation and feelings of heightened awareness of visual, auditory, and tactile sensations. It also causes impairment of coordination, performance, perception, attention, and short-term memory. Problems associated with long-term use include restlessness, irritability, loss of motivation, sleep disturbances, and possible damage to the lungs.

Cocaine. Cocaine has become one of the most popular drugs of abuse during recent years. Cocaine is a stimulant with effects of short duration. Cocaine use produces immediate feelings of euphoria, excitement, decreased sense of fatigue, and heightened sexual drive. Cocaine may be snorted, taken intravenously, or smoked ("free-based"). Crack is a rocklike crystalline form of cocaine that is heated in a small pipe and then inhaled, producing an immediate rush. The initial effects are extremely intense, and because they are pleasurable, strong psychological dependence is developed rapidly by users, regardless of whether they can afford this expensive habit.

Long-term effects include nasal congestion and damage to the membranes and cartilage of the nose if snorted, bronchitis, loss of appetite leading to nutritional deficiencies, convulsions, impotence, and cocaine psychosis with paranoia, depression, hallucinations, and

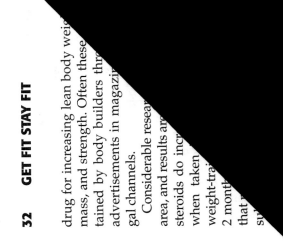

drug for increasing lean body wei... mass, and strength. Often these tained by body builders thr... advertisements in magazi... gal channels.

Considerable resea... area, and results ar... steroids do inc... when taken... 2 month... that... su...

behavior. Physical reactions can include loss of appetite, nausea, vomiting, blurred vision, increased heart rate and blood pressure, muscle tension, faintness, chills, sweating, tremors, insomnia, convulsions, and loss of control over voluntary body movements. Some reactions have been reported to persist up to 14 days after taking Ecstasy.

▶ Anabolic Steroids

The unfortunate use of anabolic steroids by persons attempting to develop high levels of strength is becoming commonplace (strength training itself is discussed in Chapter 5). **Anabolic steroids** are organic compounds that contain primarily sterols and sex hormones (testosterone). These drugs are prescribed and used therapeutically in the treatment of diseases in which protein synthesis is an essential component of the healing process. Some individuals, not necessarily only athletes, use the

> **anabolic steroids:** organic compounds that primarily contain sterols and sex hormones and are used for increasing lean body weight, muscle mass, and strength

...ht, muscle
...drugs are ob-
...ugh mail order
...es or through ille-

...ch has taken place in this
...e at best conflicting. Anabolic
...ease muscle size and strength
...in conjunction with an intense
...ning program over a period of 1 to
...s. However, it has also been proposed
...prolonged use of anabolic steroids may re-
...it in harmful side effects such as liver dysfunction and cancer, sterility, reduced testicular function and loss of sexual interest, headaches, nausea, acne, baldness, unpredictable aggressive behavior, increased blood pressure and risk of coronary heart disease, kidney tumors, and so on. Death is an all too common consequence of long-term anabolic steroid abuse. For this reason, using anabolic steroids for the purpose of strength improvement cannot be recommended and has in fact been banned by the International Olympic Committee.

Despite the uncertainty about the long-range effects of these drugs, anabolic steroid use is a continuing problem affecting many persons involved with heavy weight training at all levels.

Androstenedione is classified by the FDA as a dietary supplement and thus can be purchased over the counter. It has been suggested that this "anabolic-steroid-like" drug has some of the same effects but is safer than steroids. Currently, there is no definitive research to support its use.

ALCOHOL ABUSE

The consumption of alcohol in our American society is commonplace. The reasons some people abstain, some drink moderately, while others imbibe heavily have never been completely explained. The studies seem to indicate that alcohol meets individual need patterns. It is felt that situations and environmental conditions that produce tension and insecurity may cause some to resort to drinking.

People who are uncomfortable and lack poise at social gatherings use drinking as a social lubricant. The alcohol gives them courage and helps them feel at ease. Unfortunately, some people have failed to develop wholesome interpersonal relationships. Alcohol provides a temporary means of escape from those experiences that frustrate and worry them. Drinking does not solve the problem but instead offers a temporary means of escape from reality. Although there are some conflicting views as to its cause, there appears to be agreement that some of the causes are psychological. Some psychologists believe that individuals who are emotionally disturbed, have compulsive personalities, or exhibit obsessive-compulsive behavior are more prone to alcoholism.

▶What Is Alcoholism

Alcoholism is called a disease because an alcoholic is sick, totally dependent on the substance and the abuse of it. The National Council on Alcoholism defines an alcoholic as "a person who is powerless to stop drinking, and whose drinking seriously alters his (or her) normal living pattern." Many persons may ask, "Why do some people become alcoholics while others in the same situation or environment do not?" Why is it that only 10 to 15 percent of the more than 100 million drinkers become alcoholics? These are valid questions for which there are no absolute answers. There are many potential alcoholics who do not become alcoholics. Unfortunately, alcoholism is a chronic condition that does not go away. It is progressive and incurable as long as the

alcoholism: a disease in which a person is powerless to stop drinking and drinking seriously alters his or her normal living pattern

alcoholic keeps on drinking. If he or she stops drinking, the disease can be arrested. But most experts believe that the alcoholic must not drink again. Otherwise that person will be right back where he or she was when the decision was made to stop drinking. Alcoholics are sensitive to alcohol and all other sedatives. The brain of an alcoholic produces a substance called THIQ, which is extremely addicting. Years of abstinence will not eliminate the ability to produce THIQ. It is always present and renders the alcoholic powerless to quit once she or he begins drinking.

▶ What Are the Effects of Alcohol?

Alcohol is classified as a drug that depresses the central nervous system. Alcohol is absorbed from the digestive system into the bloodstream very rapidly. Factors that affect how rapidly absorption takes place include the number of drinks consumed, the rate of consumption, the alcohol concentration of the beverage, and the amount of food in the stomach. Some alcohol is absorbed into the blood through the stomach, but the greater part is absorbed through the small intestine. Alcohol is transported through the blood to the liver, where it can be metabolized at a rate of 2/3 ounce per hour. An excess causes an increase in the level of alcohol circulating in the blood. As blood alcohol content (BAC) levels continue to increase, predictable signs of intoxication appear. At 0.1 percent the person loses motor coordination, and from 0.2 to 0.5 percent the symptoms become progressively more profound and perhaps even life threatening. Women tend to absorb more alcohol and at a faster rate than do men of the same body weight. Intoxication persists until the remainder of the alcohol can be metabolized by the liver. There is no way to accelerate the liver's metabolism of alcohol ("sober up"); it just takes time.

▶ Alcohol-Related Diseases

Alcohol consumption can directly or indirectly cause numerous physical problems. Gastritis, an inflammation of the stomach, can result from excessive alcohol consumption. Alcoholics suffer from malnutrition because they lose interest in food and are unable to purchase proper foods. Also, alcohol provides considerable calories but lacks important nutrients.

Alcohol is poisonous to cells. The most common cause of liver disorders, cirrhosis (a scarring and hardening of liver tissue), is a result of chronic alcoholism. Over the years there has been some linkage of alcohol to cancer, especially cancer of the liver, larynx, esophagus, and tongue. These represent only a few of the diseases caused when excessive amounts of alcohol are consumed for extended periods of time.

How can you tell whether you currently have or are developing a drinking problem? You must identify the warning signs that let you know that the potential for such a problem exists. Health Link 2-5 will give you some idea of the warning signs.

TOBACCO USE

The number of deaths caused by **tobacco use** is alarming, and the impact of tobacco use on healthcare cost is almost mind-boggling. The United States government is currently waging an all-out war against tobacco. Over the years many steps have been taken to educate the nation's 53 million smokers about the dangers of tobacco. Yet millions of Americans continue to smoke.

▶ Why Do People Smoke?

The pleasure derived from smoking may be due as much to the social ritual that is associated with it as to the physiologic effects.

tobacco use: the use of cigarettes, cigars, pipes, or smokeless tobacco

HEALTH LINK 2-5

Warning Signs for Excessive Alcohol Use

Do you:

- Drink more frequently than you did a year ago?
- Drink more heavily than you did a year ago?
- Plan to drink, sometimes days in advance?
- Gulp or "chug" your drinks, perhaps in a contest?
- Set personal limits on the amount you plan to drink but then consistently disregard these limits?
- Drink at a rate greater than two drinks per hour?
- Encourage or even pressure others to drink with you?
- Frequently want a nonalcoholic beverage but then end up drinking an alcoholic drink?
- Drive your car while under the influence of alcohol or ride with another person who has been drinking?
- Use alcoholic beverages while taking prescription or over-the-counter medications?
- Forget what happened while you were drinking?
- Have a tendency to disregard information about the effects of drinking?
- Find your reputation fading because of alcohol use?

National Institute on Alcohol Abuse and Alcoholism, www.niaaa.nih.gov

Certainly, many young people who begin to smoke do so because they regard it as symbolic of adulthood. Some use smoking as a form of rebellion. Still others use smoking as a form of weight control. It has been suggested that the habit-forming nature of tobacco is to a large extent psychologically and socially determined. As millions of smokers know, smoking is a habit that becomes more difficult to break the more and the longer one smokes. It is known that nicotine is physically addictive. Although a smoker does not suffer the harsh withdrawal symptoms typical of certain addictive drugs, nervousness and irritability are commonly experienced when smoking is stopped.

▶ What Is In Tobacco Smoke?

The major components of tobacco smoke are carbon monoxide, nicotine, and tars, all of which have harmful effects on the body. The more deeply the smoker inhales and the shorter the length to which the cigarette is smoked, the more nicotine is absorbed.

Nicotine. Nicotine, a colorless, oily compound, is extremely poisonous in concentrated form. Nicotine affects the body in a variety of ways. Small doses have a stimulating effect upon various brain centers. It constricts the blood vessels of the skin, resulting in a clammy, pallid appearance and a reduction of skin temperature. Nicotine also increases the blood pressure and the heart rate. It has a numbing effect on the taste receptors of the tongue, hence the loss of interest in food by many heavy smokers. Beginning smokers may experience some slight toxic effects such as nausea and vomiting, but, as the smoker builds up a tolerance, these generally disappear.

Carbon Monoxide. Approximately 1 percent of cigarette smoke is composed of carbon monoxide. A highly poisonous gas, carbon monoxide is also a component of automobile exhaust. Many individuals are killed each year by the inhalation of this gas in closed areas such as garages. The carbon monoxide in cigarette smoke reduces the oxygen carrying capacity of the red blood cells and therefore causes a reduction of oxygen in the body. This is one of the reasons why smokers complain of "shortness of breath" after mild exercise.

Tar. Tobacco tar is a dark, sticky substance that can be condensed from cigarette smoke. It is the substance discussed in advertisements concerning "low tar and nicotine." Certainly "low tar" is not better than "no tar." Tar is extremely toxic and is carcinogenic (causing cancerous lesions) on test animals. The chemicals in cigarette tar are believed to contribute to the development of lung cancer.

▶ Passive Smoke

There are dangers associated with the passive inhalation of smoke ("secondhand") by nonsmokers. Both smokers and nonsmokers are exposed to smoke containing carbon monoxide, nicotine, ammonia, and cyanide. Obviously smokers inhale the greater quantity of contaminated air. However, it has been estimated that for each pack of cigarettes smoked, the nonsmoker, sharing a common air supply, will inhale the equivalent of three to five cigarettes. According to a review of passive smoking research, passive smoking may be responsible for as many as 15,000 premature deaths among exposed nonsmokers. It is also true that significant numbers of individuals exposed to passive smoke develop nasal symptoms, eye irritation, headaches, cough, and in some cases allergies to smoke. For these reasons and others, many state, local, and private sector policies have been established that restrict or ban smoking in public areas. There is little doubt that passive smoking poses a significant health threat to the nonsmoker.

▶ Smokeless Tobacco

Unfortunately, the use of smokeless chewing tobacco has seen a tremendous increase in recent years. Once a pinch or pouch of chewing tobacco is placed "between the cheek and gum," nicotine is absorbed through the mucous membranes, and within a short period of time the level of nicotine in the blood is equivalent to that of a cigarette smoker. The user of chewing tobacco experiences the nicotine effects without exposure to the tar and carbon monoxide associated with a burning cigarette. Certainly the use of smokeless tobacco has eliminated many of the risks associated with cigarette smoking. However, inadvertently swallowed saliva contains carcinogens that must be eliminated through the digestive and urinary systems, thus predisposing the user to the risks of cancer. Additionally, the use of chewing tobacco increases the risk of periodontal disease in the gums, destroys the enamel on teeth, and causes the development of white blotches on the mucous membranes of the mouth, which are thought to be associated with development of cancer in the mouth.

▶ Curbing the Use of Tobacco

Many steps have been taken to caution the nation's 53 million smokers about the dangers of tobacco. A warning from the U.S. surgeon general is printed on each package of cigarettes. Television commercials for cigarettes have been banned. Group therapy sessions have been organized to help people stop smoking. Patches that deliver nicotine through the skin are often prescribed along with group sessions to help smokers "kick the habit." Special cigarette holders and filter tips have been devised to cut down on tar and nicotine. Some states have outlawed smoking in all public buildings. Municipalities are acting to ban smoking altogether in public places. In many states it is illegal to sell tobacco products to individuals under 18 years of age. Yet millions of Americans, including many college students, continue to smoke. Many adults belong to the hard core group of smokers who will never quit the habit. However, a major focus is educational efforts to prevent young people from choosing to begin to smoke.

CREATING A HEALTHY LIFESTYLE: YOUR PERSONAL RESPONSIBILITY

Some people today think of health as the responsibility of doctors, hospitals, clinics, insurance companies, and the government. It is important to realize, however, that health cannot be purchased or the responsibility relegated to some other person or agency. Health is an obligation on the part of each individual, and it is erroneous to equate more health services with better health. Instead, individuals must take responsibility for their own health.

The decisions that people make relative to their lifestyle have an effect on their health. They are the ones who decide what to eat and when and whether to exercise, drink, engage in drug abuse, smoke, or see a doctor. Thus the decisions they make leave an imprint on their health and well-being. In many cases people who become sick have only themselves to blame.

The call to attain the optimal level of health for ourselves and our loved ones is a lifetime challenge. No one can do the job for us, nor should they. This is a responsibility each person should assume to the extent he or she is able, with pride and conviction. Lab Activity 2–2 will help you determine whether you are living a healthy lifestyle.

of life and for growth and development. Stress involves physiological and psychological responses.

- Coping skills to ward off stress are those procedures that allow a person to deal with reality in a positive way. Several relaxation techniques for coping with stress exist, including the progressive relaxation technique, biofeedback, yoga, breathing exercises, meditation, imagery, massage, and autogenic training.
- Coronary artery disease (CAD) accounts for half of all the deaths in the United States each year. The major risk factors, which cannot be changed, that predispose a person to CAD are family history, age, gender and race. Risk factors that can be changed include cigarette smoking, hypertension, lack of physical activity and high blood-cholesterol levels. Obesity, diabetes, and stressful living would be considered contributing risk factors.
- Cancer is the second leading cause of death in adult Americans. Early detection and treatment are critical for reducing the likelihood of death.
- It is important to recognize that using alcohol, tobacco, or other drugs is a deterrent to health and wellness.
- Sexually transmitted infections (STIs) are extremely common and have a negative impact on wellness. AIDS and other STIs are life-threatening diseases.
- Creating a healthy style of living is a personal responsibility.

SUMMARY

- Creating a healthy lifestyle incorporates aspects of intellectual, physical, social, emotional, and spiritual health in a manner that allows you to enjoy the highest level of health and well-being possible.
- Everyone experiences stress, and some stress is needed to perform the daily tasks

SUGGESTED READINGS

American Cancer Society. 2002. *2002 cancer facts and figures.* Atlanta: American Cancer Society.
American Heart Association. 1998. *Primary prevention of coronary heart disease: Guidance from Framingham.* Dallas: American Heart Association.
Bassuk, S. S., and J. E. Manson. 2004. Preventing cardiovascular disease in women: How much physical activity is "good enough"? *President's Council on Physical Fitness and Sports research digest* 4(5):1–7, 9.

Begg, C. B. 2001. The search for cancer risk factors: When can we stop looking? *American Journal of Public Health* 91(3):360–64.

Bellenir, K. 2004. *Smoking concerns sourcebook: Basic consumer health information about nicotine addiction and smoking cessation, featuring facts about the health effects of tobacco use.* Detroit: Omnigraphics, Inc.

Brehm, B. A. 2002. Heart disease: Lifestyle is key to prevention. *Fitness Management* 18(5):30.

Brubaker, P., L. A. Kaminsky, and M. H. Whaley. 2002. *Coronary artery disease: Essentials of prevention and rehabilitation programs.* Champaign, IL: Human Kinetics.

Burak, L. J. 2001. Smokeless tobacco education for college athletes. *Journal of Physical Education, Recreation and Dance* 72(1):37–38, 53.

Cooper, C. B. 2001. Smoking and exercise. *ACSM's Health and Fitness Journal* 5(2):27, 31.

Courneya, K. S., and J. R. Mackey. 2001. Exercise during and after cancer treatment: Benefits, guidelines, and precautions. *International Sports Medicine Journal* 1(5):206–10.

Dickey, R. A., and J. J. Janick. 2001. Lifestyle modifications in the prevention and treatment of hypertension. *Endocrine Practice* 7(5):392–99.

Do Lee, C., and S. N. Blair. 2002. Cardiorespiratory fitness and smoking-related and total cancer mortality in men. *Medicine and Science in Sports and Exercise* 34(5):735–39.

Gill, J. 2004. *Personalized stress management: A manual for everyday life and work.* Otsego, Michigan: Pagefree Publishing Inc.

Green, G. A., F. D. Uryasz, T. A. Petr, and C. D. Bray. 2001. NCAA study of substance use and abuse habits of college student-athletes. *Clinical Journal of Sport Medicine* 11(1):51–56.

Greene, R. 2002. *Get with the program!: Getting real about your weight, health, and emotional well-being.* New York: Simon and Schuster Adult Publishing.

Heart disease risk high, knowledge low. 2004. *IDEA Personal Trainer* 15(2):10.

Heyward, V. H. 2002. Assessing and managing stress. In *Advanced fitness assessment and exercise prescription,* 4th ed., edited by V. H. Heyward, pp. 251–58, 347–48. Champaign, IL: Human Kinetics.

High-intensity exercise best to reduce stress. 2004. *Fitness Business Canada* 5(4):46–47.

Hildebrand, K. M., D. J. Johnson, and K. Bogle. 2001. Comparison of patterns of alcohol use between high school and college athletes and non-athletes. *College Student Journal* 35(3):358–65.

Howard-Pitney, B., and M. A. Winkleby. 2002. Chewing tobacco: Who uses and who quits? Findings from NHANES III, 1988–1994. *American Journal of Public Health* 92(2):250–56.

Iven, V. G. 1998. Recreational drugs. *Clinics in Sports Medicine* 17(2):245–59.

Kavanagh, T. 2001. Exercise in the primary prevention of coronary artery disease. *Canadian Journal of Cardiology* 17(2):155–61.

Keller, J. 2004. Nine risk factors to blame for 90% of heart attacks. *IDEA Fitness Journal* 1(5):13.

Kinney, J. 2005. *Loosening the grip: A handbook of alcohol information.* New York: McGraw-Hill.

Koehler, G. 2001. Stress management: Exercises for teachers and students. *Strategies* 15(2):7–10.

Lee, I. M., and R. S. Paffenbarger, Jr. 2001. Preventing coronary heart disease: The role of physical activity. *Physician and Sports Medicine* 29(2):37–40, 43–46, 49, 52.

Luskin, F., and K. Pelletier. 2005. *Stress free for good: 10 scientifically proven life skills for health and happiness.* New York: Harper Collins Publishers.

Meade, T. W. 2001. Cardiovascular disease: Linking pathology and epidemiology. *International Journal of Epidemiology* 30(5):1179–83.

Meyer, H. E., A. J. Sogaard, A. Tverdal, and R. M. Selmer. 2002. Body mass index and mortality: The influence of physical activity and smoking. *Medicine and Science in Sports and Exercise* 34(7):1065–70.

Nieman, D. C. 1998. *The exercise-health connection.* Champaign, IL: Human Kinetics.

Perkinson, R. 2003. *The alcohol and drug abuse patient workbook.* Thousand Oaks, CA. Sage Publications.

Pescatello, L. S., B. A. Franklin, and R. Fagard. 2004. American College of Sports Medicine position stand: Exercise and hypertension. *Medicine and Science in Sports and Exercise* 36(3):533–53.

Slattery, M. L., and J. D. Potter. 2002. Physical activity and colon cancer: Confounding or interaction? *Medicine and Science in Sports and Exercise* 34(6):913–19.

Svebak, S. 1999. *Stress and health: A reversal theory perspective.* Washington, DC: Taylor & Francis.

The war on cancer: Are we winning or losing? 2004. *Tufts University Health & Nutrition Letter* 22(2):8.

Thune, I., and A. S. Furberg. 2001. Physical activity and cancer risk: Dose-response and cancer, all sites and site-specific. *Medicine and Science in Sports and Exercise* 33(6 Suppl):S530–50.

Wannamethee, S. G., and A. G. Shaper. 2001. Physical activity in the prevention of cardiovascular disease: An epidemiological perspective. *Sports Medicine* 31(2):101–14.

Zuzanek, J., J. P. Robinson, and Y. Iwasaki. 1998. The relationships between stress, health, and physically active leisure as a function of life-cycle. *Leisure Sciences* 20(4):253–75.

SUGGESTED WEB SITES

ACSH: Tobacco

The American Council on Science and Health has been a leader in restoring scientific fact and context to health issues, in exposing both overstated and understated risks. This page covers tobacco, including what the warning label doesn't tell you.
www.acsh.org/tobacco/index.html

American Cancer Society

This is the official Web site of the American Cancer Society. The site provides information on all types of cancer, cancer

research, therapy, support groups, and local community resources for cancer patients and their families.
www.cancer.org/index_4up.html

American College Health Association

The ACHA provides health information, facts, and guidance for college students.
www.acha.org/home.htm

American Heart Association

This site is dedicated to providing you with education and information on fighting heart disease and stroke.
www.americanheart.org

CDC's TIPS: Tobacco Information and Prevention Source

The Centers for Disease Control and Prevention (CDC) presents the Tobacco Information and Prevention Source (TIPS). This Web site is maintained by the CDC's Office on Smoking and Health, which is a division of the National Center for Chronic Disease Prevention and Health Promotion (US Gov't Web site). Information covering tobacco-related issues and statistics is presented. There are also sections dedicated to youth.
www.cdc.gov/tobacco

Health Education Alliance for Life and Longevity

This site presents 10,000+ hand-picked resources that sort the wheat from the chaff on alternative medicine, Y2K, vitamins, herbs, natural product recommendation, and resource lists. Marketing coop, wellness author features, and Citizen's Action and Freedom of Choice in Medicine updates are also featured.
www.heall.com

National Institute on Alcohol Abuse and Alcoholism

The NIAAA supports and conducts biomedical and behavioral research on the causes, consequences, treatment, and prevention of alcoholism and alcohol-related problems. The NIAAA also provides leadership in the national effort to reduce the severe and often fatal consequences of these problems
www.niaaa.nih.gov

National Institute on Drug Abuse

The mission of the National Institute on Drug Abuse (NIDA) is to lead the nation in bringing the power of science to bear on drug abuse and addiction.
www.nida.nih.gov

National Wellness Association

The NWA is the Membership Division of the National Wellness Institute. NWA is a non-profit professional membership organization that serves professionals working in all areas of wellness and health promotion.
www.nationalwellness.org

National Wellness Institute—NationalWellness.org

Search the Wellness Resource Directory! The National Wellness Institute helps professionals interested in wellness and health promotion.
www.wellnesswi.org/index.htm

Stress Management and Relaxation Central

Take control of your stress response and learn to relax, yet retain alertness and energy.
www.futurehealth.org/stresscn.htm

Tobacco BBS—Resources on Tobacco, Smoking, Cigarettes

Tobacco BBS presents tobacco issues, tobacco and smoking-related news, addresses, tobacco history, quitting, and a great quote-of-the-day section.
www.tobacco.org

Wellness Institute

This site provides the community with services that promote health, prevent illness and disability, and restore wellness of body, mind, and spirit.
www.wellnessinstitute.mb.ca

4Addictions—A Guide to Addictions from 4Anything

Get the support and information you need. Here you can anonymously learn all about addictions to alcohol, drugs, tobacco, food, sex, and other things. You can find support groups and counseling, prevention organizations, or just someone to talk to.
www.4addictions.com

Starting Your Own **Fitness** Program

Objectives

After completing this chapter, you should be able to do the following:

- Identify the basic principles of a fitness program.
- Discuss the importance of the warm-up and cool-down periods.
- Determine your individual goals for your fitness program.
- Identify precautions for beginning a fitness program.

A t this point, you should have some idea about why you need to get fit. Your individual reasons and motivations have been identified in Chapter 1. Beginning a fitness program is simple. In addition, you can do several things to ensure that your program is successful and yet fun and enjoyable.

THE PROGRAM SHOULD BE FUN AND ENJOYABLE

Enjoying yourself may be one of the most critical factors for a successful fitness program over the long run. The activity you select must be one that you enjoy and that provides motivation to continue for a lifetime (Figure 3-1). For example, a quick look at the streets on a sunny day will show that running is a popular form of physical activity. There is no question that a running program eventually will result in significant improvement in cardiorespiratory endurance. Personally, I hate to run and would prefer to do any other activity. If I were

to select running as my fitness activity because it is "in" and not because I enjoy doing it, then chances are that I would not stick with it for long. You should enjoy getting into good physical condition, and a successful fitness program will be considered fun rather than work.

ADHERING TO AN EXERCISE PROGRAM

Motivation plays an important role in your ability to stick with an exercise program. You should select the type of activity that will allow you to do two things: (1) achieve the ultimate

KEY TERMS

overload	*specificity*
SAID principle	*warm-up*
progression	*cool-down*
consistency	

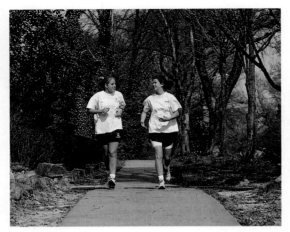

FIGURE 3-1.
An exercise program should be fun and enjoyable.

goals of physical fitness improvement that you have established for yourself, and (2) maintain your interest and motivation for a long time (weeks, months, even years). Fit List 3-1 provides some suggestions that can make your program fun and enjoyable.

FIT LIST 3-1

Suggestions for Making Physical Activity Fun

Some students find physical activity dull. Here are some ways to make it more inviting.

- Exercise to music.
- Exercise with classmates.
- Keep your program simple.
- Instill variety into activity: for example, dancing, hiking, tennis, and swimming.
- Reward yourself when fitness goals are met.
- Don't become upset when goals are not met and benefits are not immediate.
- Keep a record of things such as your weight and the distance you jog.
- Take a break whenever you wish.
- Plan the program to fit into your daily life.

WHAT ARE THE BASIC PRINCIPLES OF A FITNESS PROGRAM?

Regardless of the type of physical activity in which you choose to participate, certain principles should be incorporated into every program. These principles and guidelines apply to anyone who is physically active. Paying attention to these basic principles will help to create an effective yet safe environment for physical activities. Fit List 3-2 summarizes these principles.

OVERLOAD

To achieve the greatest benefits from an exercise program, you should recognize the principle of **overload** (Figure 3-2). For a physical component of fitness to improve, the system must work harder than it is used to working. The system must experience stress so that over a period of time it will improve to the point where it can easily accommodate additional stress. The **SAID principle** (an acronym for *specific adaptation to imposed demands*) states that when the body is subjected to stresses and overloads of varying intensities, it will gradually adapt, over time, to overcome whatever demands are placed on it. Even though overload

FIT LIST 3-2

The Basic Principles of a Fitness Program

- Overload
- Progression
- Consistency
- Specificity
- Diminishing Returns
- Reversibility
- Individuality
- Safety

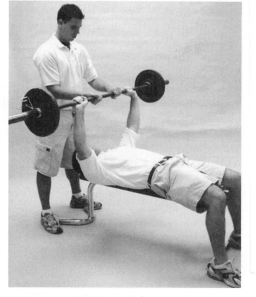

FIGURE 3-2. OVERLOAD.
To see improvement you must use the principle of overload.

is a critical factor for getting fit, the stress must not be great enough to produce damage or injury. The body needs to have a chance to adjust to the imposed demands. Therefore overload is a gradual increase in the frequency, intensity, time or duration, and type (FITT) of the physical activity that is a part of the fitness program. (The FITT formula will be discussed in detail in Chapter 4.) This is one of the most critical factors in any activities program. For example, if you are on a jogging program to improve cardiorespiratory endurance and you

> **overload:** exercising at a higher level than normal

> **SAID principle:** when the body is subjected to stresses and overloads of varying intensities, it will gradually adapt, over time, to overcome whatever demands are placed on it

your physical ability. Even though creases may be minimal in streng progression of even 1 pound is maintain interest and motiv

CONSISTENCY

One of the bigg fitness prog day to fit particul dem

nificant improvement in that system's ability to handle a stressful exercise session.

PROGRESSION

A little today and a little more tomorrow is a good principle to follow in any fitness program. You should start gradually and add a little each day. The rate of **progression** should be within your capabilities to adapt physically. In other words, the workout should gradually become a little longer or more intense until you reach the desired level of physical fitness. If you try to progress too rapidly, it is likely that you may develop some type of injury (see Chapter 9). There comes a time in many fitness programs when *improving* fitness levels becomes less important than *maintaining* fitness levels. Progression is closely related to overload. Without overloading the system, progression does not occur. Progression is also important for motivation. Interest level in an activity remains high as long as you continue to see improvement in

> **progression:** gradually increasing the level and intensity of exercise

weight in-
...th training, a
...often enough to
...tion.

...st problems with beginning a
...am is finding time during the
...n an hour or so of activity. This is
...arly true for students who have many
...ands on their time. Nevertheless, it is im-
...rtant to select a specific period for exercising each day and stick to it.

The best time of day for you to exercise is whenever you have the time and are motivated to do so. The important point is to set aside some time for a fitness program and make it part of your daily routine for **consistency.** The least desirable times are probably after a meal, when activity may make you uncomfortable, and just before bedtime, when the activity has been so invigorating that it is difficult to fall asleep. The number of days per week you are involved with a specific activity will vary depending on several personal factors. However, it is recommended that you try to work out at least 3 days per week to see minimal improvement.

SPECIFICITY

The type of physical changes that occur is directly related to the type of training undertaken. To realize the maximum gains desired, activities and programs should be selected and designed with **specificity** to achieve this

> **consistency:** engaging in fitness activities on a frequent and regular basis
>
> **specificity:** the type of physical changes that occur are directly related to the type of training used

Specific Workout to target
Specific bidy pass to exercise

aim. Once again, according to the SAID principle, a particular physical system will respond and adapt over time to whatever specific demands are placed on it. For example, to develop flexibility in a specific joint, stretching exercises must be incorporated that progressively lengthen the muscles and tendons that surround that joint.

DIMINISHING RETURNS

The greatest gains in fitness will be seen early on in an exercise program. After the initial increase, gains will continue, but at a slower pace. The fitness benefits that an individual acquires from exercising are only sustained with the maintenance of his or her exercise program. Therefore we should encourage people to continue to exercise throughout their lifetime to prevent these gains from being lost.

REVERSIBILITY

In adults, it is likely that some or all of the gains made in strength, flexibility, cardiorespiratory endurance, etc., during an exercise program will be lost if the program is stopped. However, in children and teenagers who are still growing, it is possible that some of the gains achieved from increased loading during an exercise program may be retained after the exercise program is discontinued.

INDIVIDUALITY

When you become involved in a fitness program, it is important to remember that no two persons are exactly the same. People have different ideas about their goals for a fitness program, motivation, and state of physical fitness. A fitness program for one person will not necessarily satisfy the needs of another person. Furthermore, not all people involved in similar activities will progress at the same rate, nor will they be able to overload their systems to the same degree. Exercise is good, but it must be adapted to individual needs and abilities. Just as a medical prescription must be related to a person's health needs, so should a physical fitness prescription. A person's exercise prescription needs to be based on his or her objectives, needs, functional capacity, and interests.

SAFETY

Another factor to consider when planning a fitness program is safety. The purpose of your fitness program should be to improve selected components of fitness through physical exercise. Unfortunately, injuries often occur as the result of poorly planned activity programs. The rule of thumb to follow is to start out slowly and progress according to your own capabilities. Adhering to the rule "train—don't strain" can certainly reduce the likelihood of injury. If you are unsure of how to get started or perhaps of how quickly to progress in a personal fitness program, seek professional advice from persons with some expertise in fitness.

SHOULD YOU DO A WARM-UP ROUTINE BEFORE YOU EXERCISE?

Absolutely! It is important for you to **warm up** before you begin any type of workout for several reasons. The warm-up routine increases body core temperature, stretches ligaments and muscles, and increases flexibility. Warm-up routines have been found to be important in

> **warm-up:** designed to increase body temperature, stretch ligaments and muscles, and increase flexibility

reducing injury and muscle soreness. It appears that muscle injury can result when vigorous exercises are not preceded by a related warm-up routine. A good, short warm-up routine can also be an effective motivator. If you get satisfaction from warming up, you probably will have a stronger desire to participate in an activity. By contrast, a poor warm-up routine can lead to fatigue and boredom, limiting your attention and ultimately resulting in a poor program. Also, there is some evidence that a good warm-up routine may improve certain aspects of performance.

The function of the warm-up routine is to prepare your body physically for a workout. Most professionals view the warm-up period as a precaution against unnecessary muscle injury and possible muscle soreness. The purpose is to gradually stimulate the cardiorespiratory system to a moderate degree. This produces an increased blood flow to exercising muscles and results in an increase in muscle temperature.

Moderate activity speeds up your metabolism, producing an increase in your body temperature. Furthermore, an increase in the temperature of muscle allows the muscle to stretch to a greater degree without fear of injury.

A good warm-up routine should begin with 2 or 3 minutes of slow walking, light jogging, or cycling to increase your metabolism and warm up the muscles. Breaking into a light sweat is a good indication that the muscle temperature has increased (Figure 3-3). Although research has indicated that increasing core temperature is effective in reducing injuries, there is little or no evidence that stretching during the warm-up reduces injury. Empirically, many professionals feel that stretching should be a part of the warm-up and continue to recommend that flexibility exercises be included. There is also no evidence that stretching does any harm. The total warm-up routine should last no longer than 10 to 15 minutes, and you should begin your activity immediately following the warm-up routine.

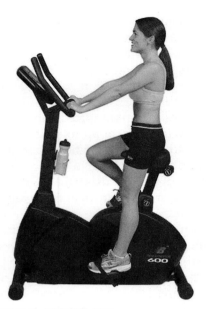

FIGURE 3-3. WARM-UP.
A warm-up routine should include an activity to increase body core temperature.

WORKOUT

The type and length of workout in which you choose to engage are determined by your reasons for engaging in a fitness program and by the goals you have established for yourself. Thus the workout will differ significantly between individuals. Recommendations for workouts to accomplish specific fitness goals are presented throughout the text.

COOL-DOWN

After a vigorous workout, a **cool-down** period is essential. The cool-down period prevents pooling of blood in the arms and legs, thus maintaining blood pressure and enabling the body to cool and return to a resting state. The cool-down period should last about 5 to 10 minutes. During the cool-down period, you may engage in stretching activities as was done during the warm-up routine. Some people feel that stretching during the cool-down period is more effective in preventing injury than is stretching during the warm-up routine. Although the value of warm-up routine and workout periods is well accepted, the importance of a cool-down period is often ignored. Again, experience and observation indicate that people who stretch during the cool-down period tend to have fewer problems with muscle soreness after strenuous activity.

WHAT ARE THE GOALS OF YOUR FITNESS PROGRAM?

When designing an individualized physical fitness program, you must first decide what it is you are trying to accomplish and then select those specific components of fitness that ultimately help you to reach your goal. For example, the goals of fitness improvement for a person who plays Frisbee occasionally on weekends will differ considerably from those of a person preparing to compete in varsity soccer. Most people who are not athletes should be more concerned with fitness components related to good health such as cardiorespiratory endurance, flexibility, muscular strength, muscular endurance, and body composition. Improvement in these five specific areas enhance a person's ability to perform daily tasks without undue fatigue, as stated in our definition of physical fitness.

On the other hand, the soccer player must be concerned not only with the components that have been mentioned above but also with

cool-down: prevents pooling of blood and enables the body to cool and return to a resting state

components such as strength, speed, power, balance, and agility. The soccer player who does not include activities in the training regimen that specifically address these various skill-related fitness components likely will be unsuccessful in a competitive situation.

HOW SHOULD YOU EXERCISE?

It has been well documented that engaging in regular, moderate-intensity physical activity will result in substantial health benefits. Recommendations from various organizations as to exactly how people should exercise seem to be constantly evolving. For years, an exercise period of 30 to 60 minutes' duration at an intensity of 60 to 90 percent of maximum heart rate performed three or more times per week was the recommended standard for promoting good health and preventing disease according to the American College of Sports Medicine. In 1995 the Centers for Disease Control and Prevention and the American College of Sports Medicine issued a revised joint recommendation that everyone should try to engage in a minimum of 30 minutes of physical activity on most days—ideally, every day. This 30-minute total did not have to consist solely of what has traditionally been considered exercise (walking, swimming, cycling, etc.). It could involve a series of short bouts of physical activity that collectively accumulate to a total of at least 30 minutes of moderate-intensity physical exercise and that may include more intermittent activities such as walking up or down stairs, doing lawn work or gardening, and cleaning the house. (See the Activity Pyramid in Figure 3-4.)

This recommendation relative to the quantity and quality of exercise was substantially less formal than what had been recommended in the past. Research had indicated that many health benefits could be achieved by engaging in moderate-intensity physical activities not typically associated with formal exercise. The total amount of activity appeared to be more critical to improving health than the specific type of activity performed.

The total amount of activity could be measured either in minutes of physical activity performed or in the number of calories expended. Moderate-intensity activity expends about 150 calories over a total of 30 minutes of exercise (which can be performed periodically over the course of a day). The intensity of the activities should correspond to walking at a pace of 3 to 4 miles per hour. Engaging in this amount of activity can decrease the risk of coronary artery disease by 50 percent and the risk of colon cancer, diabetes, and hypertension by 30 percent.

The most recent recommendation came in 2002 from the National Academies of Science Institute of Medicine. This newest recommendation states that to maintain cardiovascular health at a maximal level, regardless of weight, adults and children should spend a total of at least 1 hour each day in moderately intense physical activity, which is double the daily minimum goal set by the 1996 Surgeon General's Report. The new goal of 1 hour per day of total activity stems from studies of how much energy is expended on average each day by individuals who maintain a healthy weight. Energy expenditure is cumulative, including both low-intensity activities of daily life, such as stair climbing and housecleaning, and more vigorous exercise like swimming and cycling. Someone in a largely sedentary occupation can achieve the new exercise goal by engaging in a moderate-intensity activity (such as walking at 4 miles per hour) for a total of 60 minutes every day, or engaging in a high-intensity activity (such as jogging at 6 miles per hour), for 20 to 30 minutes, 4 to 7 days per week.

It has been estimated that the majority of Americans do not meet this minimum standard for daily physical activity. Thus it is recommended that everyone make an effort to gradually incorporate physical activity into

FIGURE 3-4. THE PHYSICAL ACTIVITY PYRAMID.

Exercises or activities are divided into 4 groups and are put on different level of the Physical Activity Pyramid. The requirement of each type of activity is proportional to the area of the corresponding level of the pyramid:

From Corbin CB, Welk GJ, Corbin WR, Welk KA: *Concepts of Fitness and Wellness: A Comprehensive Lifestyle Approach*, ed. 6, New York: McGraw-Hill, 2006

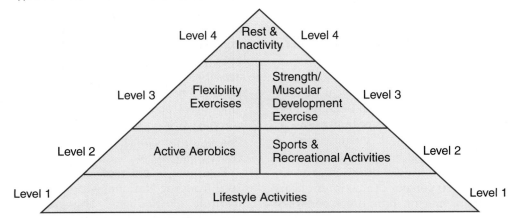

Bottom Level 1: Lifestyle Activities—Do everyday

- Climbing stairs rather than using elevator, walking to or from school, active play at playground, etc.

Level 2: Active Aerobics, Sports & Recreational Activities—Do more

- Aerobic exercises, such as swimming, cycling, jogging, brisk walking, playing basketball, badminton, football, etc.

Level 3: Flexibility Exercise, Strength/Muscular Development Exercise—Do

- Leisure activities, such as dancing, martial arts and fishing, etc.
- Exercises for flexibility and strength, such as push-ups, sit-ups, weight lifting, stretching, etc.

Level 4: Rest & Inactivity—Do less

- Watching television, playing video or computer games, sitting for more than 30 minutes, etc.

their daily routine, eventually increasing to a minimum total of 60 minutes on a consistent basis.

It must be pointed out that the recommendations from the American College of Sports Medicine were made with the idea of reducing risks for chronic diseases, while the recommendations from the Institute of Medicine were primarily referring to avoiding weight gain.

WHERE DO YOU BEGIN?

Just as you are never too sedentary to begin a fitness program, you are also never too old. It is wise to start a fitness program early in life, but all of us can benefit from exercise no matter when we begin. Long-term success in staying with an exercise program undoubtedly has some basis in your underlying motivation for beginning such a program in the first place.

PRECAUTIONS IN BEGINNING A FITNESS PROGRAM

For most high school and college students, chances are that overall health is pretty good. In the normal healthy individual, there is virtually no reason to expect that participation in any type of fitness activity will pose a threat to health or well-being. Generally, exercise is considered a safe activity for most individuals. Nevertheless, it is always a good idea to assess your medical history by identifying any pre-existing medical conditions that should be considered before beginning an exercise program. For non-traditional students, this is especially true for anyone over 30 years of age. If your medical history identifies any health-related problem, it is advisable to consult appropriate medical personnel before engaging in any type of activity. Lab Activity 3-1 will help you to assess your current medical history and may indicate a reason for you to seek additional medical advice.

Paying attention to the principles and guidelines of fitness as detailed earlier in this chapter can markedly reduce your chances of suffering injuries associated with exercise. Many of the injuries that occur with exercise can be eliminated by an awareness of the way you exercise, by "listening" to what your body is telling you through aches and pains.

READY TO BEGIN?

At this point you have been given the basic guidelines and considerations for beginning a fitness program. The chapters that follow will provide you with knowledge about and understanding of the various aspects of fitness. The chapters are designed to show the importance of fitness's essential ingredients, and they will explain how you can assess, develop, and maintain fitness. Finally, the rest of this text will demonstrate how to plan, develop, and implement a personalized fitness program based on your individual interests. Lab Activity 3-2 will help you begin planning your physical activity program.

SUMMARY

- The type of physical activity that you choose to engage in should be fun and enjoyable.
- The basic considerations of any training and conditioning program should include the following principles: overload; progression; consistency; diminishing returns; reversibility; specificity; individuality; and safety.
- The three basic elements of any training and conditioning program are the warm-up routine, the workout or conditioning activity, and the cool-down period.
- As a precaution, before you begin an exercise program, you should complete a medical history questionnaire to identify any problems.

SUGGESTED READINGS

American College of Sports Medicine. 1990. Position stand on recommended quantity and quality of exercise for developing and maintaining cardiorespiratory and muscular fitness in healthy adults. *Medicine and Science in Sports and Exercise* 22:265–74.

American College of Sports Medicine. 2001. *ACSM's resource manual: For guidelines for exercise testing and prescription.* Baltimore: Lippincott, Williams & Wilkins.

American College of Sports Medicine. 2003. *ACSM fitness book.* 2nd ed. Champaign, IL: Human Kinetics.

Bouchard, C., R. Shepard, and T. Stephens. 1994. *Physical activity, fitness and health.* Champaign, IL: Human Kinetics.

Dupont, G., W. Moalla, and C. Guinhouya. 2004. Passive versus active recovery during high-intensity intermittent exercises. *Medicine and Science in Sports and Exercise* 36(2):302–8.

Gray, S., and M. Nimmo. 2001. Effects of active, passive or no warm-up on metabolism and performance during high-intensity exercise. *Journal of Sports Sciences* 19(9):693–700.

Harris, J. 2002. *Warming up and cooling down.* 2nd ed. Champaign, IL: Human Kinetics.

Heyward, V. 2002. *Advanced fitness assessment and exercise perscription.* Champaign, IL: Human Kinetics.

Howley, E., D. Franks, and W. Westcott. 2003. *Health fitness instructor's handbook.* Champaign, IL: Human Kinetics.

Mannie, K. 2004. Dynamic warm-up/flexibility. *Coach and Athletic Director* 73(6):8–10.

Mannie, K. 2004. Overloading without overtraining. *Coach and Athletic Director* 74(4):9–12.

Middlesworth, M. 2002. More than ergonomics: Warm-up and stretching key to injury prevention. *Athletic Therapy Today* 7(2):32–34.

Molkin, M. 2004. Warming up, cooling down and stretching: Preparing for a workout and recovering afterward deserve a lot more attention than many believe. *Fitness Management* 20(2):30–32.

National Academies of Science Institute of Medicine. 2002. *Dietary reference intakes for energy, carbohydrates, fiber, fat, protein and amino acids (macronutrients).* Washington, DC: National Academies Press.

Pate, R. et al. 1995. Physical activity and public health: A recommendation from the Centers for Disease Control and Prevention and the American College of Sports Medicine. *Journal of the American Medical Association* 273(5):402–7.

Stewart, I. B., and G. G. Sleivert. 1998. The effect of warm up intensity on range of motion and anaerobic performance. *Journal of Orthopedic and Sports Physical Therapy* 27(2):154–61.

Sweet, S., and P. Hagerman. 2001. Warm-up or no warm-up. *Strength and Conditioning Journal* 23(6):36.

Suggested Web Sites

Aerobics and Fitness Association of America

AFAA, the world's largest fitness educator, links members, consumers, corporate subscribers, and allied professionals throughout the world with a revolutionary group of dynamic fitness services. Whether you're looking for aerobics certification, a personal trainer, or just some fitness facts, this is the place to be.
www.afaa.com

American Alliance for Health, Physical Education, Recreation and Dance

This site is sponsored by the national organization of physical education, health, and fitness professionals.
www.aahperd.org

American Fitness Professionals and Associates

Provides a list of fitness and nutrition certifications as well as a list of providers of continuing education and resources.
www.afpafitness.com

Health: Fitness

Search the contents of 2,000,000 reviewed sites available on the Internet.
http://gocrawl.com/web/Health/Fitness

International Dance Exercise Association

The IDEA supports the world's leading health and fitness professionals with credible information, education, career development, and leadership.
www.ideafit.com

Internet's Fitness Resource

The primary purpose of this site is the dissemination of information on exercise and nutrition. IFR offers a comprehensive listing of fitness related sites as well as the Fitness Instructor FAQ, the Fitness Plan, guest editorials, fitness classifications and more.
www.netsweat.com

International Health, Racquet and Sportsclub Association

This organization promotes fitness through education and sport club membership.
www.ihrsa.org

National Academy of Sports Medicine

This site addresses fitness, sports performance, and sports medicine, and provides live, online, and home-study courses.
www.nasm.org

National Association for Health and Fitness

This not-for-profit organization exists to improve the quality of life of every individual in the United States through the promotion of physical fitness and healthy lifestyles and by fostering and supporting councils for physical activity, health, and sports.
www.physicalfitness.org

National Center on Physical Activity and Disability

The NCPAD encourages persons with disabilities to participate in regular physical activity to promote healthy lifestyles and prevent secondary conditions.
www.ncpad.org

National Institute for Fitness and Sport

This nonprofit organization is committed to enhancing human health, physical fitness, and athletic performance through research, education, and service.
www.nifs.org

The Fitness Zone

This site includes an extensive collection of articles, tips, and recommendations for engaging in a fitness program.
www.fitnesszone.com

www.fitness.com

Fitness.com includes everything about fitness: chat, discussion board, links, shopping.
www.fitness.com/e_index.htm

Developing **Cardiorespiratory** Fitness

Objectives

After completing this chapter, you should be able to do the following:

- Relate the importance of cardiorespiratory endurance to overall fitness and health.
- Contrast aerobic and anaerobic activity.
- Explain how maximum aerobic capacity determines your level of cardiorespiratory endurance.
- Describe the principles of continuous, interval and fartlek training and the potential of each technique for improving cardiorespiratory endurance.
- Analyze specific aerobic activities that can be used to improve cardiorespiratory endurance.
- Identify methods for assessment of cardiorespiratory endurance.

WHY IS CARDIORESPIRATORY FITNESS IMPORTANT FOR YOU?

Of all the components of physical fitness listed in Chapter 1, none is more important than cardiorespiratory endurance, also referred to as cardiovascular endurance. Cardiorespiratory endurance is the ability to perform whole-body activities and continue movement for extended periods without undue fatigue. We rely on the cardiorespiratory system to transport and supply the oxygen needed by the various tissues within our bodies. It is the basic life-support system of the body. Without oxygen, the cells within the human body cannot function, and ultimately death occurs.

Everyone needs some degree of cardiorespiratory endurance to carry out normal daily activities. If you are engaged in exercise, the cardiorespiratory system must work harder to deliver enough oxygen to sustain that activity. Thus as the cardiorespiratory system becomes more efficient at supplying the needed oxygen,

KEY TERMS

aerobic activity
anaerobic activity
stroke volume
cardiac output
aerobic capacity
maximum aerobic
  capacity
fast-twitch muscle
  fibers

slow-twitch muscle
  fibers
FITT principle
continuous training
target heart rate
rating of perceived
  exertion
interval training
fartlek

your level of cardiorespiratory fitness improves and you are likely to be more resistant to fatigue.

For the older individuals such as nontraditional college students, the health benefits of improving cardiorespiratory endurance may be more important than the fitness benefits.

Engaging in regular exercise will also improve your cardiovascular health and can greatly reduce your chance of heart disease. If you have low levels of cardiorespiratory endurance, your risk of developing heart disease is higher than normal.

WHAT IS THE DIFFERENCE BETWEEN AEROBIC VERSUS ANAEROBIC ACTIVITIES?

Without oxygen, the body is incapable of producing energy for an extended period of time. Muscles must generate energy to move. Two energy-generating systems function in muscle tissue: aerobic metabolism and anaerobic metabolism. Each of these systems produces a chemical compound called *adenosine triphosphate (ATP)*, which is the ultimate usable form of energy for muscular activity. During sudden outbursts of activity in intense, short-term exercise, ATP can be rapidly used to meet energy needs. After a few seconds of intensive exercise, however, the small stores of ATP are used up. Glucose found in the muscle can be used to generate small amounts of ATP energy without the need for oxygen. This energy system is referred to as *anaerobic metabolism* (occurring in the absence of oxygen).

As exercise continues, the body has to rely on using both carbohydrate and fat metabolism to generate ATP. This second energy system requires oxygen and is therefore referred to as *aerobic metabolism* (occurring in the presence of oxygen). The aerobic system of producing energy generates considerably more ATP than the anaerobic one.

In most activities both aerobic and anaerobic systems function simultaneously. The degree to which the two major energy systems are involved is determined by the intensity and duration of the activity. If that intensity of the activity is such that sufficient oxygen can be supplied to meet the demands of working tissues, the activity is considered to be **aerobic.** Conversely, if the activity is of high enough intensity or the duration is such that there is insufficient oxygen available to meet energy demands, the activity becomes **anaerobic.**

Table 4-1 provides a comparison summary between aerobic and anaerobic activities.

TABLE 4-1
COMPARISON OF AEROBIC VERSUS ANAEROBIC ACTIVITIES

	Mode	Relative Intensity	Performance	Frequency	Duration
Aerobic Activities	Continuous, long-duration, sustained activities	Less intense	60% to 85% of maximum range	At least 3 but no more than 6 times per week	20 to 60 minutes
Anaerobic Activities	Explosive, short-duration, burst-type activities	More intense	85% to 100% range	3 to 4 days per week	10 seconds to 2 minutes

HOW DOES EXERCISE AFFECT THE FUNCTION OF THE HEART?

The capacity of the cardiorespiratory system to carry oxygen throughout the body depends on the coordinated function of four components: (1) the heart, (2) the blood vessels, (3) the blood, and (4) the lungs. Improvement of cardiorespiratory endurance through exercise occurs because of an increase in the capability of each of these four components in providing necessary oxygen to the working tissues. A basic discussion of what occurs in the heart in response to training and exercise should make it easier for you to understand why the training techniques discussed later are effective in improving cardiorespiratory endurance.

The heart is the main pumping mechanism and circulates oxygenated blood throughout the body to the various tissues. The heart receives oxygen-poor blood from the venous system and then pumps the blood through the pulmonary vessels to the lungs, where carbon dioxide is exchanged for oxygen. The oxygen-rich blood then returns to the heart, from which it exits through the aorta to the arterial system and is circulated throughout the body, supplying oxygen to the tissues (Figure 4-1).

As you begin to exercise, your muscles use the oxygen at a much higher rate, and thus your heart must pump more oxygenated blood to meet this increased demand. Like any other muscle, the heart will adapt to the increased demands placed on it over a period of time. The heart is capable of adapting to this increased demand through three mechanisms, as listed below.

1. *Increased heart rate.* As the intensity of the exercise increases, the heart rate also increases, reaching a plateau at a given level after about 2 to 3 minutes. At rest, the heart beats about 70 times per minute. The maximal heart rate is different in everybody, but it can be estimated by subtracting the person's age (in years) from 220.

2. *Increased stroke volume.* The volume of blood being pumped out of the heart with each beat is called the **stroke volume.** At rest, the heart pumps out approximately 70 ml of blood per beat. During acute exercise, stroke volume increases. Stroke volume can continue to increase only to a point (about 110 ml/beat) at which there is simply not enough time between beats for the heart to fill up. The long term effects of exercise produce an increase in maximum stroke volume during exercise, particularly in individuals who are sedentary.

3. *Increased cardiac output.* **Cardiac output** indicates how much blood the heart is capable of pumping in exactly 1 minute. It is determined by heart rate (the rate of pumping) and stroke volume (the quantity of blood ejected with each heartbeat).

aerobic activity: an activity in which the intensity of the activity is low enough that the cardiovascular system can supply enough oxygen to continue the activity for long periods

anaerobic activity: an activity in which the intensity is so great that the demand for oxygen is greater than the body's ability to deliver oxygen

stroke volume: the volume of blood being pumped out of the heart with each beat

cardiac output: indicates how much blood the heart is capable of pumping in exactly 1 minute

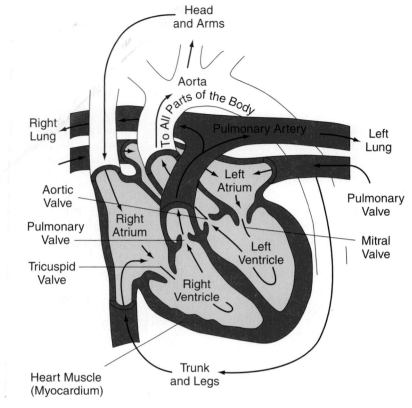

Head
and Arms

Aorta

To All Parts of the Body

Right
Lung

Pulmonary Artery

Left
Lung

Aortic
Valve

Left
Atrium

Pulmonary
Valve

Right
Atrium

Pulmonary
Valve

Mitral
Valve

Tricuspid
Valve

Left
Ventricle

Right
Ventricle

Heart Muscle
(Myocardium)

Trunk
and Legs

FIGURE 4-1.
Anatomy of the Heart and Blood Flow.

Cardiac output is the primary determinant of the maximal rate at which oxygen can be used. Approximately 5 liters (L) of blood are pumped through the heart during each minute at rest. During exercise, cardiac output increases to approximately four times that experienced during rest (about 20L) in the normal individual and may increase as much as six times in the elite endurance athlete (about 30L). As your level of fitness improves, the heart becomes more efficient because it is capable of pumping more blood with each stroke and thus heart rate during exercise will be lower.

WHAT DETERMINES HOW EFFICIENTLY THE BODY IS USING OXYGEN?

The greatest rate at which oxygen can be taken in and used during exercise is referred to as **aerobic capacity,** or as your **maximum aerobic capacity.** Maximum aerobic capacity is measured in a laboratory to determine how much oxygen can be used during 1 minute of maximal exercise. It is most often presented in terms of the volume of oxygen used relative to body weight per unit of time (ml/kg/min). Normal maximal aerobic capacity for most men and women ages 15 to 25 years would fall in the range of 38 to 46 ml/kg/min. However, a world-class male marathon runner may have a maximum aerobic capacity in the 70 to 80 ml/kg/min range, and a female marathoner may have a 60 to 70 ml/kg/min range.

The performance of any activity requires a certain rate of oxygen utilization that is about the same for everybody. Generally, the greater the rate or intensity of the activity, the greater the oxygen demands. Each person has his or her own maximal rate of oxygen utilization, and his or her ability to perform an activity is closely related to the amount of oxygen required by that activity.

The maximal rate at which oxygen can be used is largely a genetically determined characteristic. Each person's maximal aerobic capacity falls within a given range. The more active you are, the higher the existing maximum aerobic capacity will be within that range. The less active you are, the lower your maximum aerobic capacity will be in that range. Thus, by engaging in a training program, it is possible to increase your aerobic capacity to its highest limit within your range.

The range of maximal aerobic capacity that you inherit is determined in large part by the types of muscle fibers that you have. **Fast-twitch muscle fibers** (FT), or fast-contracting fibers, are not as dependent on the presence of oxygen for contraction and tend to tire very rapidly. Fast-twitch fibers are responsible for speed or power activities such as sprinting or weight lifting. **Slow-twitch muscle fibers** (ST) are slow-contracting fibers that require large amounts of oxygen for contraction and are more resistant to fatigue. Slow-twitch fibers are more useful in long-term, endurance activities such as marathon running or cross-country skiing. If you have a greater percentage of slow-twitch muscle fibers than fast-twitch fibers throughout your body, you will be able to use oxygen more efficiently and thus your maximum aerobic capacity will be higher. It appears that different forms of training can to some extent selectively hypertrophy one type of fiber more than the others.

Fatigue is closely related to the percentage of maximum aerobic capacity that a particular activity demands. It should be apparent that the greater the percentage of maximal aerobic capacity required during an activity, the shorter the time the activity may be performed. Fatigue partly occurs when insufficient oxygen is supplied to muscles. For example, Figure 4-2 compares two people, A and B. A has a maximum aerobic capacity of 50 ml/kg/min, whereas B has a maximum aerobic capacity of only 40 ml/kg/min. If A and B are exercising at the same intensity, then A is working at a much lower percentage of maximum aerobic capacity than is B. Consequently, A should be able to sustain his or her activity over a much longer period. Everyday activities such as walking up stairs or running to catch a bus may be adversely affected if your ability to use oxygen efficiently is impaired. Thus improvement of cardiorespiratory endurance should be an essential component of any fitness program.

aerobic capacity: the greatest rate at which oxygen can be taken in and used during exercise

maximum aerobic capacity: measured in a laboratory to determine how much oxygen can be used during 1 minute of maximal exercise

fast-twitch muscle fibers: a type of muscle fiber used for speed or power activities such as sprinting or weight lifting

slow-twitch muscle fibers: a type of muscle fiber that is resistant to fatigue and is more useful in long-term endurance activities

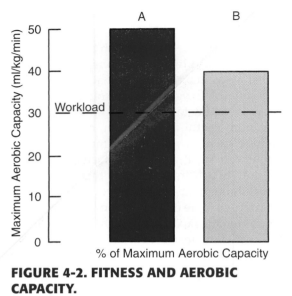

FIGURE 4-2. FITNESS AND AEROBIC CAPACITY.
Individual A should be able to work longer than can individual B as a result of lower use of maximum aerobic capacity.

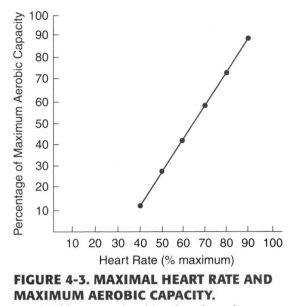

FIGURE 4-3. MAXIMAL HEART RATE AND MAXIMUM AEROBIC CAPACITY.
Maximal heart rate is achieved at about the same time as maximum aerobic capacity.

HOW DO YOU KNOW WHAT YOUR AEROBIC CAPACITY IS?

The most accurate technique for measuring aerobic capacity is done in a laboratory. It involves exercising a person on a treadmill or bicycle ergometer at a specific intensity and then monitoring heart rate and collecting samples of expired air using somewhat expensive and sophisticated equipment. Obviously, this is a somewhat impractical technique for the typical person. Therefore, what we most often do is monitor the heart rate as a means of estimating a percentage of maximum aerobic capacity.

Monitoring heart rate is an indirect method of estimating oxygen uptake. In general, heart rate and oxygen uptake have a linear relationship, although at very low intensities as well as at high intensities this linear relationship breaks down (Figure 4-3). The greater the intensity of the exercise, the higher the heart rate. Because of this existing relationship,

it should be apparent that the rate of oxygen utilization can be estimated by measuring the heart rate. The Lab Activities at the end of this chapter, which all monitor heart rates, are a means of estimating maximum aerobic capacity.

THE FITT PRINCIPLE

The **FITT principle** is a basic philosophy of what is necessary to gain a training effect from an exercise program. FITT is an acronym that stands for Frequency, Intensity, Type, and Time, all of which are factors that can be altered or modified within the context of a

FITT principle: An approach to exercise that takes into consideration Frequency, Intensity, Time, and Type of Activity

fitness program. The FITT principle is most often applied to training techniques for improving cardiorespiratory endurance and less frequently to techniques of resistance training.

WHAT TRAINING TECHNIQUES CAN BE USED TO IMPROVE CARDIORESPIRATORY ENDURANCE?

Several methods can be used to improve cardiorespiratory endurance, including (1) continuous or sustained training, (2) interval training, and (3) fartlek. The amount of improvement possible is largely determined by initial levels of cardiorespiratory endurance. The lower your endurance at the start, the more you will improve. Regardless of the training technique used for the improvement of cardiorespiratory endurance, one principal goal remains the same. You are trying to increase the ability of the cardiorespiratory system to supply a sufficient amount of oxygen to working muscles. Without oxygen, the body is incapable of producing energy for an extended period.

CONTINUOUS TRAINING

Continuous training is a technique that uses exercises performed at the same level of intensity for long periods. If the FITT Principle is applied to continuous training, we need to look at four variables:

- Frequency of activity
- Intensity of activity
- Time or duration of activity
- Type of Activity

> **continuous training:** a technique that uses exercises performed at the same level of intensity for long periods

▶ Frequency of Activity

To see at least minimal improvement in cardiorespiratory endurance, it is necessary for the average person to engage in no less than three sessions per week. If possible, you should aim for five sessions per week. A competitive athlete should be prepared to train as often as six times per week. Everyone should take off at least 1 day per week to give damaged tissues a chance to repair themselves.

▶ Intensity of Activity

The intensity of the exercise is also a critical factor, even though recommendations regarding training intensities vary. This is particularly true in the early stages of training, when the body is forced to make a lot of adjustments to increased workload demands.

Determining Exercise Intensity by Monitoring Heart Rate. There are several sites at which heart rate is easily measured. The most accurate site for measuring the pulse rate is the radial artery (located on the thumb side of the wrist joint). By placing your index and middle fingers on the thumb side of the wrist, you should be able to locate a strong pulse (Figure 4-4, *A*). Do not use your thumb to monitor pulse rate. Each pulse represents one heartbeat. You should count the number of beats that occur in 30 seconds and then multiply that number by 2 to give you an accurate heart rate. Heart rate should be monitored within 15 seconds after stopping exercise.

A heart rate monitor can also be used to monitor heart rate during exercise. There are a number of different heart rate monitors at all price ranges available. Figure 4-4 *C* provides an example of a typical heart rate monitor.

The objective of aerobic exercise is to elevate your heart rate to a specified target rate and maintain it at that level during your entire workout. Because heart rate is directly related to the intensity of the exercise as well as to the rate of oxygen use, it becomes a relatively simple process to identify a specific workload

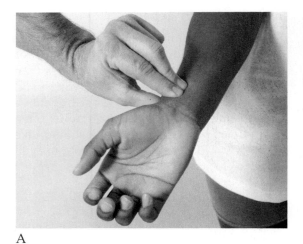

A

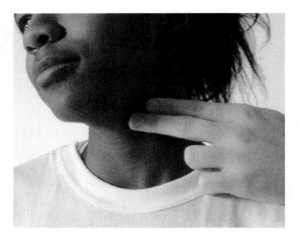

B

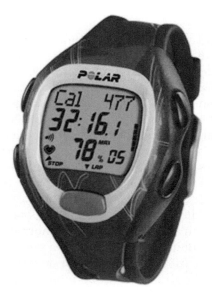

C

FIGURE 4-4. MEASURING PULSE RATE.
*Measuring pulse rate at **A**, Radial artery and **B**,
Carotid artery. **C**, Heart rate monitor. (Courtesy
Polar Electro, Inc., Lake Success, NY.)*

(pace) that will make the heart rate plateau at
the desired level. By monitoring heart rate, we
know whether the pace is too fast or too slow
to get the heart rate into a target range.

Heart rate can be increased or decreased by
speeding up or slowing down your pace. It
has already been indicated that heart rate

increases proportionately with the intensity of
the workload and will plateau after 2 to 3 minutes of activity. Thus you should be actively
engaged in the workout for 2 to 3 minutes
before measuring your pulse.

Several formulas allow you to easily identify
a training **target heart rate.** To calculate a specific target heart rate, you must first determine
your maximal heart rate. Exact determination
of maximal heart rate (HR) involves exercising
an individual at a maximal level and monitoring the HR using an electrocardiogram. This is
a difficult process outside of a laboratory. However, an approximate estimate of maximum
HR for both young boys and girls is that maximum HR is thought to be about 220 beats per
minute. However, maximum HR is related to
age, and, as you get older, your maximum HR
decreases. Thus a relatively simple estimate of
maximum HR in adults would be $HR_{max} = 220
- Age$. For a 20-year-old individual, maximum
heart rate would be about 200 beats per minute
$(220 - 20 = 200)$. Heart rate reserve is used to

target heart rate: a specific heart rate
to be achieved and maintained during
exercise

TABLE 4-2 CALCULATING HEART RATES	
Formula	Example (for a 20-year-old with a resting) heart rate of 70 beats per minute)
Maximal heart rate = 220 − Age	220 − 20 = 200 beats per minute
Heart rate reserve = maximal heart rate − resting heart rate	200 − 70 = 130
Lower limit of target heart rate range = (working heart rate × 60%) + resting heart rate	(130 × 0.6) + 70 = 148
Upper limit of target heart rate range = (working heart rate × 85%) + resting heart rate	(130 × 0.85) + 70 = 180.5

determine exercise heart rates. Heart rate reserve (HRR) is the difference between resting heart rate (HR_{rest})* and maximum heart rate (HR_{max}).

$$HRR = HR_{max} - HR_{rest}$$

The greater the difference, the larger your heart rate reserve and the greater your range of potential training heart rate intensities. The Karvonen equation is used to calculate exercise heart rate at a given percentage of training intensity. To use the Karvonen formula you need to know your HR_{max} and HR_{rest}.

Exercise HR = % of target intensity ($HR_{max} - HR_{rest}$) + HR_{rest}.

When using estimated HR_{max} or/and HR_{rest} the values are always predictions. So in a 20-year-old with a resting heart rate of 70 beats per minute the heart rate reserve is 130 (200 − 70 = 130). The heart works in a range between the lower limit and an upper limit. The lower limit is calculated by taking 60 percent of the heart rate reserve and adding the resting heart rate which would be 148 beats per minute ((130 × 0.6) + 70 = 148).

The upper limit is calculated by taking 85 percent of the heart rate reserve and adding the resting heart rate ((130 × .85) + 70 = 180.5). (See Table 4-2.)

Lab Activity 4-1 will help you calculate a Target Heart Rate.

Regardless of the formula you use, the American College of Sports Medicine recommends that young healthy individuals train with a target heart rate in the 60 to 85 percent range when training continuously. Exercising at a 70 percent level is considered a moderate level because activity can be continued for a long period with little discomfort and still produce a training effect. In a highly trained individual it is not difficult to sustain a heart rate at the 85 percent level.

Determining Exercise Intensity Through Rating of Perceived Exertion (RPE). **Rating of perceived exertion** (RPE) can be used in addition to monitoring heart rate to indicate exercise intensity. During exercise, individuals are

rating of perceived exertion: a technique used to subjectively rate exercise intensity on a numerical scale

*True resting heart rate should be monitored with the subject lying down.

TABLE 4-3
RATING OF PERCEIVED EXERTION

Scale	Verbal Rating
7	Very, very light
8	
9	Very light
10	
11	Fairly light
12	
13	Somewhat hard
14	
15	Hard
16	
17	Very hard
18	
19	Very, very hard
20	

Used with permission from Borg GA: Psychological ratings of perceived exertion, Med Sci Sports Exerc & Comm 14:377, copyright American College of Sports Medicine, 1982, Williams & Wilkins Publishing Company.

asked to rate on a numerical scale from 6 to 20 exactly how they feel relative to their level of exertion (Table 4-3). More intense exercise that requires a higher level of oxygen consumption and energy expenditure is directly related to higher subjective ratings of perceived exertion. Over a period of time, individuals can be taught to exercise at a specific RPE that relates directly to more objective measures of exercise intensity.

▶ Time or Duration of Activity

The American College of Sports Medicine (ACSM) is a professional organization whose members include physicians, exercise physiologists, biomechanists, athletic trainers, and physical therapists. The ACSM sets standards and guidelines for exercise. For minimal improvement to occur, you must participate in at least 15 minutes of continuous activity with the heart rate elevated to its working level. The ACSM recommends engaging in 15 to 60 minutes of workout/activity with the heart rate elevated to training levels. Generally, the longer the duration of the workout, the greater the improvement in cardiorespiratory endurance. The competitive athlete should train for at least 45 minutes per session.

▶ Type of Activity

The type of activity used in continuous training must be aerobic. Aerobic activities are any type that use large amounts of oxygen, elevate the heart rate, and maintain it at that level for an extended time. Aerobic activities generally involve repetitive, whole body, large-muscle movements performed over an extended time. Examples of aerobic activities are found in Fit List 4-1. The advantage of these aerobic activities as opposed to more intermittent activities, such as racquetball, squash, basketball, or tennis, is that it is easy to regulate the intensity of aerobic activities by either speeding up or slowing down the pace. Because we already know that the given intensity of the workload elicits a given heart rate, these aerobic activities allow us to

FIT LIST 4-1

Examples of Aerobic Fitness Activities

- Walking
- Jogging
- Running
- Swimming
- Cycling
- Stepping
- Aerobic dance exercise
- In-line skating
- Cross-country skiing
- Rowing

TABLE 4-4
GUIDELINES FOR CONTINUOUS

Training Level	Frequency (Sessions per Week)
Beginner	3
Intermediate	4–5
Advanced	5–6

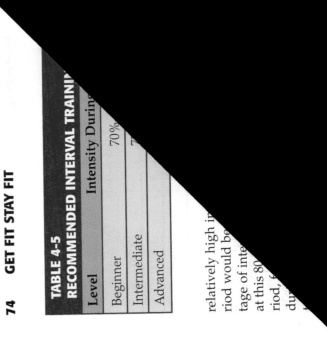

TABLE 4-5
RECOMMENDED INTERVAL TRAINI

Level	Intensity Durin
Beginner	70%
Intermediate	
Advanced	

relatively high i
riod would be
tage of inte
at this 80
riod, f
du

maintain heart rate at a specified
level. Intermittent activities involve
speeds and intensities that cause t
rate to fluctuate considerably. Althou
intermittent activities will improve ca
piratory endurance, they are much r
ficult to monitor in terms of intens
important to point out that any type
ity, from gardening to aerobic exercise, can
improve fitness and reduce the risks for developing several chronic diseases. Again, the
fact that you enjoy a specific type of activity should be an important factor in your
selection of one.

▶Guidelines for Continuous Training

In summary, when using the continuous training method, the activity selected must be aerobic and should be enjoyable. To see minimal
improvement in cardiorespiratory endurance,
training must be done for 15 to 60 minutes,
three to five times per week with the heart rate
elevated to an intensity of no less than 60 percent of its maximal rate. As mentioned in
Chapter 3, each training program should be
designed to meet individual needs and abilities. The principle of overload states that you
must stress the system if you are to see improvement and progress from one level to another. Everyone should begin slowly with the
idea that he or she will progress as quickly as
possible at his or her own rate. If you are able
to perform an activity at a given level without
undue stress and it seems that you are not

activity. Heart rate can be increased or decreased by altering the pace. The guidelines in
Table 4-4 can be applied to beginning, intermediate, and advanced levels.

INTERVAL TRAINING

Unlike continuous training, **interval training**
involves activities that are more intermittent.
Interval training consists of alternating periods of relatively intense work with periods of
active recovery. It permits you to perform
much more work at a more intense workload
over a longer period than you could if you
were working continuously. It is most desirable in continuous training to work at an intensity of about 60 to 85 percent of maximal
heart rate. Obviously, sustaining activity at a

interval training: alternating periods
of relatively intense work with periods
of active recovery

...g Training Period	Intensity During Recovery Period
...-75% of MHR	30%–35% of MHR
...5%–85% of MHR	35%–40% of MHR
85%–95% of MHR	40%–45% of MHR

...tensity over a 20-minute pe-...extremely difficult. The advan-...rval training is that it allows work ...percent or higher level for a short pe-...followed by an active period of recovery ...ing which you may be working at only 30 ...o 45 percent of maximal heart rate. Thus the intensity of the workout and its duration can be greater than with continuous training.

Most sports are anaerobic, involving short bursts of intense activity followed by a type of active recovery period (football, basketball, soccer, and tennis all qualify). Training with the interval technique allows you to be more sport-specific during the workout. With interval training you can apply the overload principle by making the training period much more intense. Several important factors should be considered in interval training. The *training period* is the amount of time that continuous activity is actually being performed, and the *recovery period* is the time between training periods. A *set* is a group of combined training and recovery periods, and a *repetition* is the number of training/recovery periods per set. *Training time* or *distance* refers to the rate or distance of the training period. The *training/recovery ratio* indicates a time ratio for training versus recovery. (Table 4-5 provides specific recommendations for an interval training workout.)

An example of interval training would be a soccer player running sprints. An interval workout would involve running ten 120-yard sprints in under 20 seconds, with a 1-minute recovery period (walking) between each sprint. During this training session the soccer player's heart rate would probably increase to 85 to 95 percent of maximal level during the sprint and should probably fall to the 35 to 45 percent level during the recovery period.

Inactive or sedentary individuals should exercise some caution when using interval training as a method for improving cardiorespiratory endurance. The intensity levels attained during the active periods may be too high for the inactive individual.

FARTLEK TRAINING

Fartlek is a training technique, a type of cross-country running, that originated in Sweden. Fartlek literally means "speed play." It is similar to interval training in that you must run for a specified period; however, specific pace and speed are not identified. The course for a fartlek workout should be some type of varied terrain including some level running, some uphill and downhill running, and some running around obstacles such as trees or rocks. The object is to put surges into a running workout, varying the length of the surges according to individual purposes. One big advantage of fartlek training is that because the pace and terrain are always changing, the training session is less regimented and allows

fartlek: a type of workout that involves jogging at varying speeds over varying terrain

TABLE 4-4
GUIDELINES FOR CONTINUOUS TRAINING

Training Level	Frequency (Sessions per Week)	Intensity of Training Heart Rate (% Maximal Heart Rate)	Time (Duration) (Minutes)
Beginner	3	60%	<20
Intermediate	4–5	70%–80%	30–45
Advanced	5–6	80%–90%	45–60

maintain heart rate at a specified or target level. Intermittent activities involve variable speeds and intensities that cause the heart rate to fluctuate considerably. Although these intermittent activities will improve cardiorespiratory endurance, they are much more difficult to monitor in terms of intensity. It is important to point out that any type of activity, from gardening to aerobic exercise, can improve fitness and reduce the risks for developing several chronic diseases. Again, the fact that you enjoy a specific type of activity should be an important factor in your selection of one.

▶Guidelines for Continuous Training

In summary, when using the continuous training method, the activity selected must be aerobic and should be enjoyable. To see minimal improvement in cardiorespiratory endurance, training must be done for 15 to 60 minutes, three to five times per week with the heart rate elevated to an intensity of no less than 60 percent of its maximal rate. As mentioned in Chapter 3, each training program should be designed to meet individual needs and abilities. The principle of overload states that you must stress the system if you are to see improvement and progress from one level to another. Everyone should begin slowly with the idea that he or she will progress as quickly as possible at his or her own rate. If you are able to perform an activity at a given level without undue stress and it seems that you are not

being "challenged" at that particular level, you may progress to the next level. Remember, however, that beginning at a level that is too high will probably produce various musculoskeletal injuries that often cause setbacks in a training program.

All training programs are based on monitoring heart rate during some type of aerobic activity. Heart rate can be increased or decreased by altering the pace. The guidelines in Table 4-4 can be applied to beginning, intermediate, and advanced levels.

INTERVAL TRAINING

Unlike continuous training, **interval training** involves activities that are more intermittent. Interval training consists of alternating periods of relatively intense work with periods of active recovery. It permits you to perform much more work at a more intense workload over a longer period than you could if you were working continuously. It is most desirable in continuous training to work at an intensity of about 60 to 85 percent of maximal heart rate. Obviously, sustaining activity at a

interval training: alternating periods of relatively intense work with periods of active recovery

TABLE 4-5 RECOMMENDED INTERVAL TRAINING WORKOUTS		
Level	Intensity During Training Period	Intensity During Recovery Period
Beginner	70%–75% of MHR	30%–35% of MHR
Intermediate	75%–85% of MHR	35%–40% of MHR
Advanced	85%–95% of MHR	40%–45% of MHR

relatively high intensity over a 20-minute period would be extremely difficult. The advantage of interval training is that it allows work at this 80 percent or higher level for a short period, followed by an active period of recovery during which you may be working at only 30 to 45 percent of maximal heart rate. Thus the intensity of the workout and its duration can be greater than with continuous training.

Most sports are anaerobic, involving short bursts of intense activity followed by a type of active recovery period (football, basketball, soccer, and tennis all qualify). Training with the interval technique allows you to be more sport-specific during the workout. With interval training you can apply the overload principle by making the training period much more intense. Several important factors should be considered in interval training. The *training period* is the amount of time that continuous activity is actually being performed, and the *recovery period* is the time between training periods. A *set* is a group of combined training and recovery periods, and a *repetition* is the number of training/recovery periods per set. *Training time* or *distance* refers to the rate or distance of the training period. The *training/recovery ratio* indicates a time ratio for training versus recovery. (Table 4-5 provides specific recommendations for an interval training workout.)

An example of interval training would be a soccer player running sprints. An interval workout would involve running ten 120-yard sprints in under 20 seconds, with a 1-minute recovery period (walking) between each sprint. During this training session the soccer player's heart rate would probably increase to 85 to 95 percent of maximal level during the sprint and should probably fall to the 35 to 45 percent level during the recovery period.

Inactive or sedentary individuals should exercise some caution when using interval training as a method for improving cardiorespiratory endurance. The intensity levels attained during the active periods may be too high for the inactive individual.

FARTLEK TRAINING

Fartlek is a training technique, a type of cross-country running, that originated in Sweden. Fartlek literally means "speed play." It is similar to interval training in that you must run for a specified period; however, specific pace and speed are not identified. The course for a fartlek workout should be some type of varied terrain including some level running, some uphill and downhill running, and some running around obstacles such as trees or rocks. The object is to put surges into a running workout, varying the length of the surges according to individual purposes. One big advantage of fartlek training is that because the pace and terrain are always changing, the training session is less regimented and allows

fartlek: a type of workout that involves jogging at varying speeds over varying terrain

for an effective alternative in the training routine. When you really think about it, most people who jog or walk are really engaging in a fartlek-type workout.

Again, if fartlek training is going to improve cardiorespiratory endurance, it must elevate the heart rate to at least minimal training levels (60 to 85 percent). Fartlek may best be used as an off-season conditioning activity or as a change-of-pace activity to counteract the boredom of a training program that uses the same activity day after day.

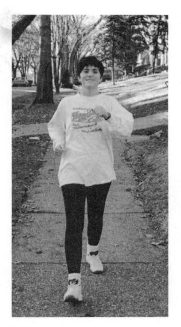

FIGURE 4-5.
Walking is the most popular aerobic activity.

GOOD AEROBIC ACTIVITIES FOR IMPROVING CARDIO-RESPIRATORY ENDURANCE

WALKING

If walking is your primary form of exercise, you're part of a large club that has become the fitness phenomenon of the new millenium. More than 60 million Americans now walk for exercise, making it the number one participation sport in the country (Figure 4-5).

There are several reasons why people are walking for fitness. It is, after all, an activity that can be pursued at almost any time, anywhere, with anyone, at no cost. Besides being fun, walking can expend a lot of energy. A walking regimen can be started easily at any age and can be worked into almost anybody's daily schedule. Although some techniques are better than others, walking demands little skill or practice. Walking is an action that is low impact which means that the chances of injury to the joints of the lower extremities are much lower than jogging or running. It does require a pair of comfortable shoes, but no other specialized clothing or equipment is really necessary. As long as you're in relatively good health, the activity presents few, if any, health hazards. As with any program involving your health, just check with your physician before you begin.

Walking's greatest value as a fitness activity is that you can just go out and walk. Like other physical activities, technique becomes a factor in developing a more effective program. In walking, the development of proper technique involves correct stride, arm swing, posture, and a steady pace. Although it's fun to experiment with techniques, it's by no means mandatory in walking. You know how to put one foot in front of the other, and there's no reason to complicate a simple activity.

RUNNING

For decades now, running has been viewed by the American public as an important fitness activity. Within the last 20 years, millions of people have taken to the streets and now run or jog on a regular basis. And the running phenomenon doesn't seem to be restricted to any one segment of the population. Young

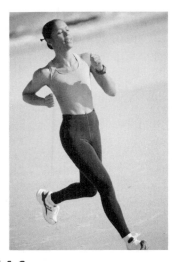

FIGURE 4-6.
Running/jogging is an excellent activity for improving cardiorespiratory endurance.

children, college students, office personnel, laborers, elderly persons, people of all backgrounds and both sexes regularly put on their running shoes and go for a run (Figure 4-6).

Although many people run to control their weight and attain a healthful physical appearance, other people run for the other physiological benefits a running program offers. Many people report that running (or jogging) is relaxing and alleviates stress, tension, and depression. They express feelings of greater self-worth and enthusiasm toward life after a run. This euphoric feeling has been called a "runner's high," and most people agree that this is both a psychological and a physiological phenomenon.

As is the case with walking, the only equipment required is a pair of running shoes and some shorts. Running offers the advantages of low cost, flexibility of time, year-round availability, and a relatively high level of benefit in return for time and effort.

However, there are some disadvantages to running. Because the feet and legs are subjected to repetitive pounding on the running surface, overuse injuries are very likely. Most of these injuries involve the muscles, tendons, ligaments, and occasionally bones of the lower extremities. Proper running and training techniques and properly fitted running shoes can reduce the number of injuries associated with running.

SWIMMING

Like running, swimming is an excellent method of developing cardiorespiratory fitness (Figure 4-7). The physiological benefits of swimming are similar to those of running; however, several differences should be addressed. The first difference is that not only must the energy of the arms and legs be used to propel the body through the water, but some energy must also be expended to keep the body afloat. For these reasons, it has been estimated that the amount of energy required to swim a given distance is approximately four times as great as running an equal distance. Energy expenditure and heart rates vary with the type of stroke. For both trained and highly skilled swimmers swimming at any given speed, the breaststroke seems to require the greatest amount of energy, then the backstroke, and last the front crawl. Monitoring heart rate is difficult in swimmers.

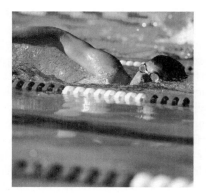

FIGURE 4-7.
Swimming is a good activity for improving cardiovascular endurance.

Swimming also eliminates many of the stresses and strains on the weight-bearing joints that are commonly experienced in running. Although the shoulder joint undergoes a significant amount of overuse-type stress, the ankle and knee joints are spared the trauma of the foot repeatedly banging into a hard surface.

A swimsuit and perhaps a pair of goggles for persons whose eyes are irritated by chlorine are all that is necessary to begin a swimming program. For many, the biggest drawback of using a swimming program for cardiorespiratory conditioning is the unavailability of a swimming pool.

AEROBIC EXERCISE

In today's terminology, the word *aerobics* is primarily used to refer specifically to aerobic exercise, which may well be the country's largest, most widespread, organized fitness endeavor (Figure 4-8). Aerobics is a combination of choreographed fitness routines set to music. In other words, it is movement to music that contributes to physical fitness by improving cardiorespiratory endurance, strength, flexibility, and muscular endurance.

As a rapidly developing participation sport, aerobics is undergoing an evolutionary process. Different styles of aerobics have been advocated over the last few years.

▶ Step Aerobics

"Stepping" uses a bench ranging between 4 and 8 inches high and slower music that makes it appropriate for all age groups. The intensity of the workout can be modified by changing the height of the bench.

▶ Low-Impact Aerobics

The impact to the lower extremities is reduced by eliminating excessive jumping and by keeping one leg slightly bent and in constant contact with the floor throughout the conditioning phase of the workout. Traveling movements rather than stationary steps are used, with an emphasis on maintaining proper body alignment at all times.

▶ Aquatic Aerobics

Aquatic aerobics are done in water to eliminate any jarring of the weight-bearing body parts while taking advantage of the water's resistance to movement during the conditioning component. Of all the types of aerobics, water aerobics will probably be the safest.

▶ Kick Boxing

Kick boxing is an exercise technique that combines kicks from the ancient martial art of Tae Kwon Do with punches from boxing performed to high-energy exercise music. It has become extremely popular in both health clubs and in home exercise videos.

▶ Circuit Aerobics

Circuit aerobics combines the use of resistance equipment with an advanced aerobic exercise class. Holding light hand weights or wearing banded wrist weights is a common practice in various forms of aerobic exercise.

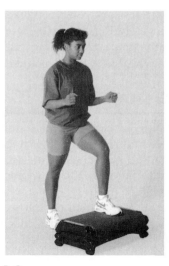

FIGURE 4-8.
Aerobic step exercise is still very popular.

Addition of these light weights increases energy expenditure during activity. Approximately 30 minutes is devoted to aerobic dance and 30 minutes to resistance training at various stations.

▶High-Impact Aerobics

This is the more traditional form in which the cardiorespiratory conditioning component consists of running, jumping, and hopping movements set to music. High-impact aerobics has produced a significant number of musculoskeletal injuries as a result of the repetitive pounding of the lower extremities against a hard surface and is almost obsolete in today's aerobics world.

CYCLING

Cycling is another aerobic activity that is excellent for improving cardiorespiratory endurance (Figure 4-9). It is also enjoyed by people of all ages, primarily because of the ease with which anyone can learn to ride without formal training. Like running and swimming, cycling produces some very desirable physiological responses in terms of strength, endurance, and weight control.

Bicycles come in thousands of different makes and models, with countless numbers of available accessories and options. The cost of purchasing an inexpensive bicycle is not much

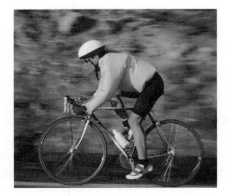

FIGURE 4-9.
Cycling can be enjoyed by people of all ages.

more than that of buying a pair of good running shoes for the average person.

Perhaps the biggest problem with cycling is locating a safe place to ride. No matter how safety conscious you are on the bicycle, there is always a danger posed by traffic. For this reason, stationary exercise bikes, or ergometers, have become popular. The stationary bike allows you to gain all the cardiovascular benefits of cycling without having to worry about dealing with traffic safety. Additionally, you can exercise in privacy, regardless of outdoor conditions, and read, watch TV, or listen to music at the same time.

SPINNING

Spinning is a new exercise technique that is basically aerobic exercise performed on stationary exercise bikes. It is being recommended as a great workout with no impact, thus minimizing chances of injury. Spinning usually involves a 40- to 45-minute workout. It is good for all levels in any class because you can get a very intense workout or a low-level workout in the same class depending on your fitness level and how hard you want to work. The workout is done to music, with the class instructor acting as a coach to work you through the routine. At this point spinning classes are found primarily in health clubs and spinning clubs. Videos are widely available to the consumer.

IN-LINE SKATING

In-line skating, also called rollerblading, is another fitness and recreational activity that has quickly gained popularity throughout the United States (Figure 4-10). However, contrary to popular belief, skating is not a new activity. In-line skating is essentially "high-tech" rollerskating. A pair of rollerblades looks like ice skates that have had the blade replaced with a series of four to six small wheels. These wheels are made for gliding on hard, smooth surfaces. In-line skaters are capable of attaining speeds approaching 25 miles per hour. For this reason,

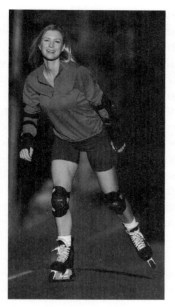

FIGURE 4-10.
Rollerblading is popular on college campuses.

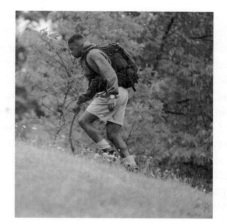

FIGURE 4-11.
Hiking or backpacking can be a relaxing activity that can also improve cardiorespiratory endurance.

pads must be worn to protect elbows, knees, and hands. It is also recommended that protective headgear, such as a cycling helmet, be worn to minimize the likelihood of injury.

The motions used with in-line skating are similar to those used in ice skating—pushing with the legs from side to side and using a side-to-side swinging motion of the arms for balance. In-line skating uses gross movements of both the arms and the legs, making it an excellent aerobic activity.

HIKING OR BACKPACKING

Hiking or backpacking is a simple way to add a little variety to a fitness or exercise routine (Figure 4-11). It is a great way to get outdoors and improve your endurance at the same time. Unlike some of the other activities discussed in this chapter, it is important that you plan ahead and take some simple safety precautions to ensure an enjoyable experience. Hiking and backpacking demand that you be prepared physically, so you should se-

lect a trail that matches your conditioning, the amount of time you have, and the type of terrain you enjoy. Initially, you should start with moderate hikes and gradually increase your endurance by progressively selecting more difficult trails. It is essential to pack the right gear (lightweight) for changing weather, dress in layers of fabric that insulates well and dries rapidly, and make sure your hiking boots fit properly to avoid developing blisters and sore spots. Always know where you are and where you are going by having a compass, a map, or a hiking guidebook. You should avoid hiking alone. If you must go by yourself, it is wise to pick more popular trails so that there are other hikers around. You must know how to take care of yourself should an emergency arise.

WHAT IS YOUR LEVEL OF CARDIO-RESPIRATORY ENDURANCE?

How fit is your cardiorespiratory system? Several tests have been developed to evaluate fitness levels. Most of these tests are based on the idea that cardiorespiratory endurance capacity is best indicated by the maximum aerobic capacity of the working tissues to use oxygen. We know from an earlier discussion that maximum aerobic capacity can be predicted or estimated by measuring heart rates at varying workloads. You can use Lab Activities 4-2 and 4-3 as tests to determine your specific levels of cardiorespiratory endurance. It must be remembered that each of these activities is based largely on one or both of the following factors: (1) the motivation of the person, and (2) the minimal level of cardiovascular endurance.

SUMMARY

- Cardiorespiratory endurance involves the coordinated function of the heart, lungs, blood, and blood vessels to supply sufficient amounts of oxygen to the working tissues.
- The best indicator of how efficiently the cardiorespiratory system functions is aerobic capacity, or the maximal rate at which oxygen can be used by the tissues.
- Heart rate is directly related to the rate of oxygen consumption. It is therefore possible to predict the intensity of the exercise in terms of a rate of oxygen use by monitoring heart rate.
- Aerobic exercise involves an activity in which the level of intensity and duration is low enough to provide a sufficient amount of oxygen to supply the demands of the working tissues.
- In anaerobic exercise the intensity of the activity is so high that oxygen is being used more quickly than it can be supplied; thus an oxygen debt is incurred that must be repaid before working tissue can return to its normal resting state.
- Continuous training for improving cardiorespiratory endurance involves selecting an activity that is aerobic in nature and training at least 3 times per week for a period of no less than 15 minutes with the heart rate elevated to 60 to 85 percent of maximal rate.

- Interval training involves alternating periods of relatively intense work followed by periods of active recovery. Interval training allows performance of more work at a relatively higher workload than does continuous training.
- Fartlek makes use of jogging or running over varying types of terrain at changing speeds.
- Walking, running, swimming, aerobic exercise, cycling, and in-line skating, and hiking and backpacking are all excellent activities for improving cardiorespiratory endurance.

SUGGESTED READINGS

American College of Sports Medicine. 1990. The recommended quantity and quality of exercise for developing and maintaining cardiorespiratory and muscular fitness in healthy adults. *Medicine and Science in Sports and Exercise* 22:265–74.

American College of Sports Medicine. 2005. *Guidelines for exercise testing and prescription.* Philadelphia: Lippincott Williams, and Wilkins.

Banks, B. 1999. *The tae bo way.* New York: Bantam, Doubleday, Dell.

Billat, L. V. 2001. Interval training for performance: A scientific and empirical practice. Special recommendations for middle- and long-distance running. Part I: Aerobic interval training. *Sports Medicine* 31(1):13–31.

Borg, G. A. 1982. Psychophysical basis of perceived exertion. *Medicine and Science in Sports and Exercise* 14:377.

Colwin, C. M. 2002. *Breakthrough swimming.* Champaign, IL: Human Kinetics.

Crouter, S.E., C. Albright, and D. R. Bassett Jr. 2004. Accuracy of Polar S410 heart rate monitor to estimate energy cost of exercise. *Medicine and Science in Sports and Exercise* 36(8):1433–1439.

Decker, J., ed. 2002. *Walking games and activities.* Champaign, IL: Human Kinetics.

Eichner, E. R. 2001. On the road: Jogging defensively. *Sports Medicine Digest* 23(4):46.

Fleck, S. J. and W. J. Kraemer. 2004. Integrating other fitness components. In *Designing resistance training programs,* 3rd ed., edited by S. J. Fleck, 129–47, 325–61. Champaign, IL: Human Kinetics.

Glidewell, S. 2004. *Inline skating.* Minneapolis: Lerner Publishing Group.

Grier, T. D., L. K. Lloyd, J. L. Walker, and T. D. Murray. 2002. Metabolic cost of aerobic dance bench stepping at varying cadences and bench heights. *Journal of Strength and Conditioning Research* 16(2):242–49.

Haywood, K. M., and N. Getchell. 2001. Development of cardiorespiratory endurance. In *Learning activities for life span motor development*, 3rd ed., edited by K. M. Haywood, 181–86, 212–23. Champaign, IL: Human Kinetics.

Hweitt, B. 2005. *Bicycling Magazine's training techniques for cyclists: Greater power, faster speed, longer endurance, better skills.* Emmaus, PA: Rodale Press Inc.

Iknoian, T. 2005. *Fitness walking.* Champaign, IL: Human Kinetics.

Jackson, A. S., J. B. Kampert, and C. E. Barlow. 2004. Longitudinal changes in cardiorespiratory fitness: Measurement error or true change? *Medicine and Science in Sports and Exercise* 36(7):1175–80.

Kemper, H. C. G., J. W. R. Twisk, L. L. J. Koppes, W. van Mechelen, and G. Bertheke Post. 2001. A 15-year physical activity pattern is positively related to aerobic fitness in young males and females (13–27 years). *European Journal of Applied Physiology* 84(5):341–48.

Kemsley, W. 2005. *The backpacker and hikers handbook: The ultimate guide.* Guilford, CT: Globe Pequot Press.

Kubukeli, Z. N., T. D. Noakes, and S. C. Dennis. 2002. Training techniques to improve endurance exercise performances. *Sports Medicine* 32(8):489–509.

Lagally, K. M., R. J. Robertson, K. I. Gallagher, R. Gearhart, and F. L. Goss. 2002. Ratings of perceived exertion during low- and high-intensity resistance exercise by young adults. *Perceptual and Motor Skills* 94(3 Part I): 723–31.

Larsen, G. E., et al. 2002. Prediction of maximum oxygen consumption from walking, jogging, or running. *Research Quarterly for Exercise and Sport* 73(1):66–72.

Laughlin, T. 2001. *Swimming made easy: The total immersion way for any swimmer to achieve fluency, ease, and speed in any stroke.* Swimwear Inc. New Paltz, NY.

Laursen, P. B., and D. G. Jenkins. 2002. The scientific basis for high-intensity interval training: Optimising training programmes and maximising performance in highly trained endurance athletes. *Sports Medicine* 32(1):53–73.

Lepretre, P. M., J. P. Koralsztein, and V. L. Billat. 2004. Effect of exercise intensity on relationship between VO2max and cardiac output. *Medicine and Science in Sports and Exercise* 36(8):1357–63.

MacNeill, I. *The beginning runner's handbook: The proven 13-week walk/run program.* Vancouver: Douglas & McIntyre Publishing Group.

Marshall, P., J. Somerville, and F. Rosato. 2002. *Walking and jogging for health and wellness.* Belmont, CA: Wadsworth.

Mazzeo, K. 2001. *Fitness through aerobics and step training.* Belmont, CA: Wadsworth.

Nealy, W. 1998. *Inline: A manual for beginning to intermediate inline skating.* Birmingham, AL: Menasha Ridge Press.

Noakes, T. D. 1998. Maximal oxygen uptake: "Classical" versus "contemporary" viewpoints: A rebuttal. *Medicine and Science in Sports and Exercise* 30(9):1381–98.

O'Connor, J. 1999. *Fitness on foot today: Walking, jogging, and running health sciences series.* Pacific Grove, CA: Brooks Cole.

Pavelka, E. 1999. *Bicycling Magazine's training techniques for cyclists: Greater power, faster speed, longer endurance, better skills.* Emmaus, PA: Rodale Press.

Powers, S., and E. Howley. 2003. *Exercise physiology: Theory and application to fitness and performance.* New York: McGraw-Hill.

Pryor, E., and M. Kraines. 1999. *Keep moving: It's aerobic dance.* Mountain View, CA: Mayfield.

Robergs, R., and S. Keteyian. 2002. *Fundamentals of exercise physiology: For fitness, performance, and health.* New York: McGraw-Hill.

Sandrock, M. 2001. Fartlek training: Mixing it up. In *Running tough*, edited by M. Sandrock. Champaign, IL: Human Kinetics.

Sharkey, B. J., ed. 2002. *Fitness and health.* 5th ed. Champaign, IL: Human Kinetics.

Sidman, C. L., C. B. Corbin, and G. Le Masurer. 2004. Promoting physical activity among sedentary women using pedometers. *Research Quarterly for Exercise and Sport* 75(2):122–29.

Smith, D. J., S. R. Norris, and J. M. Hogg. 2002. Performance evaluation of swimmers. *Sports Medicine* 32(9):539–54.

Swain, D. P., and B. C. Leutholtz. 2002. Exercise prescription for cardiorespiratory fitness. In *Exercise prescription: A case study approach to the ACSM guidelines*, edited by D. P. Swain and B. C. Leutholtz, 29–42. Champaign, IL: Human Kinetics.

Swain, D. P., J. A. Parrott, and A. R. Bennett. 2004. Validation of new method for estimating VO2max based on VO2reserve *Medicine and Science in Sports and Exercise* 36(8):1421–26.

Talbert, D. 2002. *Bicycling for fun and fitness.* Santa Barbara, CA: Daniel & Daniel.

Tomlin, D. L., and H. A. Wenger. 2001. The relationship between aerobic fitness and recovery from high intensity intermittent exercise. *Sports Medicine* 31(1):1–11.

Wendel, G., A. Schuit, and R. De Niet. 2004. Factors of the physical environment associated with walking and bicycling. *Medicine and Science in Sports and Exercise* 36(4):725–30.

Suggested Web Sites

Bicycling Life

Discusses issues, editorials, Bicycling "How-Tos," Solutions for little problems, adjustments, and repairs, practical cycling.
www.bicyclinglife.com

Bicyclopedia

This site is a comprehensive encyclopedia that covers nearly everything about bikes and cycling.
http://pwp.starnetinc.com/olderr/bcwebsite

Cooper Institute for Aerobics Research

This nonprofit research and education organization is dedicated to preventive medicine and research.
www.cooperinst.org

Endurance Training: Increasing Your Aerobic Capacity

This site presents activities related to increased aerobic fitness.
www.ama-ssn.org/insight/gen_hlth/trainer/aerobic.htm

International Inline Skating Association

The IISA is a nonprofit trade association that represents the 29 million people who are regular inline skaters. The IISA conducts educational and safety programs in inline skating and promotes the benefits and pleasures of inline skating for sport, recreation, fitness, and vitality.
www.iisa.org

Road Runners Club of America

The RRCA maintains an extensive list of programs for its clubs and individual members.
www.rrca.org

Rollerblade

This site provides several resources for in-line skaters. Tips for beginners, skate maintenance videos and instruction, information on places to skate, assistance in finding a certified instructor, and industry history are some of the resources available. In addition, there is a plethora of information on skating for fitness, with a calorie-burning chart, healthy recipes, a 10-week workout program, and information on the fitness benefits of skating.
www.rollerblade.com

Runners Web

The Runners Web is designed for runners and triathletes. It contains a variety of running and triathlon (and some cycling) information.
www.runnersweb.com/running.html

Runner's World Online

This site presents a beginner's program, marathon training, health, and fitness.
www.runnersworld.com

Swimmersworld.com

This site features competitive swimming news and information.
www.swimmersworld.com

Walking

This complete guide to walking for fitness, recreation, and competitive racewalking features new articles weekly, a comprehensive link library, chat, bulletin board, and newsletter.
walking.miningco.com

Walking for Fitnes

This site includes the best new content, relevant links, how-to's, forums, and answers to just about any question concerning walking.
http://walking.about.com/mbody.htm

WebAerobics

WebAerobics, Inc., offers aerobics enthusiasts a destination on the Internet where they can find information about aerobics.
www.webaerobics.com

Yeah! Walking

A global walking community features free e-mail, chats, message boards, links, and shopping.
www.yeahsports.com/dir/walking

4Rollerblading

This is a guide to in-line skating from 4anything.com. It is essentially a directory of links.
www.4rollerblading.com

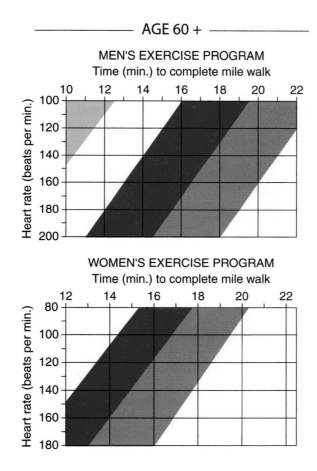

Improving Muscular **Strength,**
Endurance, and Power

Objectives

After completing this chapter, you should be able to do the following:

- Define strength, endurance, and power and indicate their relevance to health and skill of performance.
- Discuss factors that determine levels of muscular strength.
- Explain the physiological changes that occur which increase strength.
- Demonstrate proper techniques for using progressive resistance exercise to develop strength and muscular endurance in specific muscle groups.
- Discuss isometric, isokinetic, and circuit training exercises as techniques for improving muscle strength.
- Explain how functional strengthening exercises and plyometrics can be incorporated into a strength training programs.
- Demonstrate various calisthenic exercises that can be used for increasing muscular strength and endurance.
- Explain why core stabilization exercises should be a part of all strength-training programs.

WHY IS MUSCULAR STRENGTH IMPORTANT FOR EVERYONE?

The development of **muscular strength** is an essential component of fitness for anyone involved in a physical activity program. By definition, strength is the ability of a muscle to generate maximum force against some heavy resistance. The development of

muscular strength: the ability of a muscle to generate force against some resistance

KEY TERMS

muscular strength
muscular endurance
power
concentric
    contraction
eccentric contraction
hypertrophy
atrophy
motor unit
myofilaments

progressive resistance
    exercise
isometric exercise
isokinetic exercise
circuit exercise
functional strength
    training
plyometric exercise
calisthenic exercise
core stabilization
    training

muscular strength may be considered as both a health-related and a skill-related component of physical fitness. Maintenance of at least a normal level of strength in a given muscle or muscle group is important for normal healthy living. Muscle weakness or imbalance can result in abnormal movement or gait and can impair normal functional movement. Muscle weakness can also produce poor posture, which can affect appearance. One of the most common health ailments in the United States is lower back pain. In most cases lower back pain is related to lack of muscular fitness, especially lack of muscular strength in the abdominals and loss of flexibility of the hamstrings. (See Chapter 9 for more discussion of lower back pain.) Thus strength training may play a critical role not only in fitness programs but also in injury prevention and rehabilitation.

HOW ARE STRENGTH AND MUSCULAR ENDURANCE RELATED?

Muscular strength is closely associated with **muscular endurance.** Muscular endurance is the ability to perform repetitive muscular contractions against some resistance for an extended period of time. As we will see later, as muscular strength increases, there tends to be a corresponding increase in endurance. For example, suppose a person can lift a given weight 25 times. If that person's muscular strength increases by 10 percent through weight training, it is very likely that his or her maximal number of repetitions also would be increased because it is easier for the person to lift the weight. For most people, developing muscular endurance is more important than developing muscular strength, because muscular endurance is probably more critical in carrying out the everyday activities of living. It is important for anyone beginning a physical activity program to understand the need to develop muscular endurance prior to engaging in an aggressive fitness program. This

becomes increasingly true with age. However, muscular strength is essential for anyone involved in certain types of competition.

WHY IS MUSCULAR POWER IMPORTANT IN SPORT ACTIVITIES?

Most movements in sports are explosive and must include elements of both strength and speed if they are to be effective. If a large amount of force is generated quickly, the movement can be referred to as a **power** movement. Without the ability to generate power, your performance capabilities will be limited. It is difficult to hit a softball, drive a golf ball, or kick a soccer ball without generating power.

TYPES OF SKELETAL MUSCLE CONTRACTION

Skeletal muscle is capable of three different types of contraction: (1) an isometric contraction, (2) a **concentric,** or positive, **contraction,** and (3) an **eccentric,** or negative, **contraction.** An isometric contraction occurs when the muscle contracts to produce tension but there is no

muscular endurance: the ability to perform repetitive muscular contractions against some resistance for an extended period of time

power: a large amount of force is generated quickly

concentric contraction: a contraction where the muscle shortens when contracting

eccentric contraction: a contraction where the muscle lengthens when contracting

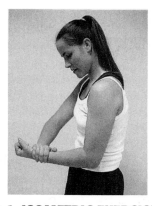

FIGURE 5-1. ISOMETRIC EXERCISE.
In isometric exercise the force is exerted against some immovable resistance and the length of the muscle does not change.

change in length of the muscle (Figure 5-1). Considerable force can be generated against some immovable resistance, even though no movement occurs. In a concentric contraction, the muscle shortens in length while tension is developed to overcome or move some resistance. In an eccentric contraction, the resistance is greater than the muscular force being produced, and the muscle lengthens while producing tension. For example, when lifting a bookbag in your hand, the biceps muscle in the upper arm is shortening as it contracts, which is a concentric contraction. As you lower the bookbag, the biceps muscle is still contracting but now it is lengthening. This is an eccentric contraction. Concentric and eccentric contractions must occur to allow most movements.

FAST-TWITCH VERSUS SLOW-TWITCH FIBERS

As mentioned in Chapter 4, all fibers in a particular muscle unit are either slow-twitch or fast-twitch fibers. Each has distinctive contractile as well as metabolic capabilities. Within a particular muscle, both types of fibers exist, and the ratio in an individual muscle varies with each person. Those muscles that function

primarily to maintain posture against the pull of gravity require more endurance and have a higher percentage of slow-twitch fibers. Muscles that produce powerful, explosive, and strength movements tend to have a much greater percentage of fast-twitch fibers.

Because this ratio is genetically determined, it may play a large role in determining ability for a given sport activity. For example, sprinters and weight lifters have a large percentage of fast-twitch fibers in relation to slow-twitch ones. One study has shown that sprinters may have as many as 95 percent fast-twitch fibers in certain muscles. Conversely, marathon runners generally have a higher percentage of slow-twitch fibers. The question of whether fiber types can change as a result of training has not been completely resolved. However, both types of fibers can improve their metabolic capabilities through specific strength and endurance training.

WHAT DETERMINES HOW MUCH STRENGTH YOU HAVE?

SIZE OF THE MUSCLE

Muscular strength is proportional to the size of a muscle as determined by the cross-sectional diameter of the muscle fibers. The greater the cross-sectional diameter or the bigger a particular muscle, the stronger it is, thus the more force it is capable of generating. The size of a muscle tends to increase in cross-sectional diameter with weight training. This increase in muscle size is referred to as **hypertrophy.** Conversely, a decrease in the size of a muscle is referred to as **atrophy.** Significant muscle

hypertrophy: an increase in muscle size in response to training

atrophy: a decrease in muscle size caused by inactivity

hypertrophy depends on the presence of an anabolic steroidal hormone called *testosterone.* Testosterone is considered a male hormone, although all females possess some testosterone in their systems. Women with higher testosterone levels tend to have the potential to develop a little more muscle bulk.

Strength is a function of the number and diameter of muscle fibers composing a given muscle. The number of fibers is an inherited characteristic; a person who inherits a large number of muscle fibers has the potential to hypertrophy to a much greater degree than does someone with relatively few fibers. However, anyone can increase strength through exercise.

NEUROMUSCULAR EFFICIENCY

Traditionally, the thinking among experts has been that change in the size of the muscle (hypertrophy) is primarily responsible for increases in strength. However in large part, increases in strength are caused by neural adaptations. Strength is directly related to the efficiency of the neuromuscular system and the function of the **motor unit** in producing muscular force. Initial increases in strength during a weight-training program can be attributed primarily to increased neuromuscular efficiency in both males and females. For a muscle to contract, an impulse must be transmitted from the nervous system to the muscle. Each muscle fiber is innervated by a specific motor unit. By overloading a particular muscle, as in weight training, the muscle is forced to work efficiently. Efficiency is achieved by getting more motor units to fire, causing a stronger contraction of the muscle.

motor unit: a group of muscle fibers innervated by a single motor nerve

BIOMECHANICAL FACTORS

Strength in a given muscle is determined not only by the physical properties of the muscle but also by biomechanical factors. Bones along with muscles and their tendons form a system of levers and pulleys that collectively generate force that can move an external object. The position of attachment of a particular muscle tendon on the bone will largely determine how much force this muscle is capable of generating.

AGE AND GENDER

The ability to generate muscular force is also related to age. Both males and females seem to be able to increase strength throughout puberty and adolescence, reaching a peak around 20 to 25 years of age. After that, this ability begins to level off and in some cases decline. It has been shown that after about age 25 a person generally loses an average of 1 percent of her or his maximal remaining strength each year. Thus at age 65 a person would have only about 60 percent of the strength he or she had at age 25.

A critical difference between men and women regarding strength developing is the ratio of strength to body weight. The reduced strength/body weight ratio in females is the result of a higher percentage of body fat. The strength/body weight ratio may be significantly improved through weight training by decreasing the percent body fat while increasing lean weight. Strength-training programs for females should follow the same guildelines as those for men.

LEVEL OF PHYSICAL ACTIVITY

Loss in muscle strength is definitely related to individual levels of physical activity. Those people who are more active, or perhaps those who continue to strength train, considerably reduce this tendency toward declining muscle strength. In addition, exercise may have an effect in slowing the decrease in cardiorespiratory endurance and flexibility, as well as in slowing increases in body fat that tend to occur with aging. Therefore strength maintenance is important for all individuals regardless of age or the level of competition if total wellness and health are an ultimate goal.

OVERTRAINING

Overtraining can have a negative effect on the development of muscular strength. The statement "if you abuse it, you will lose it" is applicable here. Overtraining can result in psychological breakdown ("staleness") or physiological breakdown, which may involve musculoskeletal injury, fatigue, or sickness. Engaging in proper and efficient resistance training, eating a proper diet, and getting appropriate rest can all minimize the potential negative effects of overtraining.

REVERSIBILITY

Gains in muscular strength resulting from resistance training are reversible. Individuals who interrupt or stop resistance training altogether will see rapid decreases in strength gains. "If you don't use it, you'll lose it."

WHAT PHYSIOLOGICAL CHANGES OCCUR TO CAUSE INCREASED STRENGTH?

There is no question that weight training to improve muscular strength results in an increased size, or hypertrophy, of a muscle. What causes a muscle to hypertrophy? Over the years, several theories have been proposed to explain this increase in muscle size; most of these have been discounted.

The primary explanation for this hypertrophy is best attributed to an increase in the size and number of small contractile protein filaments within the muscle, called **myofilaments.** Increases in both size and number of the myofilaments as a result of strength training cause the individual muscle fibers to increase in cross-sectional diameter. This increase is particularly found in males, although females will also see some increase in muscle size. More research is needed to further clarify and determine the specific causes of muscle hypertrophy. In addition to muscle hypertrophy, there are a number of other physiological adaptations to resistance training. Health Link 5-1 identifies them.

myofilaments: small protein structures that are the contractile elements in a muscle fiber

HEALTH LINK 5-1

Adaptations to Resistance Training

- The strength of noncontractile structures such as tendons and ligaments is increased.
- The mineral content of bone is increased, making the bone stronger and more resistant to fracture.
- Aerobic capacity may be improved when resistance training is done at a high

enough intensity to increase heart rate to the 60 to 85 percent range.
- There are increases in the levels of several enzymes important to aerobic and anaerobic metabolism.

www.nsca-lift.org

OVERLOAD

For a muscle to improve in strength, it must be forced to work at a higher level than that to which it is accustomed. In other words, the muscle must be *overloaded*. Without overload the muscle will be able to *maintain* strength as long as training is continued against a level of resistance to which the muscle is accustomed. However, *no additional* strength gains will be realized. This maintenance of existing levels of muscular strength may be more important in weight-training programs that emphasize muscular endurance rather than strength gains. It is certainly true that many individuals can benefit more in terms of overall health by concentrating on improving muscular endurance. However, to most effectively build muscular strength, weight training requires a consistent, increasing effort against progressively increasing resistance. Progressive resistance exercise is based primarily on the principles of overload and progression. However, the principle of overload applies to all eight training techniques which produce improvement of muscular strength over a period of time. Table 5-1 summarizes the eight techniques for improving muscular strength.

TABLE 5-1 TECHNIQUES OF IMPROVING MUSCULAR STRENGTH		
Technique	**Action**	**Equipment/Activity**
Progressive resistive exercise	Force develops while the muscle shortens or lengthens	Free weights, Free Motion, Cybex, Eagle, Body Master
Isometric exercise	Force develops while muscle length remains constant	Any immovable resistance
Isokinetic training	Force develops while muscle is contracting at a constant velocity	Kincom, Biodex
Circuit training	Used as a combination of isometric, PRE, or isokinetic exercises organized into a series of stations	May use any of the equipment listed above Calisthenics
Functional strength training	Uses concentric, eccentric, and isometric contractions in multiple planes to improve strength and neuromuscular control	Functional movements
Calisthenics	Uses body weight to provide resistance	Doesn't require special equipment
Core stabilization	Provides a stable base on which prime movers in the extremities function	Uses stability balls, machine balls, etc., to strengthen the lumbo-pelvic-hip complex
Plyometric exercise	Uses a rapid eccentric stretch of the muscle to facilitate an explosive concentric contraction	Hops, bounds, and depth jumping

WHAT ARE THE TECHNIQUES OF RESISTANCE TRAINING?

If you were to go into a weight room and ask ten different people what weight-lifting technique they thought was the most effective for improving muscular strength, you would likely get ten different responses. The key for you is to figure out which technique will best allow you to achieve the goals you have established for yourself. There are a number of different techniques of resistance training for strength improvement, including **progressive resistance exercise, isometric exercise, isokinetic exercise, circuit training, functional strength training, plyometric exercise, calisthenic exercise, and core stabilization training.**

PROGRESSIVE RESISTANCE EXERCISE

Progressive resistance exercise is perhaps the most commonly used and most popular technique for improving muscular strength. Progressive resistance exercise training uses exercises that strengthen muscles through a contraction that overcomes some fixed resistance, such as with dumbbells, barbells, or various weight machines. Progressive resistance exercise uses isotonic contractions, in which force is generated while the muscle is changing in length.

▶ Isotonic Contractions

Isotonic contractions may be either concentric or eccentric. Suppose you are going to perform a biceps curl (see Figure 5-13, page 112). To lift the weight from the starting position, the biceps muscle must contract and shorten in length (concentric or positive contraction). If the biceps muscle does not remain contracted when the weight is being lowered, gravity would cause this weight to simply fall back to the starting position. Thus to control the weight as it is being lowered, the biceps muscle must continue to contract while at the same time gradually lengthening (eccentric or negative contraction).

▶ Exercise Machines versus Free Weights

Various types of exercise equipment can be used with progressive resistive exercise, including free weights (barbells and dumbbells) or exercise machines such as Universal, Cybex, Tough Stuff, Icarian Fitness, King Fitness,

progressive resistance exercise: a technique that gradually strengthens muscles through a muscle contraction that overcomes some fixed resistance

isometric exercise: an exercise in which the muscle contracts against resistance but does not change in length

isokinetic exercise: an exercise in which the speed of movement is constant regardless of the strength of a contraction

circuit training: a series of exercise stations that consist of various combinations of weight training, flexibility, calisthenics, and brief aerobic exercises

functional strength training: uses integrated exercises designed to improve functional movement patterns for increasing strength and neuromuscular control by using eccentric, concentric, or isometric contractions in three planes of motion simultaneously

plyometric exercise: a technique of exercise that involves a rapid eccentric (lengthening) stretch of a muscle, followed immediately by a rapid concentric contraction of that muscle for the purpose of producing a forceful explosive movement

calisthenic exercises: exercises done using body weight as resistance

Body Solid, Pro-Elite, Life Fitness, Nautilus, BodyCraft, Yukon, Flex, Cam-Bar, GymPros, Nugym, Body Works, DP, Soloflex, Eagle, Free Motion Fitness, and Body Master, to name a few (Figure 5-2, *A*). Dumbbells and barbells require the use of iron plates of varying weights that can be easily changed by adding or subtracting equal amounts of weight to both sides of the bar. The exercise machines have a stack of weights that is lifted through a series of levers or pulleys. The stack of weights slides up and down on a pair of bars that restrict the movement to only one plane (Figure 5-2, *B*). Weight can be increased or decreased simply by changing the position of a weight key.

There are advantages and disadvantages to both the free weights and the machines. The machines are relatively safe to use in comparison with free weights. For example, if you are doing a bench press with free weights, it is essential to have someone "spot" you (help you lift the weights back onto the support racks if you don't have enough strength to complete the lift). If you don't, you may end up dropping the weight on your chest. A spotter has three functions: to protect the lifter from injury, to make recommendations on proper lifting technique, and to motivate the lifter. See Safe Tip 5-1 for proper spotting techniques.

With the exercise machines, you can easily and safely drop the weight without fear of injury. It is also a simple process to increase or decrease the weight with the exercise machines by moving a single weight key, although changes can generally be made only in increments of 10 or 15 pounds. With free weights, iron plates must be added or removed from each side of the barbell.

Persons who have strength-trained using both free weights and the exercise machines realize the difference in the amount of weight that

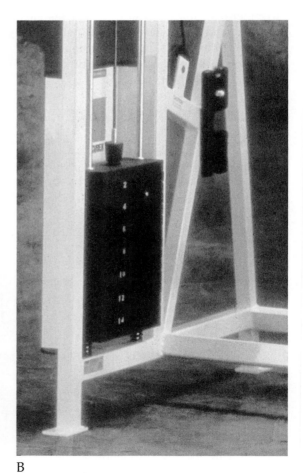

B

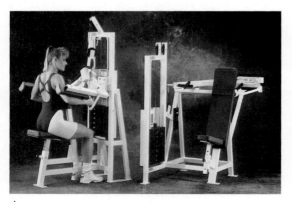

A

FIGURE 5-2. ISOTONIC EXERCISE EQUIPMENT.
*A, This Cybex equipment is isotonic. **B,** Resistance may be easily altered by changing the key in the stack of weights. (Courtesy CYBEX, Division of LUMEX Inc, New York.)*

SAFE TIP 5-1

Proper spotting techniques

- Make sure the lifter uses the proper grip.
- Check to see that the lifter is in a safe, stable position.
- Make sure the lifter moves through a complete range of motion at the appropriate speed.
- Make sure the lifter inhales and exhales during the lift.
- When spotting dumbbell exercises, spot as close to the dumbbells as possible above the elbow joint.
- Make sure the lifter understands how to get out of the way of missed attempts, particularly with overhead techniques.
- Stand behind the lifter.
- If heavy weights exceed the limits of your ability to control the weight, use a second spotter.
- Communicate with the lifter to know how many reps are to be done, whether a liftoff is needed, and how much help the lifter wants in completing a rep.
- Always be in a position to protect both the lifter and yourself from injury.

can be lifted. Unlike the machines, free weights have no restricted motion and can thus move in many different directions, depending on the forces applied. Also, with free weights, an element of muscular control on the part of the lifter is required to prevent the weight from moving in any direction other than vertically. This control will usually decrease the amount of weight that can be lifted. Regardless of which type of equipment is used, the same principles of isotonic training may be applied.

▶Using both Concentric and Eccentric Contractions

In progressive resistance exercise, it is essential to incorporate both concentric and eccentric

contractions. It is possible to generate greater amounts of force against resistance with an eccentric contraction than with a concentric contraction. Eccentric contractions are more resistant to fatigue than are concentric contractions. The mechanical efficiency of eccentric exercise may be several times higher than that of concentric exercise. Research has clearly demonstrated that the muscle should be overloaded and fatigued both concentrically and eccentrically for the greatest strength improvement to occur.

When training specifically for the development of muscular strength, the concentric or positive portion of the exercise should require 1 to 2 seconds, while the eccentric or negative portion of the lift should require 2 to 4 seconds. The ratio of negative to positive should be approximately two to one. Physiologically, the muscle will fatigue much more rapidly concentrically than eccentrically. For many years the importance of using both positive and negative contractions in strength training programs has been stressed, regardless of which brand of equipment is being used.

▶Accomodating Resistance

It has been argued that a disadvantage of any type of isotonic exercise is that the force required to move the resistance is constantly changing throughout the range of movement. One manufacturer attempted to alleviate this problem of changing force capabilities by using a cam in its pulley system (Figure 5-3). The cam was individually designed for each piece of equipment so that the resistance is variable throughout the movement. This change in resistance at different points in the range has been labeled *accommodating resistance* or variable resistance. Whether this design does what it claims to do is debatable. It must be remembered that in real-life situations it does not matter whether the resistance is changing. What is important is that you develop enough strength to move objects from one place to another. The amount of strength necessary for

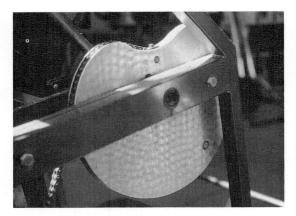

FIGURE 5-3.
A cam has been used in an attempt to equalize resistance throughout the full range of motion.

each person largely depends on his or her lifestyle and occupation.

▶ Progressive Resistance Exercise Techniques

Perhaps the most confusing aspect of progressive resistance exercise is the terminology used to describe specific programs. Fit List 5-1, which identifies specific terms with their operational definitions, may provide some clarification.

There are probably as many fallacies and misconceptions associated with resistance training as with any other component of fitness. It seems that everyone has his or her own ideas about the best techniques for increasing muscular strength. A considerable amount of research has been done in the area of resistance training to determine optimal techniques in terms of (1) the intensity or the amount of weight to be used, (2) the number of repetitions, (3) the number of sets, (4) the recovery period, and (5) the frequency of training. The FITT principle as described in Chapter 4 can also be applied to progressive resistance exercise.

There is no such thing as an optimal strength-training program. Achieving total agreement on a program of resistance training that includes specific recommendations relative to repetitions, sets, intensity, and frequency is impossible. However, the following general

FIT LIST 5-1

Progressive Resistance Exercise Terminology	
Repetition	Number of times you repeat a specific movement
Repetition maximum	Number of maximum repetitions at a given weight
One repetition maximum*	The absolute maximum weight you can lift in an exercise only one time
Set	A particular number of repetitions
Intensity	The amount of weight or resistance lifted
Recovery	The rest interval between sets
Frequency	The number of times an exercise is done in a week's period

*It should be emphasized that a one repetition maximum test can potentially cause unnecessary injury and is therefore not recommended.

recommendations will provide you with an effective resistance training program.

Selecting a starting weight. For any given exercise, the amount of weight selected should be sufficient to allow 6 to 8 repetitions maximum (RM) in each of the 3 sets with a recovery period of 60 to 90 seconds between sets. Initial selection of a starting weight may require some trial and error to achieve this 6 to 8 RM range. If at least 3 sets of 6 repetitions cannot be completed, the weight is too heavy and should be reduced. If it is possible to do more than 3 sets of eight repetitions, the weight is too light and should be increased.

Progression. progression to heavier weights is determined by the ability to perform at least 8 repetitions maximum in each of 3 sets. When progressing weight, an increase of about 10 percent of the current weight being lifted should still allow at least 6 RM in each of 3 sets.

Frequency. A particular muscle or muscle group should be exercised consistently every other day. Thus the frequency of weight training should be at least three times per week but no more than four times per week. It is common for serious weight trainers to lift every day; however, they exercise different muscle groups on successive days. For example, Monday, Wednesday, and Friday may be used for upper-body muscles, whereas Tuesday, Thursday, and Saturday are used for lower-body muscles (Figure 5-4).

It is important to realize that there are many effective techniques and training regimens that weight lifters and body builders can use. One may decide from looking at the size of a muscle or seeing the amount of weight these people are able to lift that they are doing something right even though their training regimens may not always follow the recommendations of researchers.

Regardless of specific techniques used, to improve strength the muscle must be overloaded in a progressive manner. This is the basis of progressive resistance exercise. The amount of weight used and the number of repetitions performed must be sufficient to make the muscle work at a higher intensity than it is used to. This is the single most critical factor in any strength-training program. It is also essential to design the strength-training program to meet the specific needs of a person, whether he or she is a competitive athlete or an individual interested in improving total-body health and fitness.

▶ Should You Exercise Differently to Improve Muscular Endurance

Muscular endurance was defined as the ability to perform repeated muscle contractions against resistance for an extended period of time. Most weight-training experts believe that muscular strength and muscular endurance are closely related. As one improves, there is a tendency for the other to improve also. It is generally accepted that when one is weight training for strength, heavier weights with a lower number of repetitions should be used. Conversely, endurance training uses relatively lighter weights with a greater number of repetitions.

It has been suggested that endurance training should consist of three sets of 10 to 15 repetitions, using the same criteria for weight selection progression and frequency as recommended for progressive resistive exercise. Thus suggested training regimens for both muscular strength and endurance are similar in terms of sets and numbers of repetitions. Persons who have great strength levels tend to also exhibit greater muscular endurance when asked to perform repeated contractions against resistance.

▶ Specific Progressive Resistance Exercises

To say that a *person* is strong is probably incorrect. We should instead refer to a specific muscle, muscle group, or movement as being strong because increases in strength occur only in muscles that are regularly subjected to overload. Because muscle contractions result in joint movement, the goal of weight training should be to increase strength in every movement possible about a given joint. Exercises must be designed to place stress on those groups of muscles collectively to produce a specific joint movement.

For this reason our approach to specific strength-training exercises deviates from the traditional approach. The following illustrations are organized to show exercises for all motions about a particular joint rather than for each specific muscle. These exercises are demonstrated using free weights (barbells, dumbbells, weights, and some machine weights). Any of the exercises described may be applied to various commercial exercise machines such as Universal or Nautilus. Positions may differ slightly when different pieces of equipment are used. However, the joint motions that affect the various muscles indicated are still the same.

Figures 5-5 to 5-27 describe exercises for strength improvement of shoulder, hip, knee, and ankle joint movements. The reader should refer to Figure 5-4 to see the anatomic location at the muscles that are referred to with specific

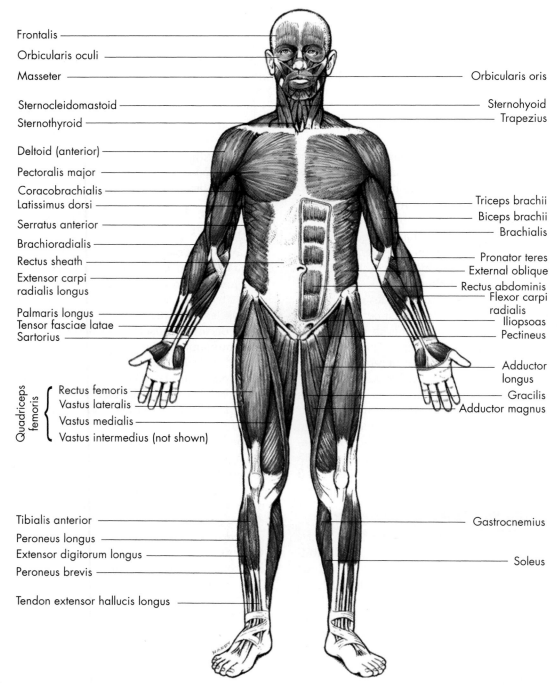

FIGURE 5-4.

A, Superficial muscles of the human body, anterior view from anatomical position.

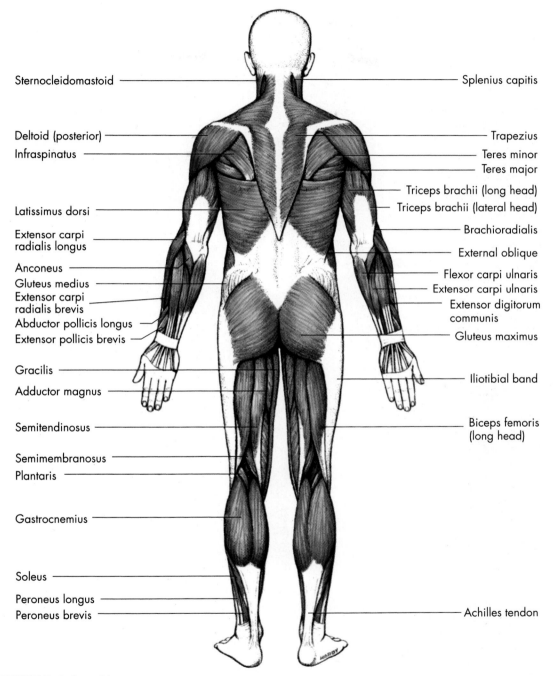

FIGURE 5-4. (cont.)

B, Superficial muscles of the human body, posterior view.

From Thompson CW and Floyd RT: *Manual of Structural Kinesiology*, ed. 15, New York: McGraw-Hill, 2004.

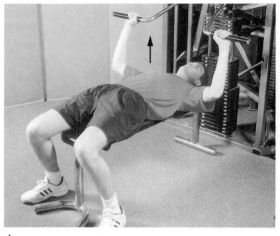

A

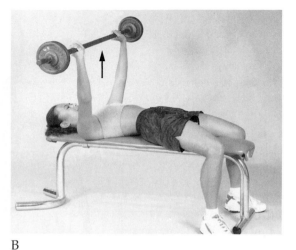

B

FIGURE 5-5. BENCH PRESS.
A, Machine. B, Free weights.
Joints affected: shoulder, elbow.
Movement: pushing away.
Position: supine, feet flat on bench or floor, back flat on bench.
Primary muscles: pectoralis major, triceps.

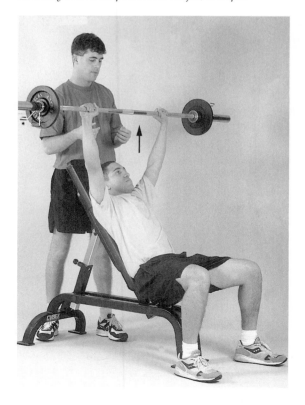

FIGURE 5-6. INCLINE PRESS.
Joints affected: shoulder, elbow.
Movement: pushing upward and away.
Position: supine at an inclined angle, feet flat on floor, back flat against bench.
Primary muscles: pectoralis major, triceps.

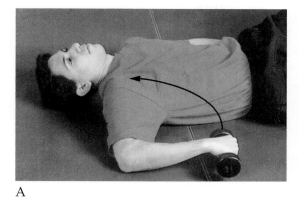

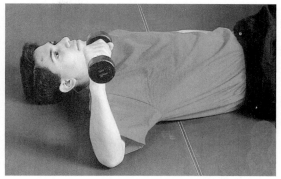

A   B

FIGURE 5-7. SHOULDER LATERAL ROTATION.

Joints affected: shoulder.
Movement: external rotation.
Position: supine, shoulder at 90-degree angle and elbow flexed at 90-degree angle.
Primary muscles: infraspinatus, teres minor.

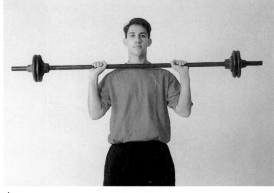
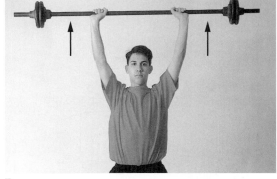

A   B

FIGURE 5-8. MILITARY PRESS.

Joints affected: shoulder, elbow. Movement: pressing the weight overhead.
Position: standing, back straight.
Primary muscles: deltoid, trapezius, triceps.

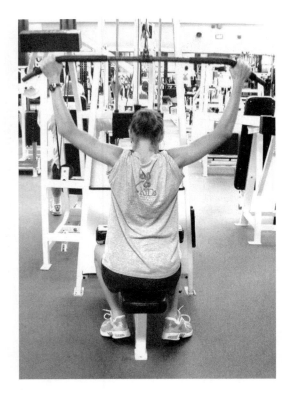

FIGURE 5-9. LAT PULL-DOWNS.
Joints affected: shoulder, elbow.
Movement: pulling the bar down behind the neck.
Position: kneeling, back straight, head up.
Primary muscles: latissimus dorsi, biceps.

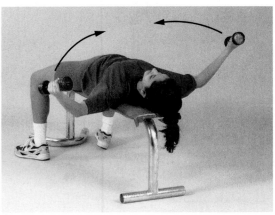

A

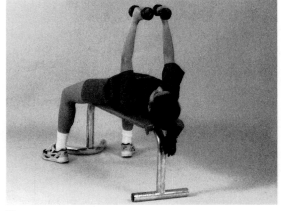

B

FIGURE 5-10. FLYS.
Joint affected: shoulder.
Movement: horizontal flexion. Bring arms together over head.
Position: lying on back, feet flat on floor, back flat on bench.
Primary muscles: deltoid, pectoralis major.

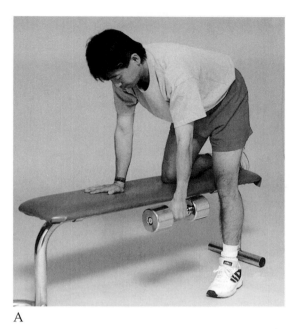
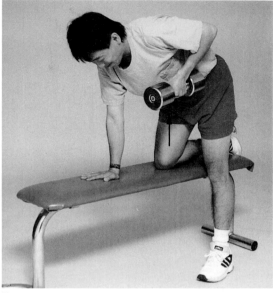

A   B

FIGURE 5-11. BENT-OVER ROWS.
Joint affected: shoulder.
Movement: adduction of scapula.
Position: standing, bent over at waist.
Primary muscles: trapezius, rhomboids.

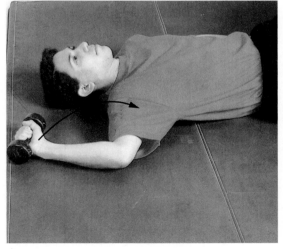
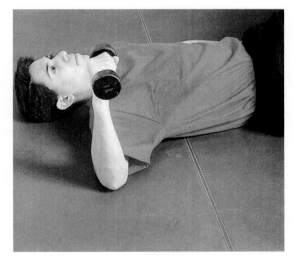

A   B

FIGURE 5-12. SHOULDER MEDIAL ROTATION.
Joint affected: shoulder. Movement: internal rotation.
Lifting weight off the floor.
Position: supine, shoulder abducted and elbow flexed.
Primary muscles: subscapularis.

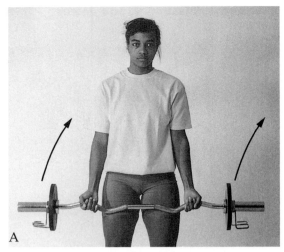
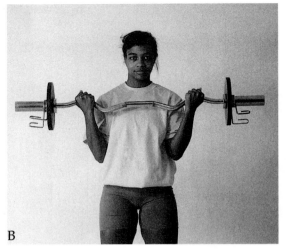

FIGURE 5-13. BICEPS CURLS.
Joint affected: elbow.
Movement: elbow flexion. Curling the weight up to the shoulder.
Position: standing feet front and back rather than side to side, back straight, arms extended.
Primary muscles: biceps.

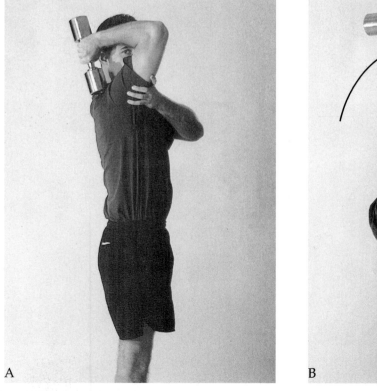
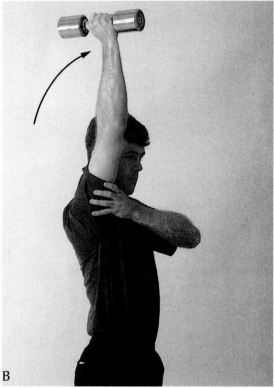

FIGURE 5-14. TRICEPS EXTENSIONS.
Joint affected: elbow.
Movement: elbow extension. Pressing weight toward ceiling.
Position: standing, elbows pointing directly forward beside ears.
Primary muscles: triceps.

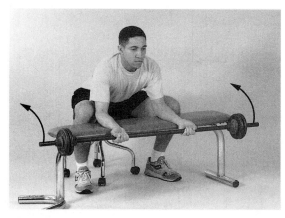

FIGURE 5-15. WRIST CURLS.
Joint affected: wrist.
Movement: wrist flexion. Curling weight upward.
Position: seated, forearms on table, palms up.
Primary muscles: long flexors of forearm.

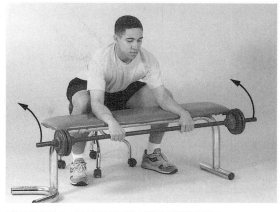

FIGURE 5-16. WRIST EXTENSIONS.
Joint affected: wrist.
Movement: extension. Curling weight upward.
Position: seated, forearms on table, palms down.
Primary muscles: long extensors of forearm.

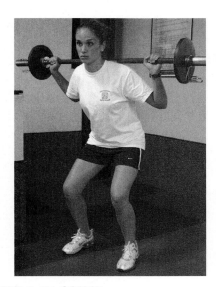

FIGURE 5-17. SQUAT.
Joint affected: hips and knees.
Movement: hip flexion and knee extension.
Position: standing, feet shoulder width apart, back straight, barbell resting on shoulders, bend knees to lower to either 3/4 or 1/2 squat position then stand up.
Muscles: hip extensors, quadriceps.

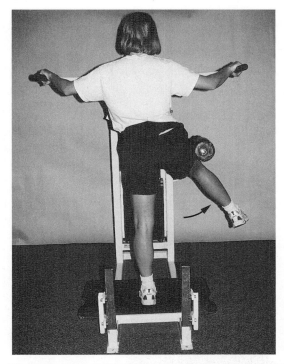

FIGURE 5-18. HIP ABDUCTION ON MACHINE.
Joint affected: hip.
Movement: hip abduction. Lifting leg up.
Position: standing, leg under resistance arm.
Primary muscles: hip abductors.

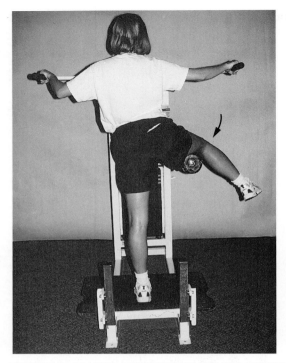

FIGURE 5-19. HIP ADDUCTION ON MACHINE.
Joint affected: hip.
Movement: hip adduction. Pulling leg toward midline of body.
Position: standing leg on top of resistance arm.
Primary muscles: hip adductors.

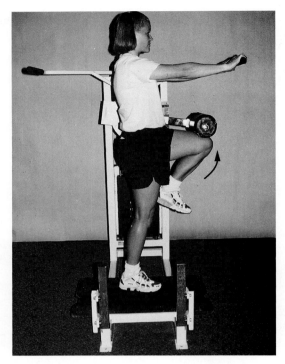

FIGURE 5-20. BENT-KNEE LEG LIFTS ON MACHINE.
Joint affected: hip.
Movement: hip flexion. Lifting knee up.
Position: Standing, knee flexed, Knee under resistance arm.
Primary muscles: iliopsoas.

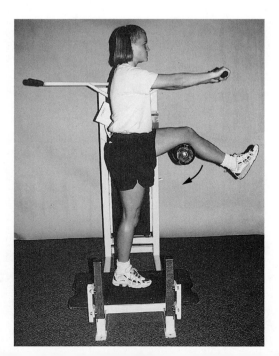

FIGURE 5-21. HIP EXTENSIONS ON MACHINE.
Joint affected: hip.
Movement: hip extension. Pulling leg downward.
Position: Standing, knee extended, resistance arm under thigh.
Primary muscles: gluteus maximus, hamstrings.

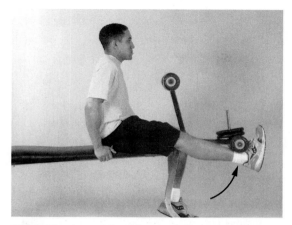

FIGURE 5-22. QUADRICEPS EXTENSIONS.
Joint affected: knee.
Movement: extension. Straightening knee.
Position: sitting, on knee machine.
Primary muscles: quadriceps group.

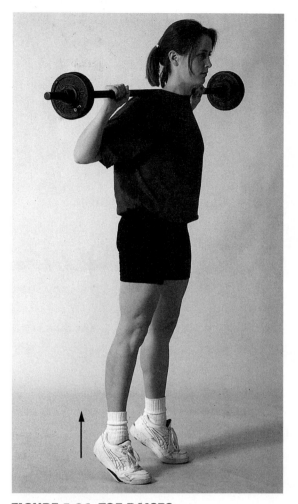

FIGURE 5-24. TOE RAISES.
Joint affected: ankle.
Movement: plantar flexion. Pressing up on toes.
Position: standing and lifting body weight.
Primary muscles: gastrocnemius, soleus.

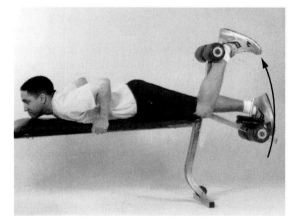

FIGURE 5-23. HAMSTRING CURLS.
Joint affected: knee.
Movement: flexion. Bending knee and lifting the weight up.
Position: prone, on knee machine.
Primary muscles: hamstring group.

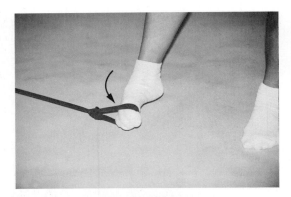

FIGURE 5-25. ANKLE INVERSION.
Joint affected: ankle.
Movement: inversion. Turning the sole of the foot up and in.
Position: sitting, resistance tubing around forefoot.
Primary muscles: anterior tibialis.

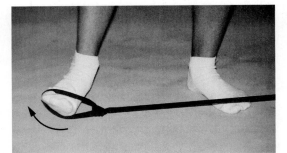

FIGURE 5-26. ANKLE EVERSION.
Joint affected: ankle.
Movement: eversion. Turning the sole of the foot up and out.
Position: sitting, resistance tubing around forefoot.
Primary muscles: peroneals.

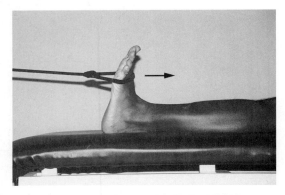

FIGURE 5-27. ANKLE DORSIFLEXION.
Joint affected: ankle.
Movement: dorsiflexion. Pulling the toes upward.
Position: sitting, resistance tubing around forefoot.
Primary muscles: dorsiflexors in shin.

exercises. Complete the worksheets in Table 5-2 to assess your progress in strength increases while doing the following exercises. Safe Tip 5-2 provides you with guidelines and precautions to be used in resistance training.

ISOMETRIC EXERCISE

An isometric exercise involves a muscle contraction in which the length of the muscle remains constant while tension develops toward a maximal force against an immovable resistance (see Figure 5-1, page 97). To develop strength, the muscle should generate a maximal force for 10 seconds at a time, and this contraction should be repeated five to ten times per day.

Isometric exercises are capable of increasing muscular strength; unfortunately, strength gains in a particular muscle will occur only in the position in which resistance is applied. At other positions in the range of motion, the strength curve drops off dramatically because of a lack of motor activity at those angles, and there is no corresponding increase in strength.

Another major disadvantage of these isometric, "sit at your desk" exercises is that they tend to produce a spike in blood pressure that can result in potentially life-threatening cardiovascular accidents. This sharp increase in blood pressure results from holding your breath and increasing pressure within the chest cavity.

TABLE 5-2
STRENGTH TRAINING WORKSHEET I: UPPER-BODY EXERCISES

Exercise	Reps	Sets	Date/Weight													
Shoulder lateral rotation	6–8	3														
Bench press	6–8	3														
Incline press	6–8	3														
Military press	6–8	3														
Lateral pull-downs	6–8	3														
Flys	6–8	3														
Reverse flys	6–8	3														
Shoulder medial rotation	6–8	3														
Biceps curls	6–8	3														
Triceps curls	6–8	3														
Wrist curls	6–8	3														
Wrist extensions	6–8	3														

Exercise	Reps	Sets	Date/Weight																
Squat	6–8	3																	
Hip abduction	6–8	3																	
Hip abduction	6–8	3																	
Bent-knee leg lifts	6–8	3																	
Hip extension	6–8	3																	
Quadriceps extensions	6–8	3																	
Hamstring curls	6–8	3																	
Toe raises	6–8	3																	
Ankle inversion	6–8	3																	
Ankle eversion	6–8	3																	
Ankle dorsiflexion	6–8	3																	

SAFE TIP 5-2

Guidelines and Precautions in Resistance Training

The following guidelines can improve your effectiveness and your safety during strength training:

- Do appropriate warm-up activities before beginning workout.
- Use proper lifting techniques as recommended on the following pages. Improper lifting techniques can result in injury.
- To ensure balanced development, exercise all muscle groups.
- Avoid doing one-repetition maximum lifts. This can result in muscle strains, especially if you are not properly warmed up.
- Always have a spotter if you are lifting free weights.
- Before using a machine (e.g., Cybex), make sure you understand how to use it properly.
- Progress gradually and within your own individual limits.
- Always train throughout a full range of motion.
- Use both concentric and eccentric contractions.
- Try to exercise the larger muscle groups first, and alternate exercises to allow previously exercised muscle groups a chance to recover.
- Do not hold your breath during a lift.
- Do not overtrain. Overtraining may result in injury.
- If you have questions about weight training, seek out an expert who can give you specific, correct advice.
- Do not try to show off; always work within your own limits.

Consequently, the heart experiences a significant increase in blood pressure. This has been referred to as the *Valsalva effect*. To avoid or minimize this effect, it is recommended that breathing be done during the maximal contraction.

Isometric exercises certainly have a place in a fitness program. There are certain instances in which an isometric contraction can greatly enhance a particular movement. A common use for isometric exercises would be for injury rehabilitation or reconditioning. A number of conditions or ailments resulting either from trauma or from overuse must be treated with strengthening exercises. Unfortunately, these problems may be aggravated with full range-of-motion strengthening exercises. It may be more desirable to make use of isometric exercises until the injury has healed to the point that full-range activities can be performed.

ISOKINETIC EXERCISE

An isokinetic exercise involves a muscle contraction in which the length of the muscle is changing while the contraction is performed at a constant velocity. In theory, maximal resistance is provided throughout the range of motion by the machine. The resistance provided by the machine will move only at some preset speed, regardless of the force applied to it by the individual. Thus the key to isokinetic exercise is not the resistance but the speed at which resistance can be moved.

Biodex and Kin-Com are among the more common isokinetic devices (Figure 5-28). In general, they rely on hydraulic, pneumatic, and mechanical pressure systems to produce this constant velocity of motion. The majority of the isokinetic devices are capable of resisting both concentric and eccentric contractions at a fixed speed to exercise a muscle.

A major disadvantage of these units is their cost. Many of them come with a computer and printing device and are used primarily as diagnostic and rehabilitative tools in the treatment of various injuries.

Isokinetic devices are designed so that regardless of the amount of force applied against a resistance, it can only be moved at a certain speed. That speed will be the same whether maximal force or only half the maximal force is applied.

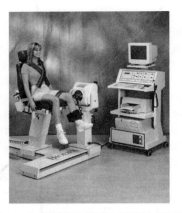

FIGURE 5-28. ISOKINETIC EXERCISE.
Isokinetic exercise works a muscle at a fixed speed of contraction.

Consequently, when training isokinetically, it is absolutely necessary to exert as much force against the resistance as possible (maximal effort) for maximal strength gains to occur. This is another one of the major problems with an isokinetic strength-training program. Anyone who has been involved in a weight-training program knows that on some days it is difficult to find the motivation to work out. Because isokinetic training requires a maximal effort, it is very easy to "cheat" and not go through the workout at a high level of intensity. In a progressive resistive exercise program, you know how much weight has to be lifted with how many repetitions. Therefore, isokinetic training is often more effective if a partner system is used primarily as a means of motivation toward a maximal effort.

Assuming that you generate a maximal effort on each repetition, a general recommendation for isokinetic training is to use three sets of 10 to 15 repetitions at whatever speed of movement you select. If you are exerting maximal effort, you should expect that fatigue will usually occur at some point within each set.

It is theoretically possible that maximal strength gains are best achieved through the isokinetic training method, in which the velocity is equal throughout the range of motion, when such training is done properly with a maximal effort. However, there is no conclusive research to support this theory.

CIRCUIT TRAINING

Circuit training uses a series of exercise stations consisting of various combinations of weight training, flexibility, calisthenics, and brief aerobic exercises. Circuits may be designed to accomplish many different training goals. With circuit training, you move rapidly from one station to the next and perform whatever exercise is to be done at that station within a specified time period. A typical circuit would consist of eight to twelve stations, and the entire circuit would be repeated three times.

Circuit training is definitely an effective technique for improving strength and flexibility. Certainly, if the pace or the time interval between stations is rapid and if the workload is maintained at a high level of intensity with heart rates at or above target training levels, the cardiorespiratory system may benefit from this circuit. It should be and most often is used as a technique for developing and improving muscular strength and endurance. Figure 5-29 provides an example of a simple circuit training setup that can be easily completed by healthy college students.

FUNCTIONAL STRENGTH TRAINING

Functional strength training is a rapidly evolving technique of improving not only muscular strength but also neuromuscular control. The strength-training techniques discussed to this point have traditionally focused on isolated, single-plane exercises used to elicit muscle hypertrophy in a specific muscle. These exercises have a very low neuromuscular demand because they are performed primarily with the rest of the body artificially stabilized on stable pieces of equipment. The central nervous system controls the ability to integrate the proprioceptive function of a number of individual

▶ Station 1 Push-ups: 30 repetitions
▶ Station 2 Hamstring: low back
   stretching
▶ Station 3 Bent-knee sit-ups (25 repetitions)
▶ Station 4 Bench press (10 repetitions at
   75% maximal weight)
▶ Station 5 Rope skipping (100 repetitions)
▶ Station 6 Knee extensions (15 repetitions
   at 80% maximal weight)
▶ Station 7 Shoulder adduction (15 repetitions)
▶ Station 8 Knee flexions (15 repetitions
   at 80% maximal weight)

There would be 60 seconds to complete
each station, and the entire circuit would
be repeated three times in succession.

**FIGURE 5-29. EXAMPLE OF CIRCUIT
TRAINING SETUP.**

muscles that must act simultaneously to produce a specific movement pattern that occurs in three planes of motion. If the body is designed to move in three planes of motion, then isolated training does little to improve functional ability. When strength training using isolated, single-plane, artificially stabilized exercises, the entire body is not being prepared to deal with the imposed demands of normal daily activities (walking up/down stairs, getting groceries out of the trunk, etc.).

Earlier in this chapter it was stated that muscles are capable of three different types of contraction: concentric, eccentric, and isometric. During functional movements, some muscles are contracting concentrically (shortening) to produce movement, others contracting eccentrically (lengthening) to allow movement to occur, and still other muscles contracting isometrically to create a stable base on which the functional movement occurs.

Since all muscles involved in a movement function either eccentrically, concentrically, or isometrically in three planes of motion simultaneously, functional strength training uses integratred exercises designed to improve functional movement patterns in terms of both increased strength and improved neuromuscular control. When using functional strengthening exercises, individuals not only develop functional strength and neuromuscular control, but also high levels of core stabilization strength and flexibility. Figures 5-30 and 5-31 provide examples of functional strengthening exercises.

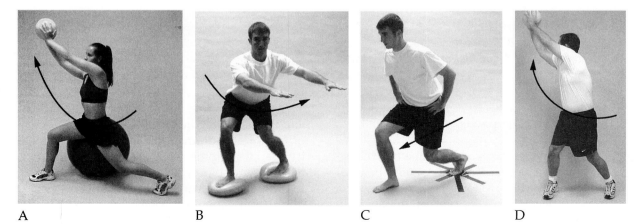

A   B   C   D

FIGURE 5-30. FUNCTIONAL STRENGTHENING EXERCISES.
A, Upper trunk and shoulder rotations with a medicine ball seated on a stability ball; B, Standing rotations on dynadisc; C, Multiplanar lunges; D, Standing rotations with medicine ball.

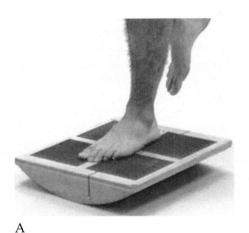

A

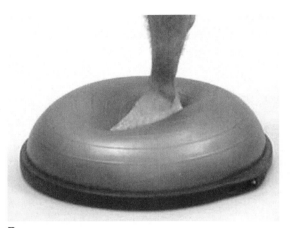

B

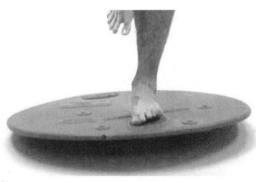

C

**FIGURE 5-31. FUNCTIONAL STRENGTH-
TRAINING EXERCISES TO ENHANCE
STRENGTHENING NEUROMUSCULAR
CONTROL FOR THE ANKLE ON DIFFERENT
PIECES OF EQUIPMENT.**
A, Rocker board. *B,* Bosu balance trainer.
C, Biomechanical Ankle Platform (BAPS) board.
D, Dynadisc.

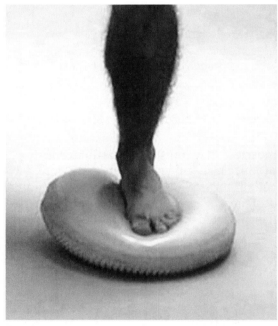

D

PLYOMETRIC EXERCISE

Plyometric exercise is a technique of exercise
that involves a rapid eccentric (lengthening)
stretch of a muscle, followed immediately by a
rapid concentric contraction of that muscle
for the purpose of producing a forceful explosive movement over a short period of time.
Plyometric exercises involve hops, bounds,
and depth jumping for the lower extremity

and the use of medicine balls and other types
of weighted equipment for the upper extremity. Depth jumping is an example of a plyometric exercise in which an individual jumps
to the ground from a specified height and then
quickly jumps again as soon as ground contact
is made. (see Figure 5-32.)

The greater the stretch put on the muscle
from its resting length immediately before
the concentric contraction, the greater the

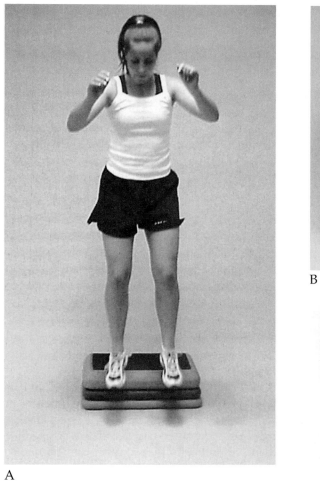

A

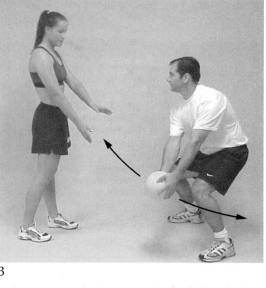

B

C

D

FIGURE 5-32. PLYOMETRIC EXERCISES.
*Plyometric Exercises. **A**, Depth jump. **B**, Medicine balltoss to partner with rotation. **C**, Shoulder rotation with rebounder. **D**, Hopping exercise.*

resistance the muscle can overcome. Plyometrics emphasize the speed of the stretch phase. The rate of stretch is more critical than the magnitude of the stretch. An advantage to using plyometric exercise is that it can help develop eccentric control in dynamic movements. Plyometrics tend to place a great deal of stress on the musculoskeletal system. The learning and perfection of specific jumping skills and other plyometric exercises must be technically correct and specific to one's age, activity, and physical and skill development. It is cautioned that plyometric exercises often cause muscle soreness in individuals who are not used to doing then. Therefore, plyometric exercises should be considered as a more advaned technique of strength training, and only be used by individuals who have experience in weight training.

Recommendations for plyometric exercise are variable. However, you should once again adhere to the three sets of six to eight repetitions rule as discussed previously.

CALISTHENIC STRENGTHENING EXERCISES

Until recently the thought of doing calisthenic exercises probably conjured up the image of a hard-nosed Marine drill instructor leading a group of recruits through a boring, regimented exercise session. But add music and bright-colored exercise clothing and change the name to aerobic exercise, aerobic dance, or tae bo and you have a multimillion-dollar industry that has swept a large segment of the American population into exercise fanaticism. This new fascination with aerobic exercise has shown that calisthenic exercise can be enjoyable without being excessively regimented.

We have already discussed weight training for the development of muscular strength. Calisthenic exercises, if done properly, can improve muscular strength and endurance, flexibility, and cardiorespiratory endurance. However, they are best suited as a supplemental activity to other previously discussed techniques rather than as a substitute for resistance-training exercises.

►Muscle Strength and Endurance

Calisthenics can help to increase muscular strength, tone, and endurance by using the weight of the body and its extremities as resistance. For example, chinning exercises (see Figure 5-41) use the weight of the body to resist the biceps and brachialis muscles in elbow flexion. The primary advantage of calisthenics over training with weights is that you do not need any expensive equipment or machines to provide resistance for you. Most of these exercises can be accomplished without the use of any equipment.

►Flexibility

Calisthenic exercises can also help to improve flexibility as long as each exercise is done through a full range of motion. The weight of a body part can assist in passively stretching a muscle to its greatest length. However, caution must be used when doing calisthenic exercise to improve flexibility. The repetitive, bouncing nature of many of these exercises causes a muscle to be stretched ballistically, which can predispose a muscle to injury, particularly in an untrained person. Through calisthenic exercises, the muscle should be progressively stretched during the set of exercises. Do not neglect a warm-up that includes flexibility exercises before engaging in calisthenics.

►Cardiorespiratory Endurance

There is some question as to whether calisthenic exercises can increase resting heart rate significantly. However, if exercise is of sufficient intensity, frequency, and duration, cardiorespiratory endurance can be improved. Anyone who has gone through a 20- to

30-minute aerobics class will agree that heart rate is elevated to training levels. Calisthenic exercises should be done at a quick pace and without much rest between sets for optimal improvement of cardiorespiratory endurance.

▶ Specific Exercises

The exercises illustrated in Figures 5-33 to 5-42 are recommended because they work on specific muscle groups and with a specific purpose. If all exercises are done, most of the major muscle groups in the body will be both stretched and contracted against resistance with the objective of improving strength, flexibility, and endurance. Each exercise can be done at your own pace, although the greater the pace, the greater the stress placed on the cardiorespiratory system. Thus it is recommended that you work quickly and move from one exercise to the next without delay. These exercises can be done to music if you so desire. Most people find it easier to exercise to fast-paced music with a hard, rhythmic beat. However, you should select the type of music most enjoyable to you.

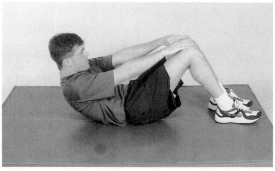

A

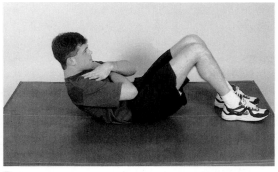

B

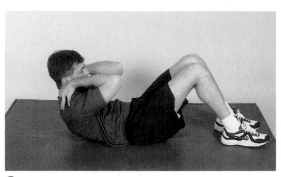

C

FIGURE 5-33. SIT-UPS.

A, Beginning; B, Intermediate; C, Advanced.
Joints affected: spinal vertebral joints.
Movement: trunk flexion.
Instructions: Lying on back, hands either on chest or behind back, knees flexed to 90-degree angle, feet on floor, curl trunk and head to approximately 45-degree angle.
Primary muscles: rectus abdominis.
Caution: *It has been suggested by some experts on low back pain that sit-up exercises done with both bent and straight legs should be avoided due to the high compressive loads on the low back and spine. This is particularly true in individuals with existing low back pain. (McGill, 2001) While this view is not universally accepted, if sit-ups, crunches, or even straight leg raises cause increased low back pain, they should be avoided.*

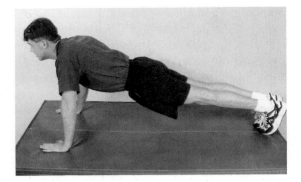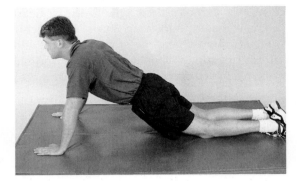
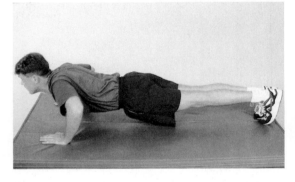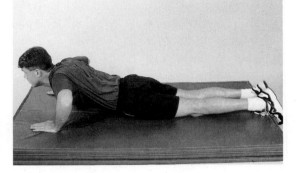

A   B

FIGURE 5-34. PUSH-UPS.

A, Push-ups. *B, Modified push-ups.*

Purpose: strengthening.

Muscles: triceps, pectoralis major.

Repetitions: beginner 10; intermediate 20; advanced 30.

Instructions: Keep the upper trunk and legs extended in a straight line. Touch floor with chest.

Caution: *Avoid hyperextending the back, especially in modified push-ups.*

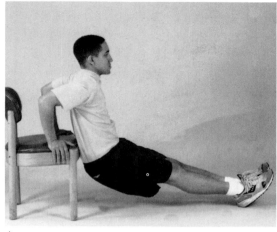
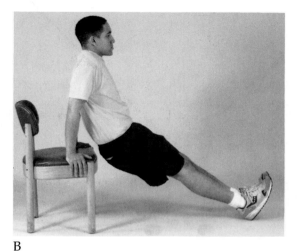

A   B

FIGURE 5-35. TRICEPS EXTENSIONS.
Purpose: strengthening and range of motion at shoulder joint.
Muscles: triceps, trapezius.
Repetitions: beginner 7; intermediate 12; advanced 18.
Instructions: Begin with arms extended and body straight. Lower buttocks until they touch the ground, then press back up.

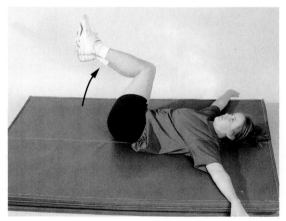
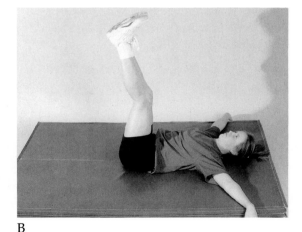

A   B

FIGURE 5-36. TRUNK ROTATION.
A, Beginner; B, Advanced.
Muscles: internal and external obliques.
Repetitions: beginner 10 each direction; intermediate 15 each direction; advanced 20 each direction.
Instructions: Rotate trunk from side to side until knees touch the floor, keeping knees slightly bent.
Caution: *This exercise should be done only by those who already have strong abdominals.*

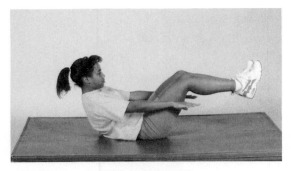

FIGURE 5-37. SITTING TUCKS.

Purpose: strengthen abdominals and stretch low back.

Muscles: rectus abdominis, erector muscles in low back.

Repetitions: beginner 10; intermediate 20; advanced 30.

Instructions: Keep legs and upper back off the ground and pull knees to chest.

Caution: *It has been suggested by some experts on low back pain that sit-up type exercises done with both bent and straight legs should be avoided due to the high compressive loads on the low back and spine. This is particularly true in individuals with existing low back pain. (McGill, 2001) While this view is not universally accepted, if sitting tucks cause increased low back pain, they should be avoided.*

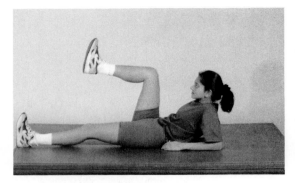

FIGURE 5-38. BICYCLE.

Purpose: strengthen hip flexors and stretch lower back.

Muscles: iliopsoas.

Repetitions: beginner 10 each side; intermediate 20 each side; advanced 30 each side.

Instructions: Alternately flex and extend legs as if you were pedaling a bicycle.

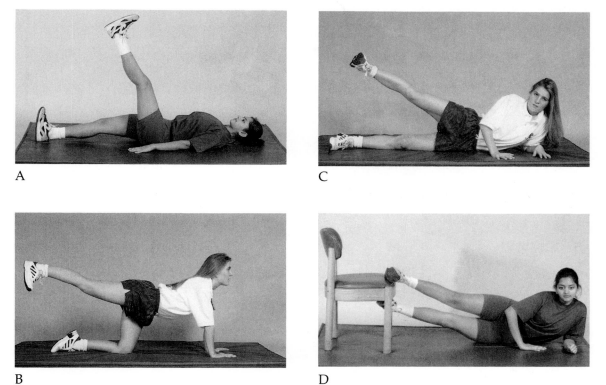

FIGURE 5-39. LEG LIFTS.

A, Front; B, Back; C, Side (leg up); D, Side (leg down).
Purpose: strengthen A, Hip flexors; B, Hip extensors; C, Hip abductors; D, Hip adductors.
Muscles: A, Iliopsoas; B, Gluteus maximus; C, Gluteus medius; D, Adductor group.
Repetitions: beginner 10 each leg; intermediate 15 each leg; advanced 20 each leg.
Instructions: Raise the exercising leg up as far as possible in each position.

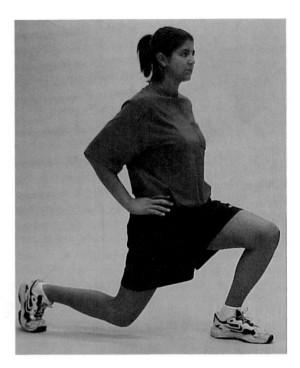

FIGURE 5-40. LUNGES.
Joints affected: hip and knee.
Movement: Forward lunge.
Position: standing, take giant step forward bend-
ing knee while holding weights in hands.
Primary muscles: gluteal, hamstrings, quadriceps.

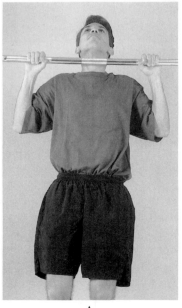

A

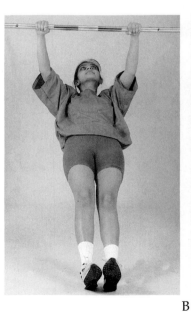 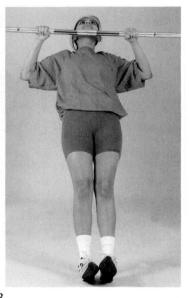

B

FIGURE 5-41. CHIN-UPS.
A, Chin-ups. B, Modified chin-ups.
Purpose: strengthening and stretch of shoulder joint.
Muscles: biceps, brachialis, and latissimus dorsi.
Repetitions: beginner 7; intermediate 10; advanced 15.
Instructions: Pull up until chin touches top of bar.

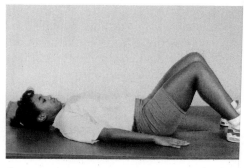

A

FIGURE 5-42. BUTTOCK TUCKS.
Purpose: strengthen muscles of buttocks.
Muscles: gluteus maximus, hamstrings.
Repetitions: beginner 10; intermediate 15; (
Instructions: Lying flat on back with knees

maximal training response. The exercises
be safe but challenging, stress multipl
incorporate a variety of resistance
(physioball, medicine ball, dumb
etc.), be derived from fundam

CORE STABILIZATION TRAINING

A dynamic **core stabilization training** program should be an important component of all
comprehensive strengthening programs. The
core is defined as the lumbo-pelvic-hip complex. The core is where the center of gravity is
located and where all movement begins. There
are 29 muscles in the lumbar spine, the abdomen, and around the hip and plevis that
have their attachment to the lumbo-pelvic-hip
complex. (See Figure 5-4 on p. 106.)

A core stabilization program will improve
dynamic postural control; ensure appropriate
muscular balance and joint movement around
the lumbo-pelvic-hip complex; allow for the

development of functional strength improve neuromuscular efficiency throughout
the entire body.

Many individuals work on developing the
strength, power, neuromuscular control, and
muscular endurance in specific muscles that
enable them to perform functional activities.
However, relatively few individuals have developed the muscles required for stabilization
of the spine. The body's stabilization system
has to be functioning optimally to effectively
utilize the strength, power, neuromuscular
control, and muscular endurance that they
have developed in their prime movers. If the
extremity muscles are strong and the core is
weak, then there will not be enough force created to produce efficient movements. A weak
core is a fundamental problem of inefficient
movements that lead to injury.

A core stabilization training program is designed to help an individual gain strength,
neuromuscular control, power, and muscle endurance of the lumbo-pelvic hip complex. A
comprehensive core stabilization training program should be systematic, progressive, and
functional. When designing a functional core
stabilization training program, you should
select the appropriate exercises to elicit a

> **core stabilization training:** A tech-
> nique for increasing the ability and effi-
> ciency of the muscles of the hip, lower
> back, pelvis, and abdomen, and for pro-
> viding stability and a base of support for
> movement of the extremities.

...must
...planes,
...equipment
...bells, tubing,
...ental movement skills, and be activity specific. Figure 5-43 shows examples of exercises that may be used to improve core stability. You should start with exercises in which you can maintain stability and optimal neuromuscular control.

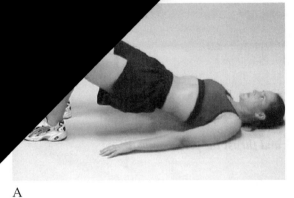

A

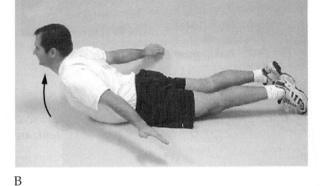

B

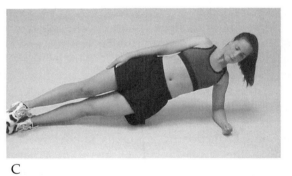

C

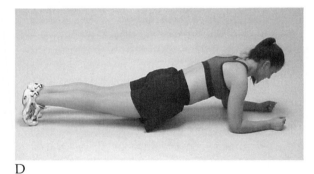

D

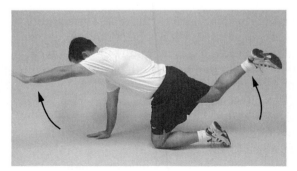

E

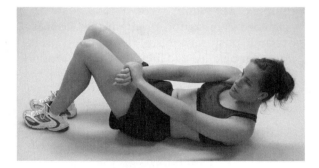

F

FIGURE 5-43. CORE STABILIZATION EXERCISES.
A, Bridging. *B*, Prone cobra. *C*, Sidelying isolated abdominal. *D*, Human arrow. *E*, Opposite arm/leg raise. *F*, Diagonal crunch.

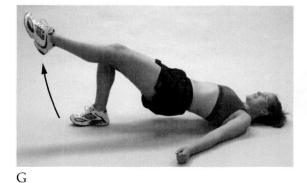

G

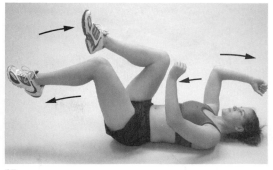

H

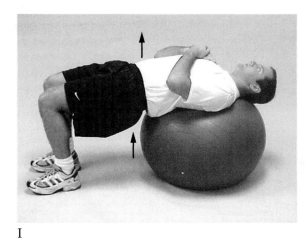

I

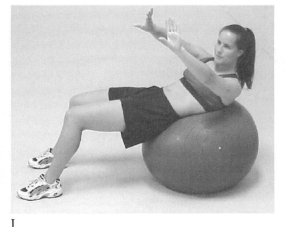

J

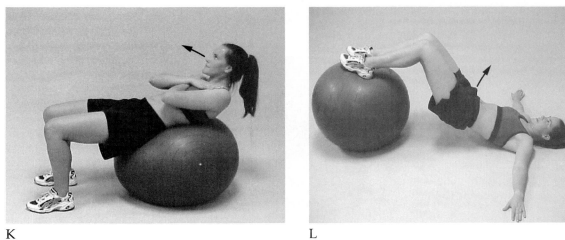

K

L

FIGURE 5-43 (cont.). CORE STABILIZATION EXERCISES.
*G, Bridge with leg extension. **H,** Dead bug. **I,** Stability ball bridging. **J,** Stability ball diagonal crunch.*
***K,** Stability ball crunch. **L,** Stability ball hamstring curl.*

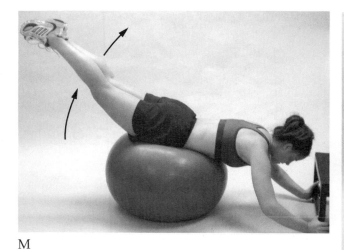

M

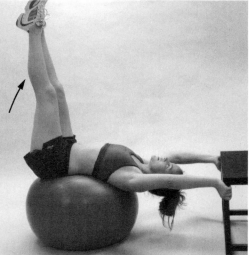

N

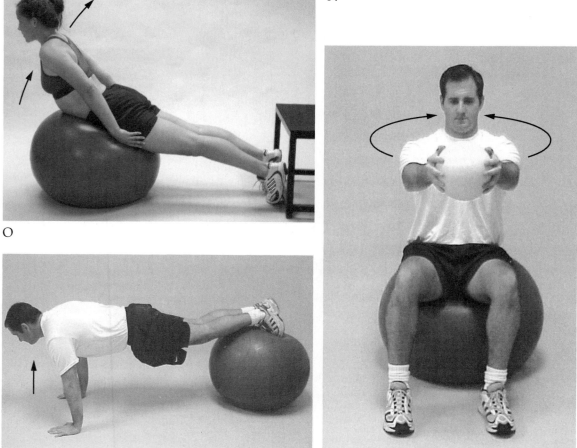

O

P

Q

FIGURE 5-43 (cont.). CORE STABILIZATION EXERCISES.
M, Stability ball hip extension. N, Stability ball straight leg raise. O, Stability ball trunk extension.
P, Stability ball push-up. Q, Stability ball rotation with medic ball.

ASSESSMENT OF MUSCULAR STRENGTH AND ENDURANCE

Lab Activities 5-1 through 5-3 will help you assess your levels of muscular strength, endurance, and power. On the worksheet on page 143 you can monitor and record your progress on each of the exercises described in this chapter.

SUMMARY

- Muscular strength and endurance are important health-related components of fitness. Power is a skill-related component of fitness.
- The ability to generate force depends on the physical properties of the muscle as well as on the mechanical factors that dictate how much force can be generated through the lever system to an external object.
- Hypertrophy of a muscle is caused by increases in the size of the protein myofilaments, which result in an increased cross-sectional diameter of the muscle.
- The key to improving strength through resistance training is using the principle of overload.
- A number of different resistance-training techniques can improve muscular strength: progressive resistive exercise, isometric exercise, isokinetic exercise, circuit training, functional strength training, plyometric training calisthenic exercises, and core stabilization exercises.
- Muscular endurance tends to improve with muscular strength; thus, training techniques for these two components are similar.

SUGGESTED READINGS

Baechle, T. R. 2000. *Essentials of strength training and conditioning.* Champaign, IL: Human Kinetics.

Bompa, T. O., and L. J. Cornacchia. 2002. *Serious strength training.* Champaign, IL: Human Kinetics.

Brown, L. E. 2000. *Isokinetics in human performance.* Champaign, IL: Human Kinetics.

Chu, D. 1996. *Explosive strength and power.* Champaign, IL: Human Kinetics.

Clark, M. 2001. *Integrated training for the new millennium.* Calabasas, CA: National Academy of Sports Medicine.

Ebben, W. P., and R. L. Jenson. 1998. Strength training for women: Debunking myths that block opportunity. *Physician and Sports Medicine* 26(5):86–88, 91–92, 97.

Ebben, W. P., and P. B. Watts. 1998. A review of combined weight training and plyometric training modes: Complex training. *Strength and Conditioning* 20(5):18–27.

Fahey, T. 2005. *Weight training basics.* New York: McGraw-Hill.

Field, R. W., and S. O. Roberts. 1999. *Weight training.* Boston: WCB/McGraw-Hill.

Flach, A., and E. O'Driscol. 2005. *The complete book of isometrics: The anywhere, anytime fitness book.* New York: Hatherleigh Press.

Fleck, S., and W. Kramer. 2004. *Designing resistance training programs.* Champaign, IL: Human Kinetics.

Garbutt, G., and N. T. Cable. 1998. Circuit weight-training. *Sports Exercise and Injury* 4(2/3):46–49.

Goldenberg, L., and P. Twist. 2001. *Strength ball training.* Champaign, IL: Human Kinetics.

Goldenberg, L., and P. Twist. 2002. Core stabilization. In *Strength ball training,* edited by L. Goldenberg. Champaign, IL: Human Kinetics.

Gravelle, B., and D. Blessing. 2000. Physiological adaptation in women concurrently training for strength and endurance. *Journal of Strength and Conditioning* 14(1):5.

Heyward, V. H. 2002. Assessing strength and muscular endurance. In *Advanced fitness assessment and exercise prescription,* 4th ed., edited by V. H. Heyward. Champaign, IL: Human Kinetics.

Knight, K. L., C. D. Ingersoll, and J. Bartholomew. 2001. Isotonic contractions might be more effective than isokinetic contractions in developing muscle strength. *Journal of Sport Rehabilitation* 10(2):124–31.

Komi, P. V. 2003. *Strength and power in sport,* 2nd ed. Oxford: Blackwell Science.

Kraemer, W. J., N. D. Duncan, and J. S. Volek. 1998. Resistence training and elite athletes: Adaptations and program considerations. *Journal of Orthopedic and Sports Physical Therapy* 28(2):110–19.

Kraemer, W., and S. Fleck. *Strength training for young athletes.* Champaign, IL: Human Kinetics.

Kraemer, W., K. Hakkinen, and W. Kraemer. 2001. *Strength training for sport.* Cambridge, MA: Blackwell Science.

Kraemer, W. J., and N. A. Ratamess, 2004. Fundamentals of resistance training: progression and exercise prescription. *Medicine and Science in Sports and Exercise* 36(4):574–688.

Leetun, D. T., M. L. Ireland, and J. D. Willson. 2004. Core stability measures as risk factors for lower extremity injury in athletes. *Medicine and Science in Sports and Exercise* 36(6):926–34.

Mannie, K. 2004. Overloading without overtraining. *Coach and Athletic Director* 74(4):9–12.

McCartney, N. 1999. Acute responses to resistance training and safety. *Medicine and Science in Sports and Exercise* 31(1):31–37.

McGill, S. 2001. Low back stability: From formal description to issues for performance and rehabilitation. *Exercise and Sport Science Reviews* 29(1):26–31.

Page, P., and T. Ellenbecker. 2004. *Strength band training.* Champaign, IL: Human Kinetics.

Plisk, S. S. 2001. Muscular strength and stamina. In *High-performance sports conditioning,* edited by B. Foran. Champaign, IL: Human Kinetics.

Radcliffe, J. C., and R. C. Farentinos. 2001. *High-powered plyometrics.* Champaign, IL: Human Kinetics.

Roetert, E. P. 1998. Facts and fallacies about strength training for women. *Strength and Conditioning* 20(6):172–78.

Schroeder, E. T., S. A. Hawkins, and S. V. Jaque. 2004. Musculoskeletal adaptations to 16 weeks of eccentric progressive resistance training in young women. *Journal of Strength and Conditioning Research* 18(2):227–35.

Stamford, B. 1998. Weight training basics. Part 1: Choosing the best options. *Physician and Sports Medicine* 26(2):115–16.

Stone, M. H., and A. C. Fry. 1998. Increased training volume in strength/power athletes. In *Overtraining in sport,* edited by R. B. Kreider et al. Champaign, IL: Human Kinetics.

Verstegen, M., and P. Williams. 2004. *Core performance: The revolutionary workout program to transform your body and your life.* Emmaus, PA: Rodale Press Inc.

Suggested Web Sites

A–Z Fitness

This site presents over 700 excellent links to fitness and bodybuilding. Five certified trainers answer your training questions. Free fitness classifieds, weekly exercise video, new online fitness articles, and more are presented.
www.atozfitness.com

International Sports Sciences Association

ISSA is the fitness certification agency of choice for personal trainers, strength coaches, aerobics instructors, and other exercise enthusiasts. ISSA-certified fitness trainers are taught the most current info on strength training, flexibility, bodybuilding, nutrition, fat loss, and lifestyle.
www.issaonline.com/certification/index.html

International Weightlifting Federation

The IWF is composed of the affiliated National Federations governing the sport of weightlifting on the basis of one federation per country and is the controlling body of all competitive lifting. The objectives of the IWF are to organize, control, and develop the sport of weightlifting on an international scale.
www.iwf.net

National Council of Strength and Fitness

The NCSF Certification Agency strives to develop the most knowledgeable professional trainers by maintaining the highest standards in the industry.
www.ncsf.org

National Strength and Conditioning Association Home Page

The NSCA sponsors this site.
www.nsca-lift.org

Plyometrics: Myths and Misconceptions

Visit this site produced by Vern Gambetta.
www.gambetta.com/articles/a97008.html

USA Weightlifting

USA Weightlifting (USAW) is the national governing body (NGB) for Olympic weightlifting in the United States. USAW is a member of the United States Olympic Committee (USOC) and a member of the International Weightlifting Federation (IWF). As the NGB, USAW is responsible for conducting Olympic weightlifting programs throughout the country.
www.usaweightlifting.org

WeightsNet—For bodybuilding, fitness, power lifting, sports, and more . . .

WeightsNet is a resource for people who work out with weights for bodybuilding, fitness, power lifting, sports, and more. It's where the 'net pumps up!
www.weightsnet.com

Weight Room Safety

"Weight Room Safety Strategic Planning" by Gary Polson is published as a 6-part article in the National Strength and Conditioning Association's Journal, *Strength and Conditioning.*
www.strengthtech.com/weight/safety.htm
www.strengthtech.com/weight/weight.htm

CHAPTER 6

Increasing Flexibility Through **Stretching**

Objectives

After completing this chapter, you should be able to do the following:

- Define flexibility and describe its importance as a health-related component of fitness.
- Identify factors that limit flexibility.
- Differentiate between active and passive range of motion.
- Explain the difference between dynamic, static, and PNF stretching.
- Describe stretching exercises that may be used to improve flexibility at specific joints throughout the body.
- Discuss pilates and yoga as two alternative stretching techniques.

WHY IS IT IMPORTANT TO HAVE GOOD FLEXIBILITY?

Flexibility may best be defined as the range of motion possible about a given joint or series of joints. Flexibility can be discussed in relation to movement involving only one joint, such as the knee, or movement involving a whole series of joints, such as the spinal vertebral joints, which must all move together to allow smooth bending, or rotation, of the trunk. Flexibility is specific to a given joint or movement. A person may have good range of motion in the ankles, knees, hips, back, and one shoulder joint. However, if the other shoulder joint lacks normal movement, then a problem exists that needs to be corrected before that person can function normally.

Flexibility was identified in Chapter 1 as a health-related as opposed to skill-related com-

ponent of fitness, although for most of us it may be considered important for both. The ability to move a joint or series of joints smoothly and

> **flexibility:** the range of motion possible about a given joint or series of joints

KEY TERMS

flexibility
active range of motion
passive range of motion
agonist muscle
antagonist muscle
dynamic (ballistic) stretching

static stretching
proprioceptive neuromuscular facilitation (PNF)
Pilates exercise
yoga

easily throughout a full range of motion is certainly essential to healthy living. The arthritic person who suffers from degeneration in one or more joints loses the capacity of painless, nonrestricted motion and is hampered in the performance of daily acts of healthful living. Lack of flexibility may result in uncoordinated or awkward movements and may predispose a person to muscle strain. Low back pain is frequently associated with tightness of the musculature in the lower spine and also of the hamstring muscles.

If you are physically active, a lack of flexibility will likely impair your performance. For example, if you are a power walker with tight, inelastic hamstring muscles, you may have a problem walking at a fast pace, because tight hamstrings restrict your ability to flex the hip joint, thus shortening your stride length. Most activities you engage in require relatively "normal" amounts of flexibility. However, some activities, such as gymnastics, ballet, diving, karate, tai chi, and yoga, require increased flexibility for superior performance (Figure 6-1). Increased flexibility may increase one's performance through improved balance and reaction time. Experts in the field of training and the development of physical fitness generally agree that good flexibility is essential to successful physical performance, although their ideas are based primarily on observation rather than on scientific research.

Most experts feel that maintaining good flexibility is important in prevention of injury to muscles and tendons, although recently some

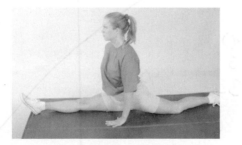

FIGURE 6-1. EXTREME FLEXIBILITY.
Certain athletic activities require extreme flexibility for successful performance.

have questioned the efficiency of stretching in both injury prevention and in improving performance. However, the majority of fitness experts will generally insist that stretching exercises be performed after the warm-up before engaging in strenuous activity. Again, little or no research evidence is available to support this contention.

WHAT STRUCTURES IN THE BODY CAN LIMIT FLEXIBILITY?

A number of different anatomical structures may limit the ability of a joint to move through a full, unrestricted range of motion.

Normal bone structure, fat, and skin or scar tissue may limit the ability to move through a full range of motion. Muscles and their tendons are most often responsible for limiting range of motion. When performing stretching exercises for the purpose of improving a particular joint's flexibility, you are attempting to take advantage of the highly elastic properties of a muscle. Over time, it is possible to increase elasticity, or the length that a given muscle can be stretched. Individuals who have a good deal of movement at a particular joint tend to have highly elastic and flexible muscles.

Ligaments function to connect bone to bone and help provide stability around a joint. If a joint is immobilized (in a cast or splint) for a period of time, ligaments will lose some of their inherent elasticity and actually shorten. This condition is most commonly seen after surgical repair of an unstable joint, but it can also result from long periods of inactivity. Stretching will have a positive effect on muscles, tendons, and ligaments.

On the other hand, it's also possible for a person to have relatively slack ligaments. These people are generally referred to as being "loose-jointed." Examples of this would be an elbow or knee that hyperextends beyond 180 degrees (beyond straight). Frequently there is instability associated with loose-jointedness that may be as great a problem in movement as a joint that is too tight.

ACTIVE AND PASSIVE RANGE OF MOTION

When a muscle actively contracts, it produces a joint movement through a specific range of motion. However, if passive pressure is applied to an extremity, it is capable of moving farther in the range of motion. **Active range of motion** refers to that portion of the total range of motion through which a joint can be moved by an active muscle contraction. Your ability to move through the active range of motion is not necessarily a good indicator of the stiffness or looseness of a joint because it applies to the ability to move a joint efficiently, with little resistance to motion. **Passive range of motion** refers to the portion of the total range of motion (beyond the active range of motion) through which a joint may be moved passively. No muscle contraction is needed to move a joint through a passive range of motion. Passive range of motion begins at the end of and continues beyond active range of motion.

It is essential in sport activities that an extremity be capable of moving through a nonrestricted range of motion. For example, a hurdler who cannot fully extend the knee joint in a normal stride is at considerable disadvantage because stride length and thus speed will be reduced significantly. Passive range of motion is important for injury prevention. There are many situations in sport in which a muscle is forced to stretch beyond its normal active limits. If the muscle does not have enough elasticity to compensate for this additional stretch, it is likely that the muscle or its tendon will be injured.

AGONIST VERSUS ANTAGONIST MUSCLES

Before discussing the three different stretching techniques, it is essential to define the terms **agonist muscle** and **antagonist muscle.**

Most joints in the body are capable of more than one movement. The knee joint, for example, is capable of flexion and extension. Contraction of the quadriceps group of muscles on the front of the thigh causes knee extension, whereas contraction of the hamstring muscles on the back of the thigh produces knee flexion. The muscle that contracts to produce a movement, in this case the quadriceps, is referred to as the agonist muscle. Conversely, the muscle being stretched in response to contraction of the agonist muscle is called the antagonist muscle. In this example of knee extension, the antagonist muscle would be the hamstring group.

Some degree of balance in strength must exist between agonist and antagonist muscle groups. This is necessary for normal, smooth, coordinated movement as well as for reducing the likelihood of muscle strain due to the muscular imbalance. Understanding the relationship between agonist and antagonist muscles is essential for a discussion of the three techniques of stretching.

active range of motion: that portion of the total range of motion through which a joint can be moved by an active muscle contraction

passive range of motion: that portion of the total range of motion (beyond active range of motion) through which a joint may be moved passively without muscle contraction producing the movement

agonist muscle: the muscle that contracts to produce a movement

antagonist muscle: the muscle being stretched in response to contraction of the agonist muscle

WHAT ARE THE DIFFERENT STRETCHING TECHNIQUES?

Maintaining a full, nonrestricted range of motion has long been recognized as an essential component of physical fitness. Flexibility is important not only for successful physical performance but also in the prevention of injury. The goal of any effective flexibility program should be to improve the range of motion around a given joint by altering the extensibility of the muscles and tendons that produce movement at that joint. It is well documented that exercises that stretch these muscles and tendons over a period of time will increase the range of movement possible about a given joint.

Stretching techniques for improving flexibility have evolved over the years. The oldest technique for stretching is called **dynamic (ballistic) stretching;** it makes use of repetitive bouncing motions. A second technique, known as **static stretching,** involves stretching a muscle to the point of discomfort and then holding it at that point for an extended time. This technique has been used for many years. In recent years, another group of stretching techniques known collectively as **proprioceptive neuromuscular facilitation (PNF),** involving alternating contractions and stretches, has also been recommended. Researchers have had considerable discussion about which of these techniques is most effective for improving range of motion.

BALLISTIC (DYNAMIC) STRETCHING

If you were to walk out to the track on any spring or fall afternoon and watch people who are warming up to run by doing their stretching exercises, you would probably see them using bouncing movements to stretch a particular muscle. This bouncing technique has been traditionally referred to as ballistic stretching, and more recently has been called the dynamic stretching technique. Repetitive contractions of the agonist muscle are used to produce quick stretches of the antagonist muscle. Over the years, many fitness experts have questioned the safety of the ballistic stretching technique. Their concerns have been primarily based on the idea that ballistic stretching creates somewhat uncontrolled forces within the muscle that can exceed the extensibility limits of the muscle fiber, thus producing small tears within the muscle. Certainly this might be true in sedentary individuals or perhaps in athletes who have sustained muscle injuries.

Most sport activities are dynamic and require ballistic-type movements. For example, forcefully kicking a soccer ball 50 times involves a repeated dynamic contraction of the agonist quadriceps muscle. The antagonist hamstrings are contracting eccentrically to decelerate the lower leg dynamic stretching of the hamstring muscle before engaging in this type of activity should allow the muscle to

dynamic (ballistic) stretching: technique involving repetitive contractions of the agonist muscle that are used to produce quick stretches of the antagonist muscle

static stretching: technique involving passively stretching a given antagonist muscle by placing it in a maximal position of stretch and holding it there for an extended time

proprioceptive neuromuscular facilitation (PNF): a group of stretching techniques including slow-reversal-hold-relax, contract-relax, and hold-relax techniques, all of which involve some combination of alternating contraction and relaxation of both agonist and antagonist muscles

gradually adapt to the imposed demands and reduce the likelihood of injury. Because ballistic stretching is more functional, it should be integrated into a flexibility program and is in fact recommended for an athlete or physically active individual who is involved in dynamic activity. However in sedentary or untrained individuals, dynamic stretching should not be used because of its potential for causing muscle soreness.

STATIC STRETCHING

The static stretching technique is an extremely effective and popular technique of stretching. This technique involves contracting the agonist muscle to passively stretch a given antagonist muscle by placing it in a maximal position of stretch and holding it there for an extended time. Recommendations for the optimal time for holding this stretched position vary, ranging from as short as 3 seconds to as long as 60 seconds. Data are inconclusive at present; however, it appears that 30 seconds may be a good time. The static stretch of each muscle should be repeated three or four times. Much research has been done comparing ballistic and static stretching techniques for the improvement of flexibility. Both static and ballistic stretching are effective in increasing flexibility, and there is no significant difference between the two. However, with static stretching there is less danger of exceeding the extensibility limits of the involved joints because the stretch is more controlled. Ballistic stretching may cause muscular soreness if performed too aggressively, whereas static stretching generally does not and is commonly used in injury rehabilitation of sore or strained muscles.

Static stretching is certainly a much safer stretching technique, especially for sedentary or untrained individuals. However, many physical activities involve dynamic movement. Thus in physically active individuals who routinely engage in dynamic activities, stretching as a warm-up should begin with static stretching and may be safely followed by ballistic stretching, which more closely resembles the dynamic activity.

PROPRIOCEPTIVE NEUROMUSCULAR FACILITATION (PNF) TECHNIQUES

PNF techniques were first used by physical therapists for treating patients who had various types of neuromuscular paralysis. Only recently have PNF stretching exercises been used as a stretching technique for increasing flexibility. A number of different PNF techniques are currently being used for stretching, including slow-reversal-hold-relax, contract-relax, and hold-relax techniques. All involve some combination of alternating contraction and relaxation of both agonist and antagonist muscles (a 10-second pushing phase followed by a 10-second relaxing phase).

Using a hamstring stretching technique as an example (Figure 6-2), the slow-reversal-hold-relax technique would be done as follows. Lying on your back with the knee extended and the ankle flexed to 90 degrees, a partner passively flexes your leg at the hip joint to the point at which you feel slight discomfort in the muscle. At this point you begin

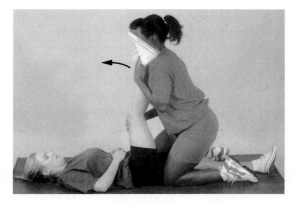

FIGURE 6-2. SLOW-REVERSAL-HOLD-RELAX TECHNIQUE.
This technique stretches hamstring muscles.

pushing against your partner's resistance by contracting the hamstring muscle. After pushing for 10 seconds, the hamstring muscles are relaxed and the agonist quadriceps muscle is contracted while your partner applies passive pressure to further stretch the antagonist hamstrings. This should move the leg so that there is increased hip joint flexion. The relaxing phase lasts for 10 seconds, at which time you again push against your partner's resistance, beginning at this new joint angle. The push-relax sequence is repeated at least three times.

The contract-relax and hold-relax techniques are variations on the slow-reversal-hold-relax method. In the contract-relax method, the hamstrings are isotonically contracted so that the leg actually moves toward the floor during the push phase. The hold-relax method involves an isometric hamstring contraction against immovable resistance during the push phase. During the relax phase, both techniques involve relaxation of hamstrings and quadriceps while the hamstrings are passively stretched. This same basic PNF technique can be used to stretch any muscle in the body. PNF stretching techniques are perhaps best performed with a partner, although they may also be done using a wall as resistance.

PRACTICAL APPLICATION

Although all three stretching techniques have been demonstrated to effectively improve flexibility, there is still considerable debate as to which technique produces the greatest increases in range of movement. The ballistic technique is seldom recommended in sedentary individuals because of the potential for causing muscle soreness. However, it must be added that most sport activities are dynamic in nature (e.g., kicking, running). In highly trained individuals, it is unlikely that ballistic stretching will result in muscle soreness. Static stretching is perhaps the most widely used technique. It is a simple technique and does not require a partner. A full nonrestricted range of

motion can be attained through static stretching over time.

PNF stretching techniques are capable of producing dramatic increases in range of motion during one stretching session. Studies comparing static and PNF stretching suggest that PNF stretching is capable of producing greater improvement in flexibility over an extended training period. The major disadvantage of PNF stretching is that a partner is required to help you stretch, although stretching with a partner may have some motivational advantages. More and more athletic teams seem to be adopting the PNF technique as the method of choice for improving flexibility. Safe Tip 6-1 offers guidelines and precautions for stretching.

ALTERNATIVE STRETCHING TECHNIQUES

Two exercise techniques, pilates exercises and yoga, integrate some elements of stretching and flexibility into their philosophies of mind/body control.

THE PILATES METHOD

The Pilates method is a somewhat different approach to improving flexibility. This method has become extremely popular and widely used among personal fitness trainers and physical therapists. Pilates is an exercise technique devised by German-born Joseph Pilates, who established the first Pilates studio in the United States before World War II. The Pilates method is a conditioning program that improves muscle control, flexibility, coordination, strength, and tone. The basic principles of **Pilates exercise** are to make people

> **Pilates exercise:** a sequence of carefully performed movements that stretch and strengthen muscles

SAFE TIP 6-1

Guidelines and Precautions for Stretching

The following guidelines and precautions should be incorporated into a sound stretching program:

- Warm up using a slow jog or fast walk before stretching vigorously.
- To increase flexibility, overload or stretch the muscle beyond its normal range but not to the point of pain.
- Stretch only to the point where you feel tightness or resistance to stretch or perhaps some discomfort. Stretching should not be painful.
- Increases in range of motion will be specific to whatever joint is being stretched.
- Exercise caution when stretching muscles that surround painful joints. Pain is an indication that something is wrong and should not be ignored.
- Avoid overstretching the ligaments that surround joints.
- Exercise caution when stretching the low back and neck. Exercises that compress the vertebrae and their discs may cause damage.
- Stretch those muscles that are tight and inflexible.
- Strengthen those muscles that are weak and loose.
- Always stretch slowly and with control.
- Be sure to continue normal breathing during a stretch. Do not hold your breath.
- Static and PNF techniques are most often recommended for individuals who want to improve their range of motion.
- Ballistic stretching should be done only by those who are already flexible and/or are accustomed to stretching and done only after static stretching.
- Stretching should be done at least three times per week to see minimal improvement. It is recommended that you stretch between five and six times per week to see maximum results.

more aware of their bodies as single integrated units, to improve alignment and breathing, and to increase efficiency of movement. Unlike other exercise programs, the Pilates method does not require the repetition of exercises but instead consists of a sequence of carefully performed movements—some of which are carried out on specially designed equipment (Figure 6-3). Each exercise is designed to stretch and strengthen the muscles involved. There is a specific breathing pattern for each exercise to help direct energy to the areas being worked while relaxing the rest of the body.

The Pilates method works many of the deeper muscles together, improving coordination and balance, to achieve efficient and graceful movement. Instead of seeking an ideal or perfect body, the goal is for the practitioner to develop a healthy self-image, through the attainment of better posture, proper coordination, and improved flexibility. This method concentrates on alignment, lengthening all of the muscles of the body into a balanced whole, and building endurance and strength without putting undue stress on the lungs and heart. Pilates instructors believe that problems such as soft-tissue injuries can cause bad posture, which can lead to pain and discomfort. Pilates exercises aim to correct this.

Normally a beginner sees a Pilates instructor on a one-to-one basis for the first session. The instructor assesses the client's physical condition and asks the client about any problems and about the client's lifestyle. The client

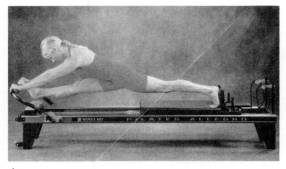

A

FIGURE 6-3. PILATES.
Pilates exercises are designed to improve muscle control, flexibility, coordination, and strength.
***A.** Machine-assisted Pilates exercise.*
***B.** Pilates exercise without equipment. (Photo courtesy Balanced Body, Inc., Sacramento, CA)*

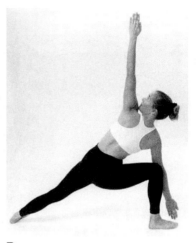

B

is then shown a series of exercises that take joints and muscles through a range of movement that is appropriate based on the client's needs. A class in a studio might involve working on specially designed equipment, primarily using resistance against tensioned springs, in order to isolate and develop specific muscle groups. Matwork classes utilize a repertoire of exercises on a floor mat only. This type of class has become very popular in health clubs and gyms and is often compared to other forms of body conditioning. In fact, the Pilates mat exercises are generally more subtle than mat exercises in most other conditioning classes.

YOGA

Yoga originated in India approximately 6,000 years ago. Its basic philosophy is that most illness is related to poor mental attitudes, posture, and diet. Practitioners of yoga maintain that stress can be reduced through combined mental and physical approaches. Yoga can help an individual cope with stress-induced behaviors like overeating, hypertension, and smoking. Yoga's meditative aspects are believed

to help alleviate psychosomatic illnesses. Yoga aims to unite the body and mind to reduce stress. Various body postures and breathing exercises are used in this activity.

Hatha-yoga uses a number of positions through which the practitioner may progress, beginning with the simplest and moving to the more complex (Figure 6-4). The various positions are intended to increase mobility and flexibility. However, caution must be used when selecting yoga positions. Some positions can be dangerous, particularly for someone who is inexperienced in yoga technique.

Slow, deep, diaphragmatic breathing is an important part of yoga. Many people breathe in a shallow fashion. However, breathing deeply—fully expanding your chest as you inhale—helps lower blood pressure and heart rate. Deep breathing has a calming effect on the body. It also increases production of endorphins, the body's own natural, morphinelike painkilling substances.

Yoga: body postures and breathing exercises used to help reduce stress

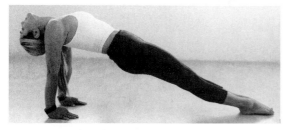

FIGURE 6-4. YOGA.
Yoga uses a variety of positions to increase flexibility in the body. (Photo courtesy International Dance Exercise Association, San Diego, CA)

IS THERE A RELATIONSHIP BETWEEN STRENGTH AND FLEXIBILITY?

We often hear about the negative effects that strength training has on flexibility. For example, someone who develops large bulk through strength training is often referred to as muscle bound. The expression muscle bound has negative connotations in terms of the ability of that person to move. We tend to think of people who have highly developed muscles as having lost much of their ability to move freely through a full range of motion.

Occasionally a person develops so much bulk that the physical size of the muscle prevents a normal range of motion. When strength training is not properly done, movement can be impaired. However, there is no reason to believe that weight training, if done properly through a full range of motion, will impair flexibility. Proper strength training probably improves dynamic flexibility and, if combined with a rigorous stretching program, can greatly enhance powerful and coordinated movements that are essential for success in many athletic activities. In all cases a heavy weight training program should be accompanied by a strong flexibility program (Figure 6-5).

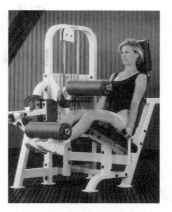

FIGURE 6-5. STRENGTH TRAINING AND FLEXIBILITY.
If strength training is combined with flexibility exercise, a full range of motion may be maintained.

STRETCHING EXERCISES

Figures 6-6 to 6-18 illustrate stretching exercises that may be used to improve flexibility at specific joints throughout the body. The exercises described may be done statically or with slight modification; they may also be done with a partner using a PNF technique.

There are many possible variations to each of these exercises. Figure 6-19 shows examples of static stretching that can be done using a stability ball. The exercises selected are those that seem to be the most effective for stretching of various muscle groups. Table 6-1 is a checklist that can help you monitor your stretching program.

Regardless of the stretching exercise or technique you are using, the same principles of overload and progression that were discussed in Chapter 5 relative to strength training must be applied to stretching. To see improvement in range of motion, the muscle must be "overloaded" or stretched to a point where there is some discomfort, but stretching should stop short of causing pain. As the muscle gradually accommodates to the demands of a stretching

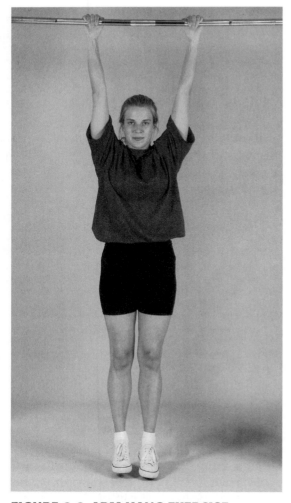

FIGURE 6-6. ARM HANG EXERCISE.
Muscles stretched: entire shoulder girdle complex.
Instructions: Using a chinning bar, simply hang
with shoulders and arms fully extended for
30 seconds. Repeat five times.

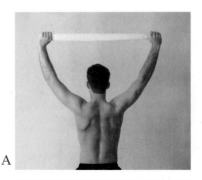

A

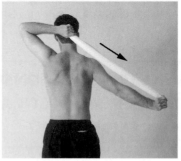

B

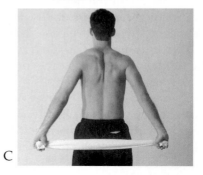

C

**FIGURE 6-7. SHOULDER TOWEL STRETCH
EXERCISE.**
Muscles stretched: internal and external rotators.
Instructions: A, Begin by holding towel above
head shoulder-width apart. B, Try to pull towel
down behind back, first with left hand then with
right; you should end up in position C. Reverse
order to get back to position A. Repeat five times
on each side.

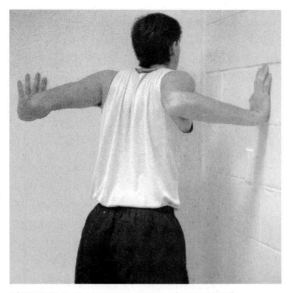

FIGURE 6-8. CHEST AND SHOULDER STRETCH EXERCISE.
Muscles stretched: pectoralis, deltoid.
Instructions: Stand in a corner, hands on walls, and lean forward. Repeat three times, hold for 30 seconds.

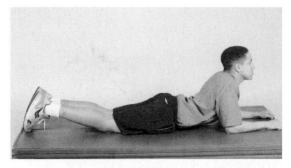

FIGURE 6-9. ABDOMINAL AND ANTERIOR CHEST WALL STRETCH EXERCISE.
Muscles stretched: muscles of respiration in thorax, abdominal muscles.
Instructions: Extend upper trunk, support weight on elbows, keeping pelvis on the floor. Repeat three times, hold for 30 seconds.
Caution: *Do not perform this exercise if you have increased back pain.*

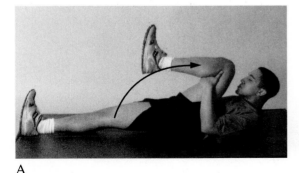

A

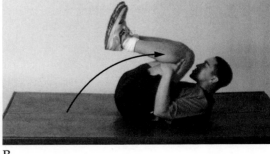

B

FIGURE 6-10. WILLIAM'S FLEXION EXERCISE.
Muscles stretched: low back and hip extensors.
Instructions:
A, *Touch chin to right knee and hold, then to left knee and hold.*
B, *Touch chin to both knees and hold. Hold each position for 30 seconds.*

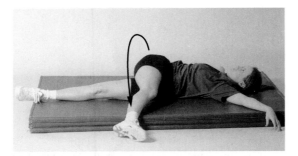

FIGURE 6-11. LOW BACK TWISTER EXERCISE.

Muscles stretched: rotators of lower back, sacrum, and hip abductors.

Instructions: Lie on back on edge of bed or table. Keep shoulders and arms flat on surface. Cross leg farthest from edge over the top and let it hang off the side of bed, keeping knee straight; repeat with other leg. Repeat three times with each leg, hold for 30 seconds.

***Caution:** If keeping the leg straight produces pain, do this exercise with the leg bent. Be sure to exercise caution in returning the leg to the starting position.*

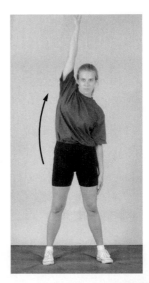

FIGURE 6-13. LATERAL TRUNK STRETCH EXERCISE.

Muscles stretched: lateral abdominals, intercostals.

Instructions: Standing with feet spread at shoulder width, extend one arm above head and "reach for the sky." Hold for 30 seconds and repeat three times on each side.

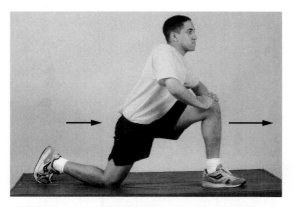

FIGURE 6-12. FORWARD LUNGE EXERCISE.

Muscles stretched: hip flexors, quadriceps.

Instructions: Assume a kneeling position with one knee on the ground; thrust pelvis forward. Repeat three times; hold for 30 seconds.

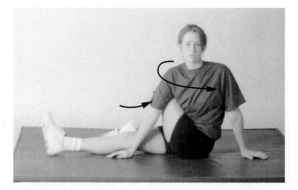

FIGURE 6-14. TRUNK TWISTER EXERCISE.

Muscles stretched: trunk and hip rotators.

Instructions: Place one foot over opposite knee. Rotate trunk to bent knee side.

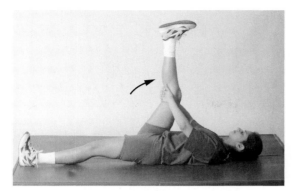

FIGURE 6-15. HAMSTRING STRETCH EXERCISE.

Muscles stretched: hip extensors, knee flexors.
Instructions: Lie flat on back. Raise one leg straight up with knee extended and ankle flexed to 90 degrees. Grasp leg around calf and pull toward head; repeat with opposite leg. Repeat three times with each leg; hold for 30 seconds.

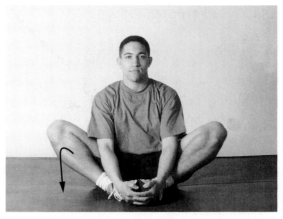

FIGURE 6-16. GROIN STRETCH EXERCISES.

Muscles stretched: hip adductors in groin.
Instructions: Sit with knees flexed and soles of feet together. Try to press knees flat on the floor; if they are flat to begin with, try to touch face to floor. Repeat three times; hold for 30 seconds.

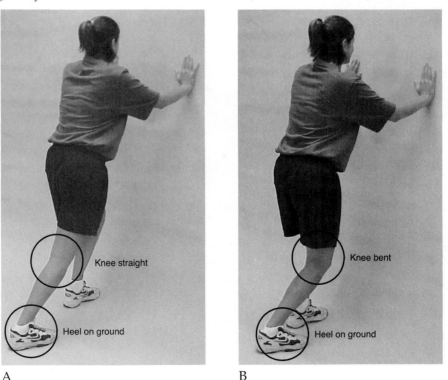

A

B

FIGURE 6-17. ACHILLES HEEL CORD STRETCH EXERCISE.

*Muscles stretched: foot plantar flexors. **A**, Gastrocnemius; **B**, Soleus.*
*Instructions: **A**, Stand facing wall with toes pointing straight ahead and knees straight. Lean forward toward wall, keeping heels flat on floor. You should feel stretching high in calf. **B**, Stand facing wall with toes pointing straight ahead and knees flexed. Lean forward toward wall, keeping heels flat on floor. You should feel stretching low in calf. Repeat each position three times; hold each for 30 seconds.*

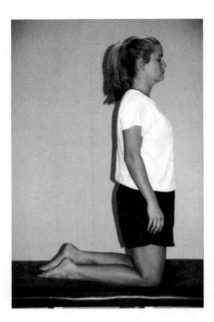

FIGURE 6-18. TOE POINTER EXERCISE.

Muscles stretched: foot dorsiflexors.
Instructions: Kneel with knees flexed and feet pointed.
Repeat three times; hold for 30 seconds.

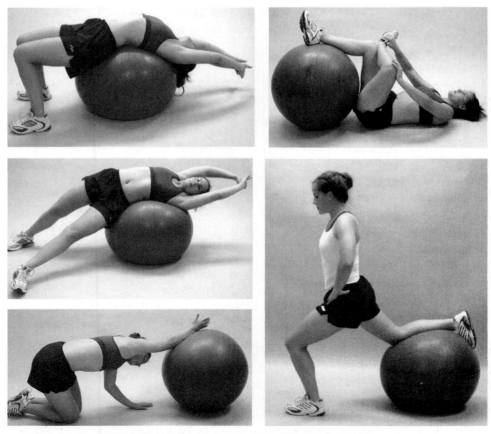

FIGURE 6-19. STATIC STRETCHING USING A STABILITY BALL.

TABLE 6-1
CHECKLIST FOR A INDIVIDUALIZED STRETCHING PROGRAM

Exercise	Hold Time (sec)	Repetitions	Date Month/Day**															
Arm hang	30	5																
Shoulder towel stretch	10	5																
Abdominal and anterior chest wall stretch	30	3																
Chest and shoulder stretch	30	3																
William's flexion exercise	30*	3																
Low back twister	30	3																
Pelvic thrust	30	3																
Lateral trunk stretch	30	3																
Quadriceps stretch	30	3																
Hamstring stretch	30	3																
Groin stretch	30	3																
Achilles heel cord stretch	30	3*																
Toe pointer	30	3																

*In each position.
**Place a check under the date when you have completed the exercise.

exercise, the intensity of the stretch should be progressively increased. Over time, this gradual progression will lead to an increase in the range of motion.

HOW DO YOU KNOW IF YOU HAVE GOOD FLEXIBILITY?

Accurate measurement of the range of joint motion is difficult. Various devices have been designed to accommodate variations in the sizes of the joints as well as the complexity of movements in articulations that involve more than one joint. Of these devices, the simplest and most widely used is the goniometer (Figure 6-20).

A goniometer is a large protractor with measurements in degrees. By aligning the two arms parallel to the longitudinal axis of the two segments involved in motion about a specific joint, it is possible to obtain relatively accurate measures of range of movement. The goniometer has its place in a rehabilitation setting, where it is essential to assess improvement in joint flexibility for the purpose

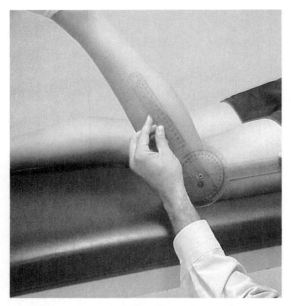

FIGURE 6-20. GONIOMETRIC MEASURE-MENT OF KNEE JOINT FLEXION.

of modifying injury rehabilitation programs. Because it is most appropriate to talk about flexibility as being specific to a given joint or movement, there is no doubt that the most accurate method for assessing joint movement is through the use of a goniometer. However, for the average person, it is not practical to assess joint movement using goniometry. Lab Activities 6-1 through 6-3 will help you to assess your existing flexibility.

Summary

- Flexibility is the ability to move a joint or a series of joints smoothly through a full range of motion.
- Flexibility may be limited by fat or defects in bone structure, skin, connective tissue, ligaments, or muscles and tendons.
- Passive range of motion refers to the degree to which a joint may be passively moved to the end points in the range of motion, whereas active range of motion refers to movement through a portion of the range of motion resulting from active contraction.
- An agonist muscle is one that contracts to produce joint motion; the antagonist muscle is stretched with contraction of the agonist.
- Ballistic (Dynamic), static, and proprioceptive neuromuscular facilitation (PNF) techniques have all been used as stretching techniques for improving flexibility.
- Pilates exercise and yoga offer two alternative approaches to stretching for improving flexibility.
- Strength training, if done correctly through a full range of motion, will probably improve flexibility.
- Measurement of joint flexibility is accomplished through the use of a goniometer.

Suggested Readings

Alter, M. J. 2004. *The science of flexibility*, 3rd ed. Champaign, IL: Human Kinetics.

Anderson, B. 2000. *Stretching*. Bolinas, CA: Shelter.

Bandy, W. D., J. M. Orion, and M. Briggler. 1998. The effect of static stretch and dynamic range of motion training on the flexibility of the hamstring muscles. *Journal of Orthopedic and Sports Physical Therapy* 27(4):295–300.

Blahnik, J. 2004. *Full body flexibility*. Champaign, IL: Human Kinetics.

Burke, D. G., C. J. Culligan, and L. E. Holt. 2000. The theoretical basis of proprioceptive neuromuscular facilitation. *Journal of Strength and Conditioning Research* 14(4):496–500.

Clark, A. 1999. *The complete illustrated guide to tai chi: The practical approach to the ancient Chinese movement for health and well-being*. Rockport, MA: Element.

De Deyne, P. G. 2001. Application of passive stretch and its implications for muscle fibers. *Physical Therapy* 81(2):819–27.

Fitzgerald, M. 2001. Strength, endurance, flexibility: A Pilates home workout will leave you all three. *Men's Fitness* 17(10):74–79.

Hedrick, A. 2000. Dynamic flexibility training. *Strength and Conditioning Journal* 22(5):33–38.

Heyward, V. H. 2002. Assessing flexibility and designing stretching programs. In *Advanced fitness assessment and exercise prescription*, 4th ed., edited by V. H. Heyward. Champaign, IL: Human Kinetics.

Iyengar, B. 2001. *Yoga: The path to holistic health*. New York: Dorling Kindersley.

Kent, H. 1999. *The complete illustrated guide to yoga: A practical approach to achieving optimum health for mind, body and spirit*. Rockport, MA: Element.

Knudson, D. 1998. Stretching: From science to practice. *Journal of Physical Education, Recreation and Dance* 69(3):38–42.

Kurz, T. 2003. *Stretching scientifically: A guide to flexibility training.* Island Port, VT: Stadion.

Lemay, M. 2003. *Essential stretch.* New York: Perigee Trade.

Mann, D., and C. Whedon. 2001. Functional stretching: Implementing a dynamic stretching program. *Athletic Therapy Today* 6(3):10–13.

McAtee, R. E. 1999. *Facilitated stretching.* Champaign, IL: Human Kinetics.

Moffat, M. 1999. *American Physical Therapy Association book of body repair and maintenence: Hundreds of stretches for every part of the human body.* New York: Henry Holt Company.

Mueller, D. 2002. Yoga therapy. *ACSM's Health and Fitness Journal* 6(1):18–24.

Nelson, R. T. and W. D. Bandy. 2004. Eccentric training and static stretching improve hamstring flexibility of high school males. *Journal of Athletic Training* 39(3):254–58.

Norris, C. 1999. *The complete guide to stretching.* London: Black.

Parragon Publishing complete guide to pilates, yoga, meditation & stress relief. 2004. New York: Parragon Publishing.

Power, K., D. Behm, and F. Cahill. 2004. An acute bout of static stretching: Effects on force and jumping performance. *Medicine and Science in Sports and Exercise* 36(8):1389–96.

Riewald, S. 2004. Stretching the limits of our knowledge on stretching. *Strength and Conditioning Journal* 26(5):58–59.

Santana, J. C. 2004. Flexibility: More is not necessarily better. *Strength and Conditioning Journal* 26(1):14–15.

Shaw, B., ed. 2001. *Beth Shaw's yogafit.* Champaign, IL: Human Kinetics.

Spernoga, S. G., T. L. Uhl, B. L. Arnold, and B. M. Gansneder. 2001. Duration of maintained hamstring flexibility after a one-time, modified hold-relax stretching protocol. *Journal of Athletic Training* 36(1):44–48.

Stewart, K. 2001. Pilates for beginners. New York: Harper Resource.

Tracker, S. B., D. F. Gilchrist, D. F. Stroup, and C. D. Kimsey Jr. 2004. The impact of *stretching* on sports injury risk: A systematic review of the literature. *Medicine and Science in Sports and Exercise* 36(3):371–78.

Tubecki, E. 2002. The world of Pilates. *Women's Fitness and Sport* 8(2):31–32.

Ungaro, A., and R. Sadur. 2002. *Pilates: Body In Motion.* New York: DK Publishing, Inc.

Ungaro, A., and R. Sadur. 2003. *Pilates: Body in motion.* New York: Dorling Kindersley.

Yeager, D. 1999. PNF: A new way to stretch! *Hughston health alert* 11(1):6–37.

Young, W., and S. Elliott. 2001. Acute effects of static stretching, proprioceptive neuromuscular facilitation stretching, and maximum voluntary contractions on explosive force production and jumping performance. *Research Quarterly for Exercise and Sport* 72(3):273–79.

SUGGESTED WEB SITES

Brad Appleton's Stretching and Flexibility FAQ

This site presents frequently asked questions with answers on flexibility and stretching. It tells you everything you ever wanted to know. www.enteract.com/~bradapp/docs/rec/stretching

Practical Tai Chi Chuan

This is an introduction to tai chi chuan with extensive text on tai chi history and principles. www.taichichuan.co.uk

References on Stretching

This site presents a list of books and articles on stretching and flexibility. www.fitabc.com/stretch/stretch6.htm

SportStretch

This new stretching aid helps improve flexibility by the practice of active isolated stretching. www.sportstretch.com

STOTT PILATES the contemporary approach to . . . pilates exercise

This site provides information on pilates equipment, educational programs, registered instructors, and a forum for posing questions about pilates. www.stottpilates.com

Stretching

This site presents stretching for everyday fitness and for running, tennis, racquetball, cycling, swimming, golf, and other sports. www.shelterpub.com/_fitness/_stretching/stretching.ht . . .

Stretching and Flexibility

This is an essay on types and uses of stretching. www.bath.ac.uk~masrjb/Stretch/stretching_l.html

The Physician and Sportsmedicine: Myths and Truths of Stretching

Myths and truths of stretching provides individualized recommendations for healthy muscles. Proposes stretching benefits. www.physsportsmed.com/issues/2

The Yoga Site—Web site directory

This online yoga resource center features a free teacher directory, posture info, Yoga Therapy Report, style guide, Q and A, retreats, books, links, and more. www.yogasite.com

Welcome to Pilates

The Pilates Method is a conditioning program that improves muscle control, flexibility, coordination, strength and tone. www.pilates.com

CHAPTER 7

Eating Right

Objectives

After completing this chapter, you should be able to do the following:

- Identify the six classes of nutrients.
- Describe the major function of the nutrients.
- Analyze your diet for nutritional quality using U.S. Dietary Guidelines and MyPyramid.
- Explain the relationship of nutrition to physical performance.

WHY DO YOU NEED TO KNOW ABOUT NUTRITION?

"**S**ports drinks," "anabolic amino acids," "antioxidants," "fat burners" —it seems that every day you read or hear about the health benefits of some nutrition-related product or service. **Nutrition** "experts" promote their latest books on radio talk shows, salespeople in health food stores praise the virtues of nutrient supplements, and friends give advice about diets that guarantee to melt pounds fast. Nutrition appears to be the key that unlocks the door to a healthy, more attractive body. How true are all of the nutrition claims about foods, nutrients, or diet plans? What role does nutrition play in maximizing fitness? Lab Activity 7-1 will help you determine how much you know about nutrition. By understanding the basics of nutrition, you will be more likely to recognize the many forms of nutritional misinformation. And,

armed with some basic nutrition information, you will be able to identify "weak" areas of your diet and work to strengthen them. Are you eating a nutritious diet now? Lab Activity 7-2 will help you assess your eating patterns and find out whether or not you are currently eating a nutritious diet.

nutrition: the science of certain food substances

KEY TERMS

nutrition	diuretics
diet	nutrient dense
nutrients	requirement
deficiencies	recommendation
overnutrition	

BASIC PRINCIPLES OF NUTRITION

What do you think of when you hear the word *diet?* Although many people think of losing weight, **diet** actually refers to your usual food selections. Everyone is on a diet! When a person eats less food in an effort to lose weight, he or she is on a weight reduction diet. Nutrition is the science of certain food substances, **nutrients,** and what they do in your body. Nutrients perform three major roles:

1. Growth, repair, and maintenance of all body cells
2. Regulation of body processes
3. Supply of energy for cells

Fit List 7-1 summarizes the various nutrients, which are categorized into six major classes: carbohydrates, fats (often called lipids), proteins, vitamins, minerals, and water. Most foods are actually mixtures of these nutrients. Although we think of bread as being a carbohydrate food, it supplies fats, proteins, and other nutrients too. Some nutrients can be made by the body; an *essential* nutrient must be supplied by the diet. Not all substances in foods are considered nutrients. For example, caffeine is found in some foods and beverages. Caffeine has definite effects on the body, but we can live without it. Furthermore, there is no such thing as a perfect food; that is, no single natural food contains all of the nutrients needed for health.

Without an adequate supply of nutrients, cells soon lose their ability to perform their jobs. Eventually the rest of the body is affected, and various health disorders called nutritional **deficiencies** develop. Thanks to our varied food supply, cases of people suffering from nutritional deficiencies are uncommon in the United States. Nevertheless, some Americans consume diets that are borderline deficient in certain nutrients. Occasionally, days with

FIT LIST 7-1

Essential Nutrients

- Carbohydrates
- Fat
- Protein
- Vitamins
- Minerals
- Water

hectic schedules often result in careless eating or skipped meals. If your usual diet is good, it is unlikely that a few "off days" will lead to the development of a nutritional deficiency disease. However, if your diet is consistently of low quality, you run the risk of not being able to function at your peak level. Also, you could develop a deficiency disorder.

Just as low levels of nutrients can lead to health problems, nutrient excesses create trouble for your body. **Overnutrition,** eating too much food or specific nutrients, is common in the United States. Eating more food than needed can lead to obesity, which will be

diet: refers to the types of food substances consumed

nutrients: perform three major roles including growth, repair, and maintenance of all body cells, regulation of body processes, and supplying energy for cells

deficiencies: consuming an inadequate supply of nutrients eventually affects the cells' ability to function and disease results

overnutrition: eating too much food or taking too many supplements can have negative effects on your body

discussed in Chapter 8. Many nutrients are toxic (poisonous) when taken in large doses. However, it is difficult to obtain toxic levels of nutrients by consuming a varied diet. Most cases of nutrient overdoses are the result of overzealous self-treatment with vitamin/mineral supplements. People think that nutrient supplements are foods and therefore perfectly safe to consume in large quantities. However, the body is designed to obtain its nutrients from foods, not supplement pills or powders.

Running your body requires energy. This energy is supplied by the carbohydrates, fats, and proteins found in foods. Alcohol also provides energy, but it is not a nutrient. The energy value of food is measured by calories. Fats are the most concentrated source of calories in our diet. A gram of fat (there are about 28 grams in an ounce) supplies 9 calories. Carbohydrates and proteins each contribute 4 calories per gram. Alcohol, the nonnutrient, supplies 7 calories per gram. Water, vitamins, and minerals do not supply any calories and therefore no energy. Most Americans eat too much fat and too little carbohydrate. Scientists recommend that we alter the proportions of fat and carbohydrate in diets (Figure 7-1). Later in this chapter, we'll focus on energy use during physical activity.

THE NUTRIENTS

▶ Carbohydrates (CHO)

The major role of carbohydrates is to provide energy for the body. Although muscles run on fats and carbohydrates, nerve tissue, especially brain cells, prefer to burn carbohydrates for energy. People should consume at least 55 percent of their total caloric needs from carbohydrates. Both children and adults should consume at least 130 grams of carbohydrate each day. Carbohydrates are classified as simple (sugars) or complex (starch, glycogen, and most forms of fiber). Let's take a closer look at some of the more important carbohydrates.

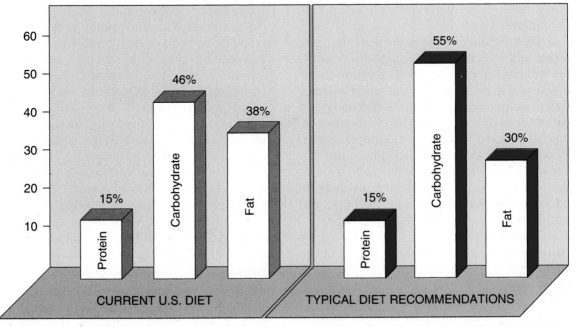

FIGURE 7-1. COMPARISON OF CALORIES FROM CARBOHYDRATES, FATS, AND PROTEINS.

Sugars. Sugars are simple carbohydrates that occur as single-sugar or double-sugar chemical units. Glucose (blood sugar) is needed for fueling all cells. It is crucial for the body to maintain normal blood sugar levels. Food sources of glucose include fruits, syrups, and honey. Fructose (fruit sugar) occurs naturally in honey and is added to processed foods. Honey is often promoted as a substitute for sugar. However, honey supplies the same simple carbohydrates as table sugar, so there is no nutritional advantage in using honey as a sweetener. Milk sugar (lactose) and table sugar (sucrose) are double sugars. Table sugar is made from sugarcane and sugar beets, and it is nearly 100 percent pure carbohydrate. Because it contributes no other nutrients besides carbohydrate, you should limit the amount of table sugar eaten to no more than 10 percent of your total calories. If too much sugar is eaten, it displaces more nutritious foods from your diet. That's why sugary foods are referred to as "empty calories." Although table sugar has been blamed for causing hyperactivity in children, criminal behavior, and allergies, the only health problem that can be actually linked to sugar consumption is dental decay.

Added sugars are those incorporated into foods and beverages during production and are different from natural sugars, such as lactose found in milk and fructose found in fruits. Major sources of added sugars are candy, soft drinks, fruit drinks, pastries, and other sweets. Added sugars should comprise no more than 10 percent of total calories consumed. The suggested maximum level stems from the evidence that people whose diets are high in added sugars have lower intakes of essential nutrients.

Sugars are often referred to as "quick" energy. However, you really don't obtain energy the instant you eat a candy bar. While it's true that it takes more time to break down starches, table sugar still has to be broken down and have its single-sugar units absorbed by the digestive tract before it can supply cells with energy.

Starches. Starches are called complex carbohydrates because they consist of long chains of glucose units. Plants make starches, such as those found in cereal grains, potatoes, and beans. During digestion, the long starch chains are broken down, releasing individual glucose units that are absorbed. Individual glucose units combine to form glycogen, which is stored in muscle and the liver. When cells need energy, glycogen is broken down to release glucose.

Fiber. Your grandparents knew the importance of eating plenty of roughage to stay "regular" (avoid constipation). We now call roughage "fiber." There are many different types of fiber, but they share the common characteristic of being from plant foods. Although most forms are complex carbohydrates, fiber cannot be digested in the small intestine, so it moves through the digestive tract relatively unchanged. Rich sources of fiber include fruits, vegetables, whole grain breads and cereals, nuts, beans, and peas.

Researchers believe that our diet does not supply enough fiber. They think that low-fiber diets may be responsible for intestinal problems, such as hemorrhoids, colon cancer, and diverticulosis. A common health problem, hemorrhoids are swollen rectal veins that can cause pain and bleeding. Colon cancer (cancer of the large intestine) is a major cause of cancer deaths in the United States. Diverticulosis is a common condition in which small "blowouts" (pouches) form in the wall of the large intestine. These pouches can become infected (diverticulitis) and cause serious health problems.

Fiber may help prevent these conditions because certain forms attract water. This helps to form large, bulky stools that are easier to eliminate during bowel movements. People consuming diets rich in fiber are not as likely to experience constipation. Therefore, instead of relying on laxatives for simple cases of constipation, just eat more fiber-rich foods!

Besides helping to prevent constipation, certain forms of fiber may help lower blood cholesterol levels. High blood cholesterol levels are a major risk factor for cardiovascular diseases. The fiber from oats, fruits, and vegetables is recommended for its cholesterol-lowering ability. These forms of fiber seem to interfere with cholesterol absorption from the intestinal tract. The less cholesterol absorbed means less enters the bloodstream and causes trouble in your arteries. The recommended daily intake for total fiber for adults 50 years and younger is set at 38 grams for men and 25 grams for women. The fiber recommendations are based on studies that show an increased risk for heart disease when diets low in fiber are consumed.

"Total fiber" is defined as the combination of "dietary" and "functional" fiber. Dietary fiber is the edible, nondigestible component of carbohydrates and lignin naturally found in plant food. Foods with dietary fiber include cereal bran, flaked corn cereal, sweet potatoes, legumes, and onions. Functional fibers are fiber sources that have been shown to have health benefits similar to those of dietary fiber, but these fibers are isolated or extracted from natural sources or are synthetic. An example would be pectin extracted from citrus peel and used as a gel as the basis for jams and jellies. The definition of functional fiber aims to exclude fiberlike products, whether extracted or synthesized, that cannot be shown to have proven health benefits.

▶Fats

Recently, fat has received a lot of negative publicity for a nutrient that is extremely important in the diet. Extra calories supplied by dietary carbohydrates, proteins, and fats may all be converted to triglyceride and stored in adipose cells as body fat for future energy needs. These body fat deposits cushion organs and give the body rounded contours (especially in women). Fat supplies a major portion of the energy used by muscles. Furthermore, certain types of fat cannot be formed by the body and are essential for health. We like to include fat in our meals because it makes eating more enjoyable by contributing flavor and texture. However, most Americans eat too much fat, a major factor in the development of obesity and cardiovascular diseases.

Saturated vs Unsaturated Fats. Depending on their chemical nature, fats may be either saturated or unsaturated. In general, unsaturated fat is from plants and is liquid at room temperature. Canola, peanut, olive oil, and vegetable oils from corn, cottonseed, sunflower, and soybean sources are rich in unsaturated fat.

Monounsaturated and polyunsaturated fatty acids reduce blood cholesterol levels and thus lower the risk of heart disease when they replace saturated fats in the diet. People must get two types of polyunsaturated fatty acids, known as omega-3 fatty acid and omega-6 fatty acid, from the foods they consume because neither is synthesized in the body. A lack of either one will result in symptoms of deficiency, including scaly skin and dermatitis. Recommended intakes for omega-3 fatty acid, which is present in high levels in vegetable oils such as safflower oil or corn oil, and in fish oil, are 17 grams per day for men and 12 grams per day for women (about 1 tablespoon) based on average intakes in the United States. For omega-6 fatty acid, which is found in milk and some vegetable oils such as soybean and flaxseed oils, the recommendations are 1.6 and 1.1 grams per day (less than ½ teaspoon) for men and women, respectively.

Saturated fats are derived mainly from animal sources. These include the fat in meats, such as beef, pork, and lamb, as well as much of the fat in eggs and dairy products—cream, butter, milk, and cheese. Coconut and palm oils, unlike most plant oils, are highly saturated.

Cholesterol. Saturated fat and cholesterol are believed to be responsible for creating blocked arteries that lead to cardiovascular diseases. Cholesterol is a fat-related substance that is only found in animal foods. People think that cholesterol is "bad," but actually it is very important. Even if you avoid all foods that contain cholesterol, your body would make what it needs. The body makes vitamin D and its own steroid hormones from cholesterol. However, when a form of blood cholesterol becomes too high, the risk of developing cardiovascular diseases also increases. Saturated fat can raise the amount of low-density lipoprotein and the level of "bad" cholesterol in the bloodstream of some individuals and heightens their risk for heart disease.

Trans fatty acids have physical properties generally resembling saturated fatty acids, and their presence tends to harden oils. Often found in cookies, crackers, dairy products, meats, and fast foods, trans fatty acids increase the risk of heart disease by boosting levels of bad cholesterol. Because they are not essential and provide no known health benefit, there is no safe level of trans fatty acids and people should eat as little of them as possible while consuming a nutritionally adequate diet.

Many studies show that eating saturated fat and cholesterol seems to increase blood cholesterol levels. Beef, milk, butter, and cheese are rich sources of saturated fat. Also, foods from animal sources, including dairy products, egg yolks, liver, and meats, contribute lots of cholesterol. Margarine made from plant fats (oils) is a good substitute for butter because all plant oils are cholesterol-free. Unsaturated fats do not raise blood cholesterol levels like saturated fats. Because certain kinds of saturated fats contribute to the development of high blood cholesterol levels, it is wise to reduce your consumption of foods made with tropical oils.

Fat Intake. Most experts believe it is more important to cut back on your total fat intake than worry about eating specific types of fats. The typical American gets about 40 percent of total calories from fat. Experts think that this is too much and recommend levels of about 25 to 30 percent. These experts also suggest that cholesterol intake be limited to around 300 milligrams a day. Considering that one egg yolk has about 250 milligrams of cholesterol, this

recommendation may be tough to meet if you like to eat eggs or products made from eggs every day. The American Heart Association recommends that you eat no more than four eggs a week. The good news is that food consumption surveys show that we have cut back on our saturated fat and cholesterol consumption. This appears to be helping to reduce the number of cardiovascular deaths, especially in younger people. Although not all of this decline is due to eating fewer eggs and drinking more skim milk, reducing overall fat consumption is believed to be partially responsible.

▶Protein

Protein is needed for growth, repair, and maintenance of all cells. Major body structures, such as bone, muscles, and organs, are made of protein. Your skin, hair, and nails are made up of protein. Proteins are needed to make the enzymes that speed up chemical reactions, certain hormones, and components of the immune system. A small amount of protein can be used for energy, too. However, the body prefers to use carbohydrate and fat for energy, conserving protein for its other important functions.

Your body's need for protein increases during periods of growth. For example, protein needs are very high in infancy, during childhood and adolescent growth spurts, and during pregnancy. Breast-feeding women need more protein to supply their nursing infant's needs. During active body-building, athletes have a greater need. However, the typical American diet contains plenty of protein to meet an athlete's needs.

The recommended amount of protein is based on body weight; the typical adult recommendation is 0.8 gram of protein per kilogram of body weight. To determine how many grams of protein are recommended for your weight, take your weight in pounds and divide by 2.2 to obtain your weight in kilograms. Multiply that number times 0.8 to obtain the grams of protein that meet recommended levels of intake. Dietary surveys show that Americans eat

more protein than needed, well over 100 gran
per day. Much of that protein is from fatty ar
mal sources. Your diet should contain about :
to 15 percent of its calories from protein.

Proteins are made up of smaller units call
amino acids. There are about 20 amino acids
the body. Nine essential amino acids must l
supplied by the diet; the remainder can l
made by the body. In order to grow, you need
have all of the essential amino acids available.
the diet is protein-deficient, growth slows
stops. During digestion, food proteins are br
ken down and amino acids are released and a
sorbed. Most animal proteins, such as tho
found in meat, fish, poultry, and eggs, conta
ample amounts of the essential amino acids ar
are called complete or high-quality proteins.

Plant proteins, such as those found in beans,
peas, nuts, seeds, and cereals, also contribute
protein to the diet. For example, a slice of bread
supplies 2 grams of protein. Plant food proteins are incomplete; that is, they are not good
sources of the essential amino acids. However,
the quality improves when they are mixed
with proteins from animal sources of food.
Many of our favorite food combinations, such
as cereal and milk, macaroni and cheese, chili
con carne, and tuna or chicken noodle casse-
role, combine small amounts of high-quality
animal proteins with larger amounts of plant
proteins. You do not have to eat large portions
of animal foods to obtain enough protein.

Vegetarianism is an alternative to the usual
American diet that is rich in animal sources of
food. All vegetarians use plant foods to form
the foundation of their diets; animal foods are
either excluded or included to varying degrees. Vegetarian diets are usually lower in fat
and higher in fiber and antioxidant nutrients
than typical American food selections.

▶ Water

Water is the most essential nutrient. You can
live for weeks, months, even years without the
other nutrients, but you will perish after a few
days without water. About 60 percent of the

Sport Drinks. Do you need to dri
sport beverages? These sport dri
popular and are widely market
ican public.

During physical activit
place fluids lost throu
lost fluids with a sp
than using water
that because
drink more
drinks
trolyt
en

your internal water levels return to normal. If
you ignore thirst signals and body water continues to decrease, dehydration results. People
who are dehydrated cannot generate energy
and feel weak. Other symptoms include nausea, vomiting, and fainting. If water losses
become too great, the individual dies.

Dehydration is more likely to occur when
you are outdoors and heavily sweating while
engaging in some strenuous activity. To prevent dehydration, make sure you replace the
lost water by drinking plenty of fluids. Don't
rely on thirst as a signal that it's time to have a
drink. Many people ignore their thirst, or, if
they do heed it, they don't drink enough.
Avoid replacing water with caffeinated beverages and alcohol; these fluids act as **diuretics,**
pulling more vital water out of your body.

Most adults can benefit from drinking more
water. You don't need to buy canned or bottled
waters. Drinking tap water may not impress
people but it will quench your thirst for a lot
less money.

diuretics: foods or chemicals that eliminate natural fluids from your body

...nk special ...nks are very ...ed to the Amer-

...y it is essential to re... ...gh sweating. Replacing ...ort drink is more effective ... alone. Research has shown ...f the flavor you are likely to ... sport drinks than water. Sport ...uickly replace both fluids and elec... ...s that are lost in sweat and also provide ...rgy to the working muscles. Water is a ...ood "thirst quencher," but it is not a good "rehydrator" because water "turns off" your thirst before you're completely rehydrated. Water also "turns on" the kidneys prematurely so you lose fluid in the form of urine much more quickly than when drinking a sport drink. A small amount of sodium allows your body to hold onto the fluid you consume rather than losing it through urine.

Not all sport drinks are the same. How a sport drink is formulated dictates how well it works in providing rapid rehydration and energy. The optimal level of carbohydrate is 14 grams per 8 ounces of water for quickest absorption and energy. It has been shown that a sport drink can be effective in improving performance during both endurance activities as well as short-term high-intensity activities such as soccer, basketball, and tennis that last from 30 minutes to an hour.

Oxygenated Bottled Water. Bottled waters with added oxygen are a recent trend in the beverage market. Athletes have touted the benefits of different brands, and such advertising attempts to persuade us that this extra oxygen will lead to improved performance. What's the reason for adding oxygen to water, and does the extra oxygen do anything for sport performance? According to manufacturers, oxygenated water delivers extra oxygen to the body to enhance metabolism and improve endurance. The bottom line is that manufac-

turers' claims have lots of theory and very little substance. Human physiology and science show us that oxygenated water won't elevate oxygen levels in the blood or muscle. Such claims are enticing, but they don't hold up when it comes to improving muscle metabolism and performance.

▶ Vitamins

Like carbohydrates, proteins, and fats, vitamins are organic compounds that are essential for health. Although required in very small amounts, vitamins perform many roles, primarily as regulators of body processes. Humans need thirteen vitamins for health. You are probably familiar with their letter names, such as vitamins A, B_1, and C. Today, many are referred to by their chemical names. For example, *thiamin* is the chemical name for vitamin B_1. During the past 50 years, no new vitamins have been discovered, but scientists are still learning about their many roles.

People mistakenly think that vitamins provide energy. In fact, the body cannot break them down to release energy. However, many of the B-vitamins participate in the various chemical steps that release energy from carbohydrate, fat, and protein. Table 7-1 provides information about vitamins, including rich food sources, deficiency symptoms, and toxicity potential from high doses.

Vitamin deficiencies are uncommon in the United States. A few groups of people, such as the elderly, alcoholics, and those who severely restrict their food intake, are at risk of developing vitamin deficiency diseases. However, nutrition experts are concerned that many people are nutritionally on the "borderline," that is, close to being deficient. We may be too busy to plan nutritious meals, and we rely too much on vending machines or fast food restaurants. Furthermore, many young people are smoking cigarettes and drinking alcoholic beverages, behaviors that increase vitamin and other nutrient needs.

TABLE 7-1 VITAMINS				
Vitamin	Major Function	Most Reliable Sources	Deficiency	Excess (Toxicity)
A	Maintains skin and other cells that line the inside of the body; bone and tooth development; growth; vision in dim light	Liver, milk, egg yolk, deep green and yellow fruits and vegetables	Night blindness, dry skin, growth failure	Headaches, nausea, loss of hair, dry skin, diarrhea
D	Normal bone growth and development; helps with absorption of calcium	Exposure to sunlight; fortified dairy products; eggs and fish liver oils	"Rickets"in children—defective bone formation leading to deformed bones	Appetite loss, weight loss, failure to grow
E	Prevents destruction of polyunsaturated fats caused by exposure to oxidizing agents; protects cell membranes from destruction	Vegetable oils, some in fruits and vegetables, whole grains	Breakage of red blood cells leading to anemia	Nausea and diarrhea; interferes with vitamin K if vitamin D is also deficient. Not as toxic as other fat-soluble vitamins
K	Production of blood-clotting substances	Green leafy vegetables; normal bacteria that live in intestines produce K that is absorbed	Increased bleeding time	
Thiamin	Needed for release of energy from carbohydrates, fats, and proteins	Cereal products, pork, peas, and dried beans	Lack of energy, nerve problem	
Riboflavin	Energy from carbohydrates, fats, and proteins	Milk, liver, fruits and vegetables, enriched breads and cereals	Dry skin, cracked lips	

Continued

**TABLE 7-1
VITAMINS—CONT'D**

Vitamin	Major Function	Most Reliable Sources	Deficiency	Excess (Toxicity)
Niacin	Energy from carbohydrates, fats, and proteins	Liver, meat, poultry, peanut butter, legumes, enriched breads and cereals	Skin problems, diarrhea, mental depression, and eventually, death (rarely occurs in U.S.)	Skin flushing, intestinal upset, nervousness, intestinal ulcers
B$_6$	Metabolism of protein; production of hemoglobin	White meats, whole grains, liver, egg yolk, bananas	Poor growth, anemia	Severe loss of coordination from nerve damage
B$_{12}$	Production of genetic material; maintains central nervous system	Foods of animal origin	Neurological problems, anemia	
Folate (Folic acid)	Production of genetic material	Wheat germ, liver, yeast, mushrooms, green leafy vegetables, fruits	Anemia	
C (Ascorbic acid)	Formation and maintenance of connective tissue; tooth and bone formation; immune function; helps with absorption of iron	Fruits and vegetables	"Scurvy" (rare); swollen joints, bleeding gums, fatigue, bruising	Kidney stones, diarrhea
Pantothenic acid	Energy from carbohydrates, fats, proteins	Widely found in foods	Not observed in humans under normal conditions	
Biotin	Use of fats	Widely found in foods	Rare under normal conditions	

Fat-Soluble Vitamins. Vitamins are grouped according to the ability to dissolve in water or fat. Vitamins A, E, D, and K dissolve in fat rather than water. Extra amounts of the fat-soluble vitamins are not easy to eliminate from the body in urine, which is mostly water. Instead they are stored in the liver or body fat until needed. This feature makes them potentially toxic, so be careful if you choose to take supplements of these vitamins. See Table 7-1 for information about the fat-soluble vitamins, including their toxicity potential.

Water-Soluble Vitamins. The water-soluble vitamins, B-complex and C, dissolve in water. This feature makes it easier for the body to eliminate excesses in urine. Many of the B-vitamins help produce energy from carbohydrates, proteins, and fats. When these vitamins are unavailable, every cell cannot generate energy to perform its numerous jobs. The result is feeling tired. Don't think that by taking extra amounts of the B-vitamins that you'll have more energy. Once your cells have enough of the B-vitamins, any additional doses will not make cells generate extra amounts of energy. Although excesses of most water-soluble vitamins are excreted in urine, high doses of certain water-soluble vitamins have been linked to toxic effects. See Table 7-1 for information about the water-soluble vitamins, including their toxicity potential.

Antioxidant Nutrients. Nutrition experts have generated excitement and controversy over reports that certain nutrients, called antioxidants, may prevent premature aging, certain cancers, heart disease, and other health problems. An antioxidant protects vital cell components from the destructive effects of certain agents, including oxygen. Vitamin C, vitamin E, and beta carotene are antioxidants. Beta carotene is a plant pigment that is found in dark green, deep yellow, or orange fruits and vegetables. The body can convert beta carotene to vitamin A. Since the early 1980s, evidence has accumulated about the benefits of a diet rich in the antioxidant nutrients. Fit List 7-2 lists foods rich in the antioxidant nutrients.

Some experts believe people should increase their intake of antioxidants, even if it means taking supplements. Others are more cautious. Excess beta carotene pigments circulate throughout the body and may turn your skin yellow. However the pigment is not believed to be toxic like its nutrient cousin, vitamin A. On the other hand, increasing your intake of vitamins C and E is not without some risk.

FIT LIST 7-2

Foods Rich in Antioxidants

Beta Carotene Foods

- Sweet potatoes
- Pumpkin
- Squash
- Carrots
- Red bell peppers
- Dark green vegetables
- Apricots
- Mango
- Cantaloupe

Vitamin C Foods

- Kiwi fruit
- Citrus fruits
- Berries
- Cantaloupe
- Honeydew
- Bell peppers
- Tomatoes
- Cabbage
- Broccoli

Vitamin E Foods

- Vegetable oils
- Nuts
- Seeds
- Margarine
- Wheat germ
- Olives
- Leafy greens
- Asparagus

Excesses of vitamin C are not well absorbed; the excess is irritating to the intestines and causes diarrhea. Although less toxic than vitamins A or D, too much vitamin E causes health problems, as indicated in Table 7-1.

▶Minerals

More than 20 mineral elements must be supplied by the diet. These include the minerals listed in Table 7-2. Other mineral elements are

TABLE 7-2
MINERALS OF MAJOR CONCERN

Vitamin	Major Function	Most Reliable Sources	Deficiency	Excess (Toxicity)
Calcium	Bone and tooth formation; blood clotting; muscle contraction; nerve function	Dairy products	May lead to osteoporosis	Calcium deposits in soft tissues
Phosphorus	Skeletal development; tooth formation	Meats, dairy products, and other protein-rich foods	Rarely seen	May contribute to the development of hypertension
Sodium	Maintenance of fluid balance	Salt (sodium chloride) added to foods and sodium-containing preservatives	Muscle cramps; fluid imbalance	Can cause death in children from supplement overdose
Iron	Formation of hemoglobin; energy from carbohydrates, fats, and proteins	Liver and red meats, enriched breads and cereals	Anemia	Nausea and vomiting
Magnesium	Strengthen bones; improves enzyme function and nerve and heart function	Wheat gram, vegetables, nuts, chocolate	Weakness, muscle pain, poor heart function, osteoporosis	Kidney failure
Copper	Formation of hemoglobin	Liver, nuts, shellfish, cherries, mushrooms, whole grain breads and cereals	Skin problems, delayed development, growth problems	Interferes with copper use; may decrease HDL levels
Zinc	Normal growth and development	Seafood and meats	Mental and growth retardation; lack of energy	
Iodine	Production of the hormone thyroxin	Iodized salt, seafood		
Fluorine	Strengthens bones and teeth	Fluoridated water	Teeth are less resistant to decay	Damage to tooth enamel

found in the body. The role of minerals is unclear. Minerals are needed for a variety of jobs, such as forming strong bones and teeth, helping to generate energy, activating enzymes, and maintaining water balance. Most minerals are stored in the body, especially in the bones and liver. Vitamins are stored in the liver, too. That explains why liver usually leads the list of most nutritious foods. Vitamins and minerals interact with one another—if you don't get enough of one, the other may not work the way it is supposed to.

Calcium. You are probably aware that calcium is needed for building strong bones and teeth, but it is also needed for nerve and muscle function. Milk products are rich in calcium, but many people do not like to drink milk. For young women, poor food choices and efforts to lose weight are believed to be responsible for low intakes of calcium. Over a lifetime, this may lead to osteoporosis, a condition in which the bones become less dense and break easily. Osteoporosis leads to loss of height, a humped-shaped upper back, and hip fractures that can result in disabling injuries and even death. Most affected bones are those in the wrist, hip, and spine. Factors contributing to osteoporosis include heredity, cigarette smoking, menopause, lack of physical activity, and a lifetime of poor calcium intake.

The calcium in milk products is well absorbed by the body. To increase your dietary calcium intake without eating too much fat, choose low-fat cheeses, milks (skim or 1 percent), or yogurt products. Although cottage cheese is made from milk, it is not a good source of calcium because the mineral is lost from the milk during processing. Vitamin D helps with the absorption of calcium, thus it is important that vitamin D intake meet the minimum recommended levels.

Iron. Iron is needed to form the oxygen-carrying pigment in red blood cells called hemoglobin. When hemoglobin picks up oxygen in the lungs, it turns the blood bright red. In cases of iron-deficiency anemia, red blood cells ar[...]
hemoglob[...]
needed to m[...]
tired and looks [...]
a fairly common d[...]
women who experien[...]
and who avoid eating[...]
can be due to a lack of iro[...]
ciency of vitamin C (which[...]
sorption of iron), or excessive[...]
Donating blood is a worthwhile ac[...]
increases the need for iron as the body[...]
red blood cells. Among the best food sou[...]
iron are red meats, which contain a type of [...]
that is well absorbed. However, some peopl[...]
need to take iron pills to treat the anemia. Furthermore, some people absorb too much iron, which causes health problems. Keep in mind that there are many possible causes of anemia; iron-deficiency anemia is just one type of the disorder. Also, if you feel fatigued, you should not automatically assume that your iron levels are low. A blood test will indicate whether you have low iron.

Others. The other minerals are just as important, but there are so many minerals needed by the body, it is beyond the scope of this text to delve further. Review Table 7-2 to learn more about calcium, iron, and several other minerals known to play important roles in the body.

PRODUCTION OF ENERGY

Energy is produced when cells break down the chemical units of glucose, fats, or amino acids to release energy stored in these compounds. Glycogen is not used directly for energy; it must first be broken down to release its supply of glucose units. This process is often referred to as "burning" the energy-supplying nutrients for energy. It is similar to burning a log, except your cells are the "fireplaces." Cellular combustion releases heat energy that maintains your body temperature and generates a form of energy that allows your cells to do work. For

smaller and do not contain enough
n. The cells cannot get the oxygen
ke energy. As a result, one feels
ale. Iron-deficiency anemia is
sorder, especially for young
ce menstrual blood losses
meat. This deficiency
n in the diet, a defi-
aids in the ab-
blood losses.
tivity, but it
replaces
ces of
iron

When sitting around watching TV or reading, oxygen needs are low, and the body runs
mostly on fat. As you can see in Figure 7-2,
carbohydrates provide the major proportion of
energy for short-term, high-intensity muscular
contractions. As the duration and the intensity
of the activity increase, breathing also increases, supplying more oxygen for the cells
and maximizing energy production. When the
activity is prolonged, such as in an endurance
type of sport, the percentage of fat and carbohydrate used for fuel is similar. Under usual
conditions, proteins supply less than about
5 percent of energy. However, when you are
engaged in an endurance type of activity, protein supplies as much as 10 to 15 percent of
your energy needs.

NUTRIENT-DENSE VS. JUNK FOODS

Foods that contain considerable amounts of
vitamins, minerals, and proteins in relation
to their caloric content are referred to being
nutrient dense. For example, a cup of orange
juice is a more nutrient-dense source of vitamin C, folate (a B-vitamin), and potassium (a
mineral) than a cup of orange drink made

n only 10 percent fruit juices. Although it
added vitamin C, the additional water
sugar make the orange drink a less nu-
ous choice. Candy, chips, doughnuts,
es, and cookies are often referred to as
k foods." These foods are not nutrient
se because they provide too many calo-
from fats and sugars in relation to vita-
s and minerals. If your overall diet is
itious, and you can "afford" the extra
ries, it's alright to eat occasional fatty or
ry foods. However, many people live on
s that are rich in these kinds of foods,
h displace more nutritious food items in
diets. This is not a healthy behavior to
tice in the long run.

NUTRIENT REQUIREMENTS AND RECOMMENDATIONS

A nutrient **requirement** is the amount of the
nutrient that is needed to prevent the nutrient's deficiency disease. Determining the precise amounts of nutrients that are needed by
individuals is not practical. However, it is
known that nutrient needs vary among individuals within a population. Some people may
require relatively small amounts of a particular vitamin or mineral. If they don't obtain that
level, over time they will start to show the
signs of that nutrient's deficiency disease.
Fortunately, the levels of nutrients present in
foods are adequate to meet the needs of most
healthy individuals.

nutrient dense: foods that contain
considerable amounts of vitamins, minerals, and proteins in relation to their
caloric content

requirement: the amount of a nutrient
needed to prevent that nutrient's deficiency disease

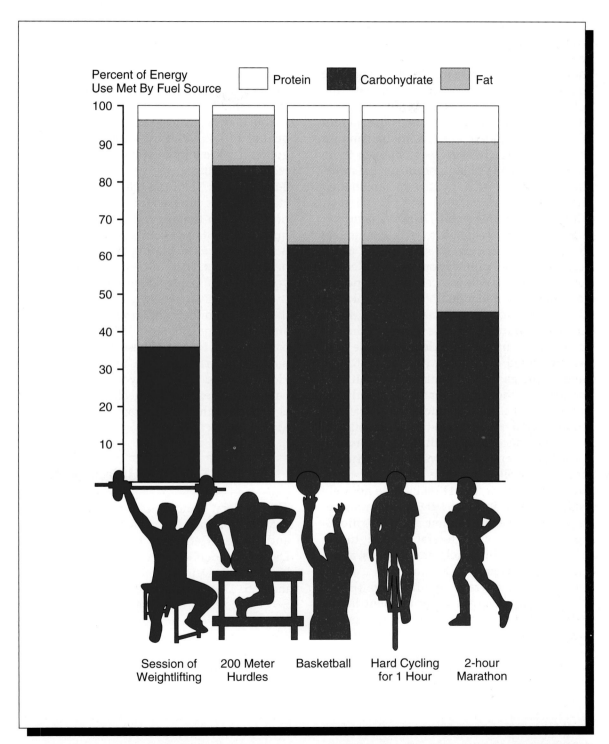

FIGURE 7-2. THE RELATIVE PROPORTIONS OF CARBOHYDRATES, FAT, AND PROTEIN FUELS USED FOR PHYSICAL ACTIVITY.

A nutritional **recommendation** for a nutrient is different from the requirement. Scientists establish recommendations for nutrients and calories. First, researchers determine the amount of the nutrient that prevents the deficiency disease for most people. Then an additional amount, referred to as the margin of safety, is included. This additional amount ensures that nearly every person, even those who have unusually high needs for the nutrient, will be covered by the recommended level.

The *U.S. Recommended Dietary Allowances (USRDA)* were designed to help consumers compare the nutritional value of food products. Since the publication of the Recommended Dietary Allowances in 1989 and the Canadian Recommended Nutrient Intakes in 1990, new information has emerged about nutrient requirements that warrants the development of updated guidelines. In the past, recommended dietary allowances, or RDAs, have served as the benchmarks of nutritional adequacy in the United States. Currently the RDAs have been changed to *Dietary Reference Intakes (DRIs)*, which are established using an expanded concept that includes indicators of good health and the prevention of chronic disease, as well as possible adverse effects of overconsumption. The DRIs include not only recommended intakes (RDA) intended to help individuals meet their daily nutritional requirements, but also tolerable upper intake levels (ULs), which help individuals avoid harm from consuming too much of a nutrient; estimated average requirements (EAR), which are the average daily nutrient intake level estimated to meet the requirement of half the healthy individuals in a particular

recommendation: the requirement plus an extra amount referred to as a "margin of safety"

age group; and adequate intake (AI), which is the recommended average daily intake level based on experimentally developed estimates of nutrient intake that are used when the RDA cannot be determined. Table 7-3 shows the latest DRIs.

You may want to estimate the nutritional quality of your diet by using the RDA as a guide. It takes a lot of work, but you need to record everything you eat and drink over a 3-day period. Then use the computerized dietary analysis program or the food composition tables in the appendices to analyze the nutritional value of your food intake. In general, if you are consuming at least two-thirds of the RDA for most nutrients on a daily basis, your diet is probably adequate (see Lab Activity 7-2). However, trying to make sense out of the RDA, with their milligram and microgram amounts of nutrients, is difficult for many consumers. How can these nutrient recommendations translate into amounts of foods? How do you know if your diet supplies enough nutrients and is healthy? The answer is to consult the U.S. Dietary Guidelines and MyPyramid.

THE DIETARY GUIDELINES*

The Dietary Guidelines are nutrition and health recommendations for healthy children and adults of any age. Every five years the Dietary Guidelines are evaluated and revised by the U.S. Department of Agriculture and the U.S. Department of Health and Human Services to ensure they are current with the latest research on nutrition and health. The most recent revision, published in 2005, places stronger emphasis on reducing calorie consumption and increasing physical activity. The Dietary Guidelines help Americans make sensible choices from every food group, get the most nutrition out of the calories

*Modified from www.healthierus.gov/dietaryguidelines

TABLE 7-3
DIETARY REFERENCE INTAKES: RECOMMENDED LEVELS FOR INDIVIDUAL INTAKE FROM THE FOOD AND NUTRITION BOARD, INSTITUTE OF MEDICINE–NATIONAL ACADEMY OF SCIENCES

Life-Stage Group	Vitamin D (μg/d)[a,b]	Thiamin (mg/d)	Riboflavin B$_2$ (mg/d)	Niacin (mg/d)[c]	B$_6$ (mg/d)	Folate (μg/d)[d]	B$_{12}$ (μg/d)	Pantothenic Acid (mg/d)	Biotin (μg/d)	Choline[e] (mg/d)	Vitamin A (μg/d)	Vitamin C (mg/d)	Vitamin E (mg/d)	Vitamin K (μg/d)
Males 14–18 yr	5*	1.2	1.3	16	1.3	400	2.4	5*	25*	550*	900	75	15	75*
19–30 yr	5*	1.2	1.3	16	1.3	400	2.4	5*	25*	550*	900	90	15	120*
31–50 yr	5*	1.2	1.3	16	1.3	400	2.4	5*	30*	550*	900	90	15	120*
51–70 yr	10*	1.2	1.3	16	1.7	400	2.4[f]	5*	30*	550*	900	90	15	120*
>70 yr	15*	1.2	1.3	16	1.7	400	2.4[f]	5*	30*	550*	900	90	15	120*
Females 14–18 yr	5*	1.0	1.0	14	1.2	400[g]	2.4	5*	25*	400*	700	65	15	75*
19–30 yr	5*	1.1	1.1	14	1.3	400[g]	2.4	5*	30*	425*	700	75	15	90*
31–50 yr	5*	1.1	1.1	14	1.3	400[g]	2.4	5*	30*	425*	700	75	15	90*
51–70 yr	10*	1.1	1.1	14	1.5	400[g]	2.4[f]	5*	30*	425*	700	75	15	90*
>70 yr	15*	1.1	1.1	14	1.5	400	2.4[f]	5*	30*	425*	700	75	15	90*
Pregnancy ≤18 yr	5*	1.4	1.4	18	1.9	600[h]	2.6	6*	30*	450*	750	80	15	75*
19–30 yr	5*	1.4	1.4	18	1.9	600[h]	2.6	6*	30*	450*	770	85	15	90*
31–50 yr	5*	1.4	1.4	18	1.9	600[h]	2.6	6*	30*	450*	770	85	15	90*
Lactation ≤18 yr	5*	1.5	1.6	17	2.0	500	2.8	7*	35*	550*	1,200	115	19	75*
19–30 yr	5*	1.5	1.6	17	2.0	500	2.8	7*	35*	550*	1,300	120	19	90*
31–50 yr	5*	1.5	1.6	17	2.0	500	2.8	7*	35*	550*	1,300	120	19	90*

Continued

TABLE 7-3
DIETARY REFERENCE INTAKES: RECOMMENDED LEVELS FOR INDIVIDUAL INTAKE FROM THE FOOD AND NUTRITION BOARD, INSTITUTE OF MEDICINE–NATIONAL ACADEMY OF SCIENCES—CON'T

Calcium (mg/d)	Phosphorus (mg/d)	Magnesium (mg/d)	Chromium (μg/d)	Copper (μg/d)	Iron (mg/d)	Iodine (μg/d)	Manganese (mg/d)	Molybdenum (μg/d)	Selenium (μg/d)	Zinc (mg/d)	Fluoride (mg/d)
1,300*	1,250	410	35*	890	11	150	2.2*	43	55	11	3*
1,000*	700	400	35*	900	8	150	2.3*	45	55	11	4*
1,000*	700	420	35*	900	8	150	2.3*	45	55	11	4*
1,200*	700	420	30*	900	8	150	2.3*	45	55	11	4*
1,200*	700	420	30*	900	8	150	2.3*	45	55	11	4*
1,300*	1,250	360	24*	890	15	150	1.5*	43	55	9	3*
1,000*	700	310	25*	900	18	150	1.8*	45	55	8	3*
1,000*	700	320	25*	900	18	150	1.8*	45	55	8	3*
1,200*	700	320	20*	900	8	150	1.8*	45	55	8	3*
1,200*	700	320	20*	900	8	150	1.8*	45	55	8	3*
1,300*	1,250	400	29*	1,000	27	220	2.0*	50	60	12	3*
1,000*	700	350	30*	1,000	27	220	2.0*	50	60	11	3*
1,000*	700	360	30*	1,000	27	220	2.0*	50	60	11	3*
1,300*	1,250	360	44*	1,300	10	290	2.6*	50	70	13	3*
1,000*	700	310	45*	1,300	9	290	2.6*	50	70	12	3*
1,000*	700	320	45*	1,300	9	290	2.5*	50	70	12	3*

NOTE: This table presents Recommended Dietary Allowances (RDAs) in bold type and Adequate Intakes (AIs) in ordinary type followed by an asterisk (*). RDAs and AIs may both be used as goals for individual intake. RDAs are set to meet the needs of almost all (97 to 98 percent) individuals in a group. For healthy breast-fed infants, the AI is the mean intake. The AI for other life-stage groups is believed to cover their needs, but lack of data or uncertainty in the data prevent clear specification of this coverage.

[a] As cholecalciferol. 1 μg cholecalciferol = 40 IU vitamin D.

[b] In the absence of adequate exposure to sunlight.

[c] As niacin equivalents. 1 mg of niacin = 60 mg of tryptohan.

[d] As dietary folate equivalents (DFE). 1 DFE = 1 μg food folate = 0.6 μg of folic acid (from fortified food or supplement) consumed with food = 0.5 μg of synthetic (supplemental) folic acid taken on an empty stomach.

[e] Although AIs have been set for choline, there are few data to assess whether a dietary supply of choline is needed at all stages of the life cycle, and it may be that the choline requirement can be met by endogenous synthesis at some of these stages.

[f] Since 10 to 30 percent of older people may malabsorb food-bound B_{12}, it is advisable for those older than 50 years to meet their RDA mainly by consuming foods fortified with B_{12} or a B_{12}-containing supplement.

[g] In view of evidence linking folate intake with neural tube defects in the fetus, it is recommended that all women capable of becoming pregnant consume 400 μg of synthetic folic acid from fortified foods and/or supplements in addition to intake of food folate from a varied diet.

[h] It is assumed that women will continue consuming 400 μg of folic acid until their pregnancy is confirmed and they enter prenatal care, which ordinarily occurs after the end of the periconceptional period—the critical time for formation of the neural tube.

consumed, find a balance between eating and physical activity to promote optimal health, and reduce the risk of certain diseases. The Dietary Guidelines describe a healthy diet based on the latest scientific medical research. Essentially the latest Dietary Guidelines describe a *healthy diet* as one that emphasizes fruits, vegetables, whole grains, and fat-free or low-fat milk and milk products; includes lean meats, poultry, fish, beans, eggs, and nuts; and is low in saturated fats, *trans* fats, cholesterol, salt (sodium), and added sugars. Health Link 7-1 on the next page, provides a list of the key recommendations from the 2005 Dietary Guidelines for Americans. Health Link 7-2 on page 189 provides additional tips for healthy cooking and food preparation.

MYPYRAMID*

The USDA's new MyPyramid, introduced in 2005, replaces the Food Guide Pyramid developed in 1992 and is part of an overall food guidance system that emphasizes the need for a more individualized approach to improving diet and lifestyle. It allows an individual to personalize his or her approach when choosing a healthier lifestyle that balances nutrition and exercise. MyPyramid incorporates recommendations from the *2005 Dietary Guidelines for Americans* and was developed to carry the messages of the dietary guidelines and to make Americans aware of the vital health benefits of simple and modest improvements in nutrition, physical activity, and lifestyle behavior. Overall health can be significantly improved by making modest changes in the diet and by incorporating regular physical activity into daily living. MyPyramid's daily food intake patterns identify amounts to consume from each food group and subgroup at a variety of energy

*Modified from United States Department of Agriculture Web site—http://www.mypyramid.gov

levels. MyPyramid represents the recommended proportion of foods from each food group and focuses on the importance of making smart food choices in every food group every day.

The MyPyramid symbol is meant to encourage consumers to make healthier food choices and to be active daily (see Figure 7-3). The MyPyramid symbol illustrates:

Gradual improvement, encouraged by the slogan, "Steps to a Healthier You." It suggests that individuals can benefit from taking small steps to improve their diet and lifestyle each day.

Physical activity, represented by the steps and the person climbing them, as a reminder of the importance of daily physical activity.

Variety, symbolized by the six color bands representing the five food groups of MyPyramid and oils. Foods from all groups are needed each day for good health.

Moderation, represented by the narrowing of each food group from bottom to top. The wider base stands for foods with little or no solid fats, added sugars, or caloric sweeteners. These should be selected more often to get the most nutrition from calories consumed.

Proportionality, shown by the different widths of the food group bands. The widths suggest how much food a person should choose from each group. The widths are just a general guide, not exact proportions.

Personalization, demonstrated by the MyPyramid Web site. To find a personalized recommendation of the kinds and amounts of food to eat each day, go to MyPyramid.gov.

Consumers can get more in-depth information from the new Web site, MyPyramid.gov, so that they can make choices to fit their own

HEALTH LINK 7-1

- Consume a variety of nutrient-dense foods and beverages within and among the basic food groups while choosing foods that limit the intake of saturated and *trans* fats, cholesterol, added sugars, salt, and alcohol.
- Meet recommended intakes within energy needs by adopting a balanced eating pattern.
- To maintain body weight in a healthy range, balance calories from foods and beverages with calories expended.
- To prevent gradual weight gain over time, make small decreases in food and beverage calories and increase physical activity.
- Consume a sufficient amount of fruits and vegetables while staying within energy needs. Two cups of fruit and 2½ cups of vegetables per day are recommended for a reference 2,000-calorie intake, with higher or lower amounts depending on the calorie level.
- Choose a variety of fruits and vegetables each day. In particular, select from all five vegetable subgroups (dark green, orange, legumes, starchy vegetables, and other vegetables) several times a week.
- Consume 3 or more ounce-equivalents of whole-grain products per day, with the rest of the recommended grains coming from enriched or whole-grain products. In general, at least half the grains should come from whole grains.
- Consume 3 cups per day of fat-free or low-fat milk or equivalent milk products.
- Consume less than 10 percent of calories from saturated fatty acids and less than 300 mg/day of cholesterol, and keep *trans* fatty acid consumption as low as possible.
- Keep total fat intake between 20 to 35 percent of calories, with most fats coming from sources of polyunsaturated and monounsaturated fatty acids, such as fish, nuts, and vegetable oils.
- When selecting and preparing meat, poultry, dry beans, and milk or milk products, make choices that are lean, low-fat, or fat-free.

- Limit intake of fats and oils high in saturated and/or *trans* fatty acids, and choose products low in such fats and oils.
- Choose fiber-rich fruits, vegetables, and whole grains often.
- Choose and prepare foods and beverages with little added sugars or caloric sweeteners.
- Reduce the incidence of dental caries by practicing good oral hygiene and consuming sugar- and starch-containing foods and beverages less frequently.
- Consume less than 2,300 mg (approximately 1 tsp of salt) of sodium per day.
- Choose and prepare foods with little salt. At the same time, consume potassium-rich foods, such as fruits and vegetables.
- Those who choose to drink alcoholic beverages should do so sensibly and in moderation—defined as the consumption of up to one drink per day for women and up to two drinks per day for men.
- Alcoholic beverages should not be consumed by some individuals, including those who cannot restrict their alcohol intake, women of childbearing age who may become pregnant, pregnant and lactating women, children and adolescents, individuals taking medications that can interact with alcohol, and those with specific medical conditions.
- Alcoholic beverages should be avoided by individuals engaging in activities that require attention, skill, or coordination, such as driving or operating machinery.
- Engage in regular physical activity and reduce sedentary activities to promote health, psychological well-being, and a healthy body weight.
- Achieve physical fitness by including cardiovascular conditioning, stretching exercises for flexibility, and resistance exercises or calisthenics for muscle strength and endurance.

*www.healthierus.gov/dietaryguidelines.
http://www.hhs.gov/news

HEALTH LINK 7-2

Healthy Cooking–Improve Your Health and Diet with These Tips

There's much you can do about healthy cooking, starting with the ingredients you use.

- Select low-fat or reduced-fat items.
- Buy polyunsaturated margarine instead of butter.
- Include as little meat as possible in your menu.
- White meat such as fish and poultry is always healthier than red meat.
- Always buy lean meat, and trim off any fat.
- When using cooking oil, try to use olive oil and canola oil.
- When you take your food out of the oven or fryer, place it on several napkins to drain the oil.

- Try cooking fewer high-fat, high-calorie foods such as burgers and pizzas, and cook healthier foods such as salads, soups, and stir-fries.
- Cooking methods such as basting, grilling, and deep-frying are less healthy than steaming, poaching, and stir-frying.
- When basting or grilling, don't use the fat from the grilled item, use vegetable oil instead.
- Eat out less, and eat less fast food.

www.healthycookingrecipes.com/cookinghealthyarticles/healthycooking.htm

needs. Health Link 7-3 summarizes the information available on the MyPyramid.gov Web site.

READING LABELS

Over the past 20 years, food labels have provided helpful nutritional information for consumers. In 1994, a new nutritional labeling format changed the look and importance of food product packaging. It was changed because people were becoming concerned over the amount of fat, cholesterol, sodium, and fiber in the typical American diet, thus producing the drive for a more health-conscious label. Health educators believe that the new format has made it easier for consumers to make more informed, healthful food selections. In 2004, the FDA mandated that *trans* fat be added to the label.

Examine the sample label shown in Figure 7-4. The manufacturer must list the total number of calories per serving, and include information about the number of total calories contributed by fat. Unfortunately, you have to do some math to figure out what percentage of total calories is fat calories. This is crucial if you are trying to limit the total amount of fat in your diet to about 25 to 30 percent of total calories. Furthermore the new format presents the information in the form of percentages that are based on "percent daily values" and a standard 2,000 calories. For example, the label shown in Figure 7-4 indicates that the 1-cup-sized serving contributes 15 percent of the percent daily value of calcium. If you are to meet 100 percent of the value for this mineral, the other foods in your daily diet should supply the remaining 85 percent of the value for calcium. Although there are a few exceptions, most packaged supermarket foods must include nutritional labels. Not everyone is satisfied with the new format; consumers will ultimately decide its usefulness.

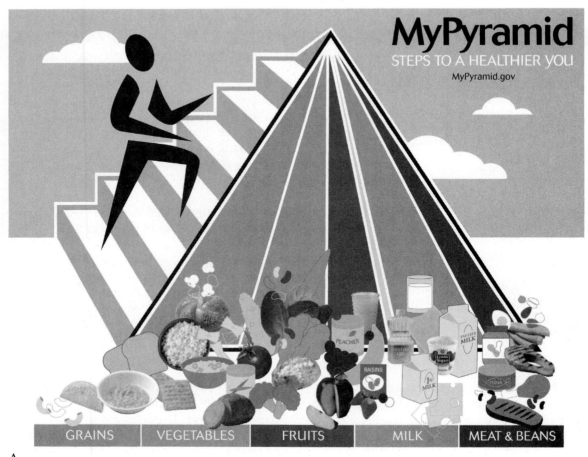

A

FIGURE 7-3. MYPYRAMID.

WHAT IS THE ROLE OF NUTRITION IN PHYSICAL ACTIVITY?

Interest in the value of nutrition to fitness is very high. Physically active people often believe that certain nutrients can help them achieve their fitness goals or a competitive edge. Depending on personal experiences and beliefs, certain foods may be valued or avoided by athletes. Let's explore some of the more common beliefs and examine what the experts have determined about the role of nutrients and foods in physical performance.

NUTRITIONAL SUPPLEMENTS

You may know people who take vitamin, mineral, and protein supplements. Every year, Americans spend millions of dollars on nutrient supplements. These products often contain amounts of nutrients that are well beyond the minimum needed and the levels recommended. Although claims about the value of

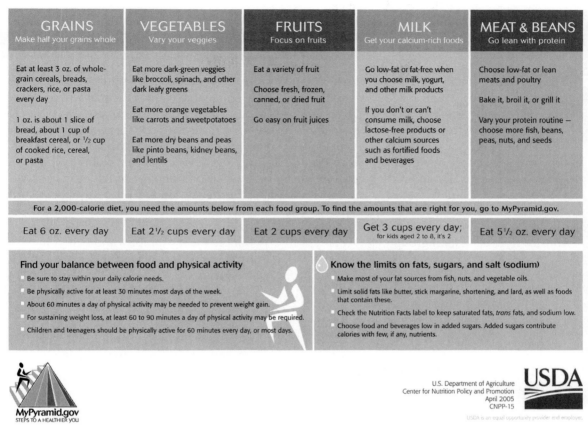

GRAINS Make half your grains whole	VEGETABLES Vary your veggies	FRUITS Focus on fruits	MILK Get your calcium-rich foods	MEAT & BEANS Go lean with protein
Eat at least 3 oz. of whole-grain cereals, breads, crackers, rice, or pasta every day 1 oz. is about 1 slice of bread, about 1 cup of breakfast cereal, or ½ cup of cooked rice, cereal, or pasta	Eat more dark-green veggies like broccoli, spinach, and other dark leafy greens Eat more orange vegetables like carrots and sweetpotatoes Eat more dry beans and peas like pinto beans, kidney beans, and lentils	Eat a variety of fruit Choose fresh, frozen, canned, or dried fruit Go easy on fruit juices	Go low-fat or fat-free when you choose milk, yogurt, and other milk products If you don't or can't consume milk, choose lactose-free products or other calcium sources such as fortified foods and beverages	Choose low-fat or lean meats and poultry Bake it, broil it, or grill it Vary your protein routine — choose more fish, beans, peas, nuts, and seeds

For a 2,000-calorie diet, you need the amounts below from each food group. To find the amounts that are right for you, go to MyPyramid.gov.

| Eat 6 oz. every day | Eat 2½ cups every day | Eat 2 cups every day | Get 3 cups every day; for kids aged 2 to 8, it's 2 | Eat 5½ oz. every day |

Find your balance between food and physical activity
- Be sure to stay within your daily calorie needs.
- Be physically active for at least 30 minutes most days of the week.
- About 60 minutes a day of physical activity may be needed to prevent weight gain.
- For sustaining weight loss, at least 60 to 90 minutes a day of physical activity may be required.
- Children and teenagers should be physically active for 60 minutes every day, or most days.

Know the limits on fats, sugars, and salt (sodium)
- Make most of your fat sources from fish, nuts, and vegetable oils.
- Limit solid fats like butter, stick margarine, shortening, and lard, as well as foods that contain these.
- Check the Nutrition Facts label to keep saturated fats, *trans* fats, and sodium low.
- Choose food and beverages low in added sugars. Added sugars contribute calories with few, if any, nutrients.

MyPyramid.gov
STEPS TO A HEALTHIER YOU

U.S. Department of Agriculture
Center for Nutrition Policy and Promotion
April 2005
CNPP-15

USDA

USDA is an equal opportunity provider and employer.

B

FIGURE 7-3. MYPYRAMID (CONTINUED)

supplements abound, there is no scientific evidence that vitamin, mineral, or protein supplements enhance physical performance or boost energy.

▶Protein Supplements

The experts do not agree on how much additional protein is needed during body building. For most, it appears that any increase in protein needs for conditioning, body building, and weight training is easily met by your usual diet. As mentioned earlier, the typical American eats over 100 grams of protein a day, so even those trying to "bulk up" are probably consuming plenty of protein. There seems to be no advantage to consuming greater amounts of

protein, especially from protein supplements. Extra proteins or amino acids are not anabolic, that is, they do not stimulate the growth of muscle cells. In fact, using amino acids supplements can be harmful. The body is designed to digest and absorb proteins from foods, not synthetic mixtures of amino acids. These protein supplements can create amino acid imbalances, can cause dehydration (loss of body water), and may increase losses of calcium.

Physical activity increases the need for energy, not protein. If the body is not supplied with enough energy, the valuable amino acids can be used for energy. Therefore, make certain that you are eating enough carbohydrates (preferably starches) to meet your body's energy

HEALTH LINK 7-3

Information Available on MyPyramid.gov Web Site

The new food guidance system utilizes interactive technology found on MyPyramid.gov. MyPyramid contains interactive activities that make it easy for individuals to key in their age, gender, and physical activity level so that they can get a more personalized recommendation on their daily calorie level based on the 2005 Dietary Guidelines for Americans. It also allows individuals to find general food guidance and suggestions for making smart choices from each food group.

MyPyramid.gov features:

- MyPyramid Plan—provides a quick estimate of what and how much food you should eat from the different food groups by entering your age, gender, and activity level.
- MyPyramid Tracker—provides more detailed information on your diet quality and physical activity status by comparing a day's worth of foods eaten with current nutrition guidance. Relevant nutrition and physical activity messages are tailored to your desire to maintain your current weight or to lose weight.
- Inside MyPyramid—provides in-depth information for every food group, including recommended daily amounts in commonly used measures, like cups and ounces, with examples and everyday tips. The section also includes recommendations for choosing healthy oils, discretionary calories, and physical activity.
- Start Today—provides tips and resources that include downloadable suggestions on all the food groups and physical activity, and a worksheet to track what you are eating.

needs and spare amino acids for other uses. The excess amino acids from foods or supplements can be converted to fat and stored for future energy needs.

▶ Vitamin and Mineral Supplements

There are people, such as the elderly or ill, who have difficulty obtaining all of the vitamins and minerals they need through the diet. These individuals often benefit from supplementation. Even for healthy people, obtaining adequate levels of antioxidant nutrients as well as calcium and iron requires careful dietary planning. Fit List 7-2 on page 179 lists foods rich in antioxidants. Although there is disagreement, some experts believe that selecting antioxidant-rich foods is not enough and taking supplements of these specific nutrients is warranted. Furthermore, supplements of the following minerals may be necessary for some people.

Calicum. Some physical activity helps to strengthen bone. However, for very active women, too much physical activity disrupts their normal hormonal levels, leading to premature osteoporosis. Extra calcium may help, but the hormonal problem needs to return to normal if bones are to be protected. These women should check with their doctors before taking calcium supplements. Recent research has indicated that magnesium is more important than calcium for preventing osteoporosis.

Iron. There have been reports of a type of anemia, sports or runner's anemia, that often occurs in those involved in training and long-distance running. It is not clear whether or not this is a true anemia. The person who is mildly anemic and experiences a reduction in

Nutrition Facts

Serving Size 1 cup (228g)
Servings Per Container 2

Amount Per Serving	
Calories 260	Calories from Fat 120

	% Daily Value*
Total Fat 13g	**20%**
Saturated Fat 5g	**25%**
Trans Fat 2g	
Cholesterol 30mg	**10%**
Sodium 660mg	**28%**
Total Carbohydrate 31g	**10%**
Dietary Fiber 0g	**0%**
Sugars 5g	
Protein 5g	

Vitamin A 4%		Vitamin C 2%
Calcium 15%		Iron 4%

*Percent Daily Values are based on a 2,000 calorie diet. Your daily values may be higher or lower depending on your calorie needs.

	Calories	2000	2500
Total Fat	Less than	65g	80g
Sat. Fat	Less than	20g	25g
Cholesterol	Less than	300mg	300mg
Sodium	Less than	2,400mg	2,400mg
Total Carbohydrate		300g	375g
Dietary Fiber		25g	30g

Calories per gram
Fat 9   Carbohydrate 4   Protein 4

FIGURE 7-4. LABEL INDICATING NUTRITION INFORMATION PER SERVING.

performance should try to increase the amounts of iron-rich foods in the diet. If the anemia is serious, a physician should be consulted for advice regarding iron supplements.

▶ Creatine Supplements

Creatine is a naturally occurring organic compound made by the kidneys, liver, and pancreas. Creatine can also be obtained from the ingestion of meat and fish. It also seems that oral supplementation with creatine may enhance muscular performance during high-intensity resistance exercise. Creatine has an integral role in energy metabolism.

There are two main types of creatine, free creatine and phosphocreatine. Phosphocreatine is stored in skeletal muscle and is used during anaerobic activity to produce energy. With creatine supplementation, phosphocreatine depletion is delayed, and performance may be enhanced through the maintenance of the normal metabolic pathways.

The positive physiological effects of creatine include allowing for increased intensity in a workout; prolonging maximal effort and improving exercise recovery time during maximal intensity activities; stimulating protein synthesis; decreasing total cholesterol; decreasing total triglycerides; and increasing fat free mass. Side effects of creatine supplementation include weight gain and occasional muscle cramping. However, there are apparently no other known long-term side effects.

▶ A Final Word About Supplements

If you choose to take a supplement, do not use it as a food, use it with food. Read the label; avoid supplements that contain more than 150 percent of the recommended levels for each of the nutrients. Do not be misled into thinking that you need to take vitamins with the words *organic* or *natural* on the label. Your body does not care if the vitamin C came from a potato, a rose "hip," or a laboratory. If it is called vitamin C (ascorbic acid), it has a specific chemical structure that cells use. Furthermore, all vitamins are organic; that is, their chemical structures include carbon atoms attached to hydrogen atoms. These terms are meant to impress average consumers and entice them into spending more for their supplements. Select the plain label or generic vitamin/

mineral supplements, which are just as effective as the highly advertised brand name ones.

Keep in mind that taking nutrient supplements is no substitute for eating food and that many nutrients are toxic in large amounts. Unlike supplements, foods usually contain nutrients in the proper forms and proportions. Therefore, take the time to analyze the nutritional quality of your diet.

SUGAR

In the past it was believed that eating large quantities of simple carbohydrates, such as those supplied by candy bars, honey, or pure sugar, immediately before physical activity had a negative impact on performance. However, recent evidence indicates that for most healthy, active people, the effects of eating carbohydrates before activity are more beneficial than negative. Some people find that large quantities of fructose lead to intestinal upset and diarrhea. (Sources of fructose include honey, fruit, and table sugar.) Therefore, it is wise to avoid fructose or, for that matter, any food that upsets your stomach, before engaging in physical activity.

CAFFEINE

Caffeine is a stimulant found in coffee, tea, chocolate, and carbonated beverages. Although small amounts of caffeine may benefit physical performance, too much can cause headaches, nervousness, irritability, and increased heart rate. Olympic officials have ruled that athletes' blood caffeine levels should not exceed the amount that results from drinking six cups of coffee.

ALCOHOL

Alcohol is a depressant drug that supplies 7 calories per gram. However, alcoholic beverages offer little nutritional value other than energy. The depressant effects of alcohol include reductions in physical coordination, slowed reaction times, and decreased mental alertness. Alcohol also has a diuretic effect, resulting in body water losses. Therefore, it is not wise to replace water losses from physical activity by using alcoholic beverages, such as beer. Too much alcohol is harmful, destroying the liver and brain cells and potentially causing negative effects in your personal life.

HERBS

The use of herbs as natural alternatives to drugs and medicines has clearly become a trend among American consumers. Most herbs, as edible plants, are safe to take as foods, and they are claimed to have few side effects. One herb that has potentially dangerous side effects is ephedrine. Ephedrine is a central nervous system stimulant that has been linked to a variety of potentially life-threatening conditions. In 2003, ephedrine was banned by the Food and Drug Administration.

Hundreds of herbs are widely available today at all quality levels. They are readily available at health food stores. However, unlike both food and medicine, there are no federal or governmental controls to regulate the sale and ensure the quality of the products being sold. Thus extreme caution must be exercised by the consumer of herbal products.

Relative to nutrition, herbs can offer the body nutrients that are reported to nourish the brain, glands, and hormones. Unlike vitamins that work best when taken with food, it is not necessary to take herbs with other foods.

Herbs in their whole form are not drugs. As medicine, herbs are essentially body balancers that work with the body functions, so that the body can heal and regulate itself. Herbal formulas can be general for overall strength and nutrient support, or specific to a particular ailment or condition.

Table 7-4 lists the most popular and widely used herbal products sold in health food stores. Some additional potent and complex herbs, such as capsicum, lobelia, sassafras,

TABLE 7-4 MOST WIDELY USED HERBS AND PURPOSES FOR USE
cayenne—used for weight loss
cascara—used as a laxative can cause dehydration
dong quai—to treat menstrual symptoms
echinacea—to promote wound healing and strengthen the immune system
fever few—to prevent and relieve migraine headaches, arthritis, and PMS
garlic—as an antibiotic, antibacterial, antifungal agent to prevent and relieve coronary artery disease by reducing total blood cholesterol and triglyceride levels and raising HDL levels
garcina cambagia—used to promote loss of fat
ginkgo biloba—to improve blood circulation especially in the brain
ginseng—to reduce impotence, weakness, lethargy, and fatigue
guarana—used as a stimulant, contains large amounts of caffeine, often in weight loss products
kava—to reduce anxiety, relax muscle tension, produce analgesic effects, act as a local anesthetic, provide antibacterial benefit
ma huang (ephedrine)—derived from the ephedra plant, it has been used in China for medicinal purposes including increased energy, appetite suppression, increased fat burning, and preservation of muscle tissue from breaking down. It is a central nervous system stimulant drug used in many diet pills. In 1995, the FDA revealed adverse reactions to ephedrine such as heart attacks, strokes, paranoid psychosis, vomiting, fever, palpitations, convulsions, and comas, and in 2003 banned its use.
mate—CNS stimulant
saw palmetto—to treat inflamed prostate; also used as a diuretic and as a sexual enhancement agent
senna—used as a laxative can cause water and electrolyte loss
St. John's wort—used as an antidepressant; also used to treat nervous disorders, depression, neuralgia, kidney problems, wounds, and burns
valerian—to treat insomnia, anxiety, stress
yohimbe—to increase libido and blood flow to sexual organs in the male

mandrake tansy, canada snake root, wormwood, woodruff, poke root, and rue, may be useful in small amounts and as catalysts but should not be used alone.

THE PROBLEM WITH EATING FAST FOODS

Eating fast food is a way of life in American society. Most Americans have grown up as fast-food "junkies." Aside from occasional problems with food flavor, the biggest concern in consuming fast foods, as can be seen in Table 7-5, is that 40 to 50 percent of the calories consumed are from fats. To compound this problem, these already sizable meals are now being "supersized" at a more affordable price for those who want maximum fat, salt, and calories in a single sitting.

On the more positive side, fast-food restaurants have broadened their menus to include

TABLE 7-5
FAST-FOOD CHOICES AND NUTRITIONAL VALUE

Food	Calories	Protein (g)	CHO (g)	Fat (g)	Calories from Fat (%)	Cholesterol (mg)	Sodium (mg)
Hamburgers							
McDonald's hamburger	263	12.4	28.3	11	38.6	29.1	506
Dairy Queen single hamburger w/cheese	410	24	33	20	43.9	50	790
Hardee's 1/4 pound cheeseburger	506	28	41	26	46.2	61	1,950
Wendy's double hamburger, white bun	560	4.1	24	34	54.6	125	575
McDonald's Big Mac	570	24.6	39.2	35	55.2	83	45
Burger King Whopper sandwich	640	27	42	41	57.6	94	842
Chicken							
Arby's chicken breast sandwich	592	28	56	27	41.0	57	1,340
Burger King chicken sandwich	688	26	56	40	52.3	82	1,423
Dairy Queen chicken sandwich	670	29	46	41	55.0	75	870
Church's Crispy Nuggets (one; regular)	55	3	4	3	49.0	—	125
Kentucky Fried Chicken Nuggets (one)	46	2.82	2.2	2.9	56.7	11.9	140
Fish							
Church's Southern Fried Catfish	67	4	4	4	53.7	—	151
Long John Silver's Fish & More	978	34	82	58	53.3	88	2,124
McDonald's Filet-O-Fish	135	14.7	35.9	25.7	53.1	45.2	799
Others							
Hardee's hot dog	346	11	26	22	57.2	42	744
Taco Bell Beef Burrito Supreme	440	17	52	18	36	35	1,220

Continued

TABLE 7-5
FAST-FOOD CHOICES AND NUTRITIONAL VALUE—CON'T

Food	Calories	Protein (g)	CHO (g)	Fat (g)	Calories from Fat (%)	Cholesterol (mg)	Sodium (mg)
Taco Bell chicken soft taco	240	14	21	11	42	45	490
Taco Bell taco salad	830	29	66	51	55	60	1,760
Arby's roast beef sandwich (regular)	350	22	32	15	38.5	39	590
Hardee's roast beef sandwich	377	21	36	17	40.5	57	1,030
French Fries							
Arby's french fries	211	2	33	8	34.1	6	30
McDonald's french fries (regular)	220	3	26.1	11.5	47.0	8.6	109
Wendy's french fries (regular)	280	4	35	14	45.0	15	95
Shakes							
Dairy Queen	710	14	120	19	24.0	50	260
McDonald's							
Vanilla	352	9.3	59.6	8.4	21.4	30.6	201
Chocolate	383	9.9	65.5	9	21.1	29.7	300
Strawberry	362	9	62.1	8.7	22.3	32.2	207
Soft Drinks							
Coca Cola	154	—	40	—	—	—	6
Diet Coke	0.9	—	0.3	—	—	—	16
Sprite	142	—	36	—	—	—	45
Tab	1	—	1	—	—	—	30
Diet Sprite	3	—	0	—	—	—	9

whole-wheat breads and rolls, salad bars, and low-fat milk products. Many of the larger fast-food restaurants provide nutritional information for consumers upon request or from well-stocked racks. Safe Tip 7-1 provides suggestions for eating more healthfully at fast-food restaurants.

PRE-EVENT MEAL

People engaging in competitive sports are often very concerned with the kinds of foods selected for pre-event meals. However, they should be more concerned with their eating patterns well before the day of the event. The

SAFE TIP 7-1

Tips for Selecting Fast Foods

- Limit deep fried foods such as fish and chicken sandwiches and chicken nuggets, which are often higher in fat than plain burgers are. If you are having fried chicken, remove some of the breading before eating.
- Order roast beef, turkey, or grilled chicken, where available, for a lower fat alternative to most burgers.
- Choose a small order of fries with your meal rather than a large one, and request no salt. Add a small amount of salt yourself if desired. If you are ordering a deep-fat-fried sandwich or one that is made with cheese and sauce, skip the fries altogether and try a plain baked potato (add butter and salt sparingly) or a dinner roll instead of a biscuit; or try a side salad to accompany your meal instead.
- Choose regular sandwiches instead of "double," "jumbo," "deluxe," or "ultimate." And order plain types rather than those with the works, such as cheese, bacon, mayonnaise, and special sauce. Pickles, mustard, ketchup, and other condiments are high in sodium. Choose lettuce, tomatoes, and onions.
- At the salad bar, load up on fresh greens, fruits, and vegetables. Be careful of salad dressings, added toppings, and creamy salads (potato salad, macaroni salad, coleslaw). These can quickly push calories and fat to the level of other menu items or higher.
- Many fast-food items contain large amounts of sodium from salt and other ingredients. Try to balance the rest of your day's sodium choices after a fast-food meal.
- Alternate water, low-fat milk, or skim milk with a soda or a shake.
- For dessert, or a sweet-on-the-run, choose low-fat frozen yogurt where available.
- Remember to balance your fast-food choices with your food selections for the whole day.

purpose of the pre-event meal is to supply the competitor with enough energy and fluids for competition. The meal should be easily digestible as well. Most experts recommend a light meal (around 300 calories) that is rich in carbohydrate about 2 to 4 hours before the event. A full stomach is uncomfortable, so avoid fatty or greasy meals that take longer to digest. Preloading on extra water is a good idea to keep well hydrated. Individuals vary in their ability to tolerate various foods, but it is advisable to avoid known gas-forming foods or any food the athlete believes contributes to intestinal upset.

VEGETARIANISM

Vegetarians use plant foods to form the foundation of their diet; animal foods are either totally excluded or included in a variety of eating patterns. People who choose to become vegetarians do so for economic, philosophical, religious, cultural, or health reasons. The U.S. Dietary Goals that recommend eating less fat, cholesterol, salt, and sugar while increasing fiber intake easily support a vegetarian eating pattern.

Types of vegetarians include the following:

- *Total vegetarians or vegans:* People who consume plant but no animal foods; meat, fish, poultry, eggs, and dairy products are excluded. This diet has been found to be adequate for most adults if they give careful consideration to obtaining enough calories; sources of vitamin B_{12}; and the minerals calcium, zinc, and iron. It is not recommended for pregnant women, infants, or children because of the difficulty in consuming the quantity of plant foods necessary to meet the caloric and nutritional needs during these life stages.

- *Lactovegetarians:* Individuals who consume milk products along with plant foods. Meat, fish, poultry, and eggs are excluded. Iron and zinc levels can be low in people who practice this form of vegetarianism.
- *Lacto-ovo-vegetarians:* People who consume dairy products and eggs in their diet, along with plant foods. Meat, fish, and poultry are excluded. Again, iron could be a problem.
- *Semivegetarians:* People who consume animal products but exclude red meats. Plant products still form an important part of the diet. This diet is usually adequate.

SUMMARY

- The classes of nutrients are carbohydrates, fats, proteins, vitamins, minerals, and water.
- Carbohydrates, fats, and proteins provide the energy required for muscular work and also play a role in the function and maintenance of body tissues.
- Protein supplementation is not necessary.
- Vitamins are substances found in foods that have no caloric value but are necessary to regulate body processes.
- Antioxidants are nutrients that protect the body against various destructive agents.
- Minerals are also involved in regulation of bodily functions and are used to form important body structures.
- Water is the most essential nutrient and should be the drink of choice.
- The 2005 U.S. Dietary Guidelines are designed to help you plan meals that are healthy.
- A nutritious diet consists of eating a variety of foods in the amounts recommended in MyPyramid. If your diet meets those

recommendations, you may not need nutrient supplements.
- Some people need extra iron and calcium.
- The pre-event meal should be (1) higher in carbohydrates, (2) easily digested, (3) eaten 2 to 4 hours before an event, and (4) acceptable to the athlete.
- Vegetarians use plant foods as the basis of their diet.

SUGGESTED READINGS

Antonio, J. 2001. *Sports supplements.* Philadelphia: Lippincott Williams & Wilkins.

Brodney, S., R. S. McPherson, R. A. Carpenter, D. Welten, and S. N. Blair. 2001. Nutrient intake of physically fit and unfit men and women. *Medicine and Science in Sports and Exercise* 33(3):459–67.

Brouns, F. 2002. *Essentials of sports nutrition,* 2nd ed. New York: John Wiley and Sons.

Brukner, P., K. Khan, K. Inge, and S. Crawford. 2002. Maximizing performance: nutrition. In *Clinical sports medicine,* 2nd rev. ed., edited by P. Brukner. New York: McGraw-Hill.

Burke, L. 2000. *Clinical sports nutrition.* 2d ed. New York: McGraw-Hill.

Burke, L. M., B. Kiens, and J. L. Ivy. 2004. Carbohydrates and fat for training and recovery. *Journal of Sports Sciences* 22(1):15–30.

Clark, N. 2003. *Nancy Clark's sports nutrition guide book.* Champaign, IL: Human Kinetics.

Coleman, E. 2001. Carbohydrate during stop-and-go sports. *Sports Medicine Digest* 23(12):142–43.

Coleman, E. 2001. Nutrition update: Position stand on nutrition and athletic performance. *Sports Medicine Digest* 23(5):54–55.

Cooper, K. 2004. *Antioxidant revolution.* Nashville: Thomas Nelson.

Daniels, D. 2000. *Exercises for osteoporosis.* New York: Hatherleigh Press.

Eberle, S. 2000. *Endurance sports nutrition.* Champaign, IL: Human Kinetics.

Eberle, S. G. 2004. Vegetarian diets for endurance athletes. *Strength and Conditioning Journal* 26(4):60–61.

Foster, S. 1998. *101 medicinal herbs.* Loveland, CO: Interweave Press.

Froiland, K., W. Koszewski, and J. Hingst. 2004. Nutritional supplement use among college athletes and their sources of information. *International Journal of Sport Nutrition and Exercise Metabolism* 14(1):104–20.

Gleeson, M., D. C. Nieman, and B. K. Pedersen. 2004. Exercise, nutrition and immune function. *Journal of Sports Sciences* 22(1):115–25.

Haas, R. 2005. *Eat to win for the 21st century: The sports nutrition bible for a new generation.* East Rutherford, NJ: Penguin Group.

Hunt, B. P., and A. Gillentine. 2001. Dietary supplement knowledge and information sources among college students. *Journal of the International Council for Health, Physical Education, Recreation, Sport, and Dance* 37(3):53–56.

Insel, P., E. Turner, and D. Ross. 2003. *Discovering Nutrition.* Sudbury, MA: Jones and Bartlett Publishers.

Izquierdo, M., J. Ibanez, J. J. Gonzalez-Badillo, and E. M. Gorostiaga. 2002. Effects of creatine supplementation on muscle power, endurance, and sprint performance. *Medicine and Science in Sports and Exercise* 34(2):332–43.

Kleiner, S. 2001. The scoop on protein supplements. *Athletic Therapy Today* 6(1): 52–53.

Kleiner, S. M., and M. Greenwood-Robinson. 2001. Performance herbs. In *Power eating,* 2d ed., edited by S. M. Kleiner. Champaign, IL: Human Kinetics.

Kleiner, S. M., and M. Greenwood-Robinson. 2001. Vitamins and minerals for strength trainers. In *Power eating,* 2d ed., edited by S. M. Kleiner. Champaign, IL: Human Kinetics.

Larson-Duyff, R. 2002. *The American Dietetic Association's complete food and nutrition guide.* New York: John Wiley.

Litt, A. (ed.) 2004. *Fuel for young athletes.* Champaign, IL: Human Kinetics.

Manore, M. M. 2004. Nutrition and physical activity: Fueling the active individual. *President's Council on Physical Fitness and Sports Research Digest* 5(1):1–8.

Maughan, R. J. 2002. *Sports nutrition.* Malden, MA: Blackwell Science.

Maughan, R., and R. Murray. 2001. *Sports drinks: Basic science and practical aspects.* Boca Raton, FL: CRC Press.

Maughan, R. J. D. S. King, and T. Lea. 2004. Dietary supplements. *Journal of Sports Sciences* 22(1):95–113.

McArdle, W. D. 2001. *Exercise physiology: Energy, nutrition, and human performance.* 5th ed. Philadelphia: Lippincott Williams & Wilkins.

National Academy of Sciences Institute of Medicine. 2002. *Dietary reference intakes for energy, carbohydrates, fiber, fat, protein, amino acids (macronutrients).* Washington, DC: National Academies Press.

Papas, A., and J. Quillen. 1998. *Antioxidant status: Diet, nutrition, and health.* Boca Raton, FL: CRC Press.

Platen, P. 2001. The importance of sport and physical exercise in the prevention and therapy of osteoporosis. *European Journal of Sport Science* 1(3):237–44

Powers, S. K. K. C. DeRuisseau, and J. Quindry. 2004. Dietary antioxidants and exercise. *Journal of Sports Sciences* 22(1):81–94.

Sen, C. K. 2001. Antioxidants in exercise nutrition. *Sports Medicine* 31(13):891–908.

Sforzo, G. A. 2002. Sports supplements [Review]. *Medicine and Science in Sports and Exercise* 34(1):183.

Sharkey, B. J. 2002. Nutrition and health. In *Fitness and health,* 5th ed., edited by B. J. Sharkey. Champaign, IL: Human Kinetics.

Spriet, L. L., and M. J. Gibala. 2004. Nutritional strategies to influence adaptations to training. *Journal of Sports Sciences* 22(1):127–41.

Stevenson, S. W., and G. A. Dudley. 2001. Creatine loading, resistance exercise performance and muscle mechanics. *Journal of Strength and Conditioning Research* 15(4):413–19.

Tribole, E. (ed.) 2004. *Eating on the run,* 3rd ed. Champaign, IL: Human Kinetics.

U.S. Department of Agriculture. 2005. *Dietary guidelines for Americans.* Washington, DC: U.S. Government Printing Office.

U.S. Department of Agriculture and U.S. Department of Health and Human Services. 2005. *Nutrition and your health: Dietary guidelines for Americans.* 6th edition. Washington, DC.

Wardlaw, G. M., and M. Kessel. 2003. *Perspectives in nutrition,* 4th ed. New York: McGraw-Hill.

Welsh, R. S., J. M. Davis, J. R. Burke, and H. G. Williams. 2002. Carbohydrates and physical/mental performance during intermittent exercise to fatigue. *Medicine and Science in Sports and Exercise* 34(4):723–31.

Williams, M. 2004. *Nutrition for health, fitness, and sport.* St. Louis: McGraw-Hill.

Williams, M., R. Kreider, and D. Branch. 1999. *Creatine: The power supplement.* Champaign, IL: Human Kinetics.

Suggested Web Sites

American Dietetic Association

This site educates individuals about how making informed food choices can help them decrease the risk of heart disease, breast cancer, osteoporosis, diabetes, and obesity; it advocates nutrition research.
www.eatright.org

American Heart Association

Complete with comprehensive nutrition guidelines, the American Heart Association is a great resource for health practitioners and laypersons.
www.americanheart.org

American Institute for Cancer Research

The latest cancer prevention research in diet and nutrition. Read the "Diet and Cancer link" and their dietary guidelines on "Reducing Your Cancer Risk" position pages.
www.aicr.org

American School Food Service Association

The ASFSA is dedicated to healthy meals for school food service, with a membership of 60,000 professionals committed to child nutrition integrity. For parents, students, and school officials.
www.asfsa.org

ASNS Publications

The American Society for Nutritional Science has a nice page on all the major vitamins and minerals, their daily requirements, sources, and toxic dosages.
www.faseb.org/asns/publications.html

Center for Food Safety and Applied Nutrition—FDA

Timely fact sheets and press releases are available from Food and Drug Administration.
http://cfsan.fda.com

CNN's Health News: Diet & Fitness

This site presents NEWS and helpful tips on topics related to diet and nutrition.
http://cnn.com/HEALTH/diet.fitness

Consumer Information Center: The Food Guide Pyramid

The Pyramid provides an outline of what to eat each day.
www.pueblo.gsa.gov/civ_text/food/food-pyramid/main.htm

Food, nutrition, exercise fact index

This site presents 450 articles and 63 medical abstracts—and it's growing! It gives very good information on 'diets' and their health effects and lots of good stuff about fats in the diet. A lot is vitamin and mineral supplement related, but the good bits are succulent.
www.afpafitness.com/factindx.htm

International Food Information Council Foundation (IFIC)

The IFIC Foundation site is an industry-sponsored foundation that steers a middle road in the debates about nutrition. This useful and cautious perspective includes some very good information on diet.
http://ificinfo.health.org

Mayo Clinic Diet and Nutrition Resource Center

Mayo Clinic nutrition experts offer practical advice, creative encouragement, and healthy recipes to cut fat, cholesterol, sodium, and calories and improve your diet. This site includes a Q&A section with Mayo dietitians.
www.mayohealth.org/mayo/common/htm/dietpage.htm

MyPyramid

This site introduces MyPyramid, a food guidance system that emphasizes the need for a more individualized approach to improving diet and lifestyle that balances nutrition and exercise.
http://www.mypyramid.gov

Nutrition: Arbor Nutrition Guide

This site presents the world's largest catalogue of nutrition resources on the Internet: food science, clinical nutrition, ancient diets, functional foods, and much more—an absolutely outstanding links page.
www.arborcom.com

The Diet Channel

Cutting-edge diet information on weight loss, sports nutrition, heart disease, cancer, and preventative nutrition is presented. You can request a professional diet analysis or browse through 600 links to reliable nutrition information on the Web.
www.thedietchannel.com

The Truth about Tufts Nutritional Navigator

Tufts University Nutrition Navigator is the LEAST reliable way to find sound nutrition information on the Web, unless you want information provided by processed food manufacturers selling junk food. The "Nutrition Navigator" is sponsored by Kraft Foods, a division of tobacco giant Phillip Morris.
www.vegsource.org/tufts_navigator.htm

U.S. Dietary Guidelines

This site details the revised 2005 U.S. Dietary Guidelines for Americans.
www.healthierus.gov/dietaryguidelines

USDA's FNIC

The USDA's Food and Nutrition Information Center is a valuable resource for any nutrition topic.
http://nutrition.about.com/gi/dynamic/offsite.htm

CHAPTER 8

Limiting Your Body Fat Through
Diet & Exercise

Objectives

After completing this chapter, you should be able to do the following:

- Explain the distinction between body weight and body composition.
- Analyze the principle of caloric balance and how imbalances lead to gain or loss of body fat.
- Identify various methods for losing body fat.
- Assess the importance of lifestyle modification for long-term weight control.
- Develop a program of weight loss or maintenance consistent with your needs.

WHY SHOULD YOU BE CONCERNED ABOUT BODY FAT?

It seems that virtually all Americans at one time or another have been concerned about their body fat. Most look in the mirror and study the "roll" of fat that spreads around their midsection or the dimpled fat on their thighs and wonder how to eliminate it. Wearing a bathing suit becomes an act of courage. Our desire to achieve a more ideal appearance makes us easy targets for those interested in profiting from our concern.

The battle against excess body fat has turned into a multibillion-dollar industry that presents various diet plans, exercise studios, and countless gimmicks and gadgets guaranteed to help you lose that extra body fat and inches. One thing they don't guarantee is that you will be able to maintain the loss of body fat. Most people who do lose body fat eventually regain it and even some extra fat. So, why bother to try and lose body fat?

Many people decide to try and lose fat because they are dissatisfied with their appearance. However, there is little question that being overweight can lead to a number of health-related problems. If you are overly fat, you run an increased risk of developing heart disease, hypertension, atherosclerosis, stroke, diabetes,

KEY TERMS

overweight	*caloric balance*
obesity	*calories*
body mass index (BMI)	*kilocalorie*
adipose cell	*basal metabolic rate*
subcutaneous fat	*set point theory*
body composition	*spot reducing*
lean body weight	*bulimia nervosa*
	anorexia nervosa

infections of the respiratory tract, cancer, and disorders of the kidneys. If you are moderately overweight, you have a 40 percent higher risk of premature death. Individuals who are obese have a death rate 70 percent higher than normal. Obviously, you must be concerned about the amount of body fat you have.

THE AMERICAN LIFESTYLE

There are many reasons why our American lifestyle makes controlling the development of body fat difficult. It is virtually impossible to do anything socially without having something to eat or drink. We associate food with dating, weddings, birthdays, and funerals.

Technology has allowed the American lifestyle to become increasingly sedentary as more "labor-saving" devices are invented. The purpose of devices such as garage door openers and remotes for video and audio equipment is to make life and work easier, but there are few associated training effects from pressing a button or moving a joystick.

We do little in our lifestyle that increases physical activity levels. We try to park as close to the entrance as possible so we don't waste time and energy walking back and forth. It is easier to hop on an elevator or escalator than to walk up flights of stairs. Most are not aware of how their behaviors conserve energy rather than burn it.

In this country the problem with people having excess body fat has reached epidemic proportions. A person who has some excess body fat relative to bone structure and height is said to be **overweight.** An individual who has a lot of excess body fat is said to be **obese.** Whether an individual with excess body fat is considered to be overweight or is considered to be obese is generally determined by their **body mass index (BMI).** BMI is determined by using a ratio of a person's body weight to height (Figure 8-1). A BMI between 18.5 and 25 is considered a range for healthy body weight. An individual with a BMI between 25 and 30

is considered overweight. If the BMI is greater than 30, that individual is considered to be obese. Lab Activity 8-1 will help you precisely calculate your BMI.

According to the Centers for Disease Control and Prevention (CDC), as of the end of 2002, about two out of three U.S. adults over age 20 (64%) have a BMI greater than 25 and thus are either overweight or obese. Thirty percent have a BMI greater than 30 and are considered to be obese. The CDC also estimates that 15 percent of children and adolescents ages 6 to 19 are overweight—almost double the rate of two decades ago. The total economic cost of obesity in the United States is about $117 billion per year, including more than $50 billion in avoidable medical costs. Clearly the problem of having excess body fat is a major health problem in the United States.

What is the best way to minimize the development of body fat? Most people tend to panic when they realize that they have put on a little extra fat. They either go on starvation diets or become exercise fanatics, neither of which is particularly enjoyable or provides a long-term solution to the problem. The key to being able to limit your body fat is to have the motivation to alter your lifestyle in ways that you can live with. You need to make a commitment to changing your lifestyle so that you burn off extra energy and consume less food. The cumulative effect of these modifications will make it easier for you to minimize the development of body fat. This approach should become an integral part of

overweight: having excess body weight relative to bone structure and height

obesity: an excessive amount of body fat

body mass index (BMI): Body mass index: ratio of body weight to height

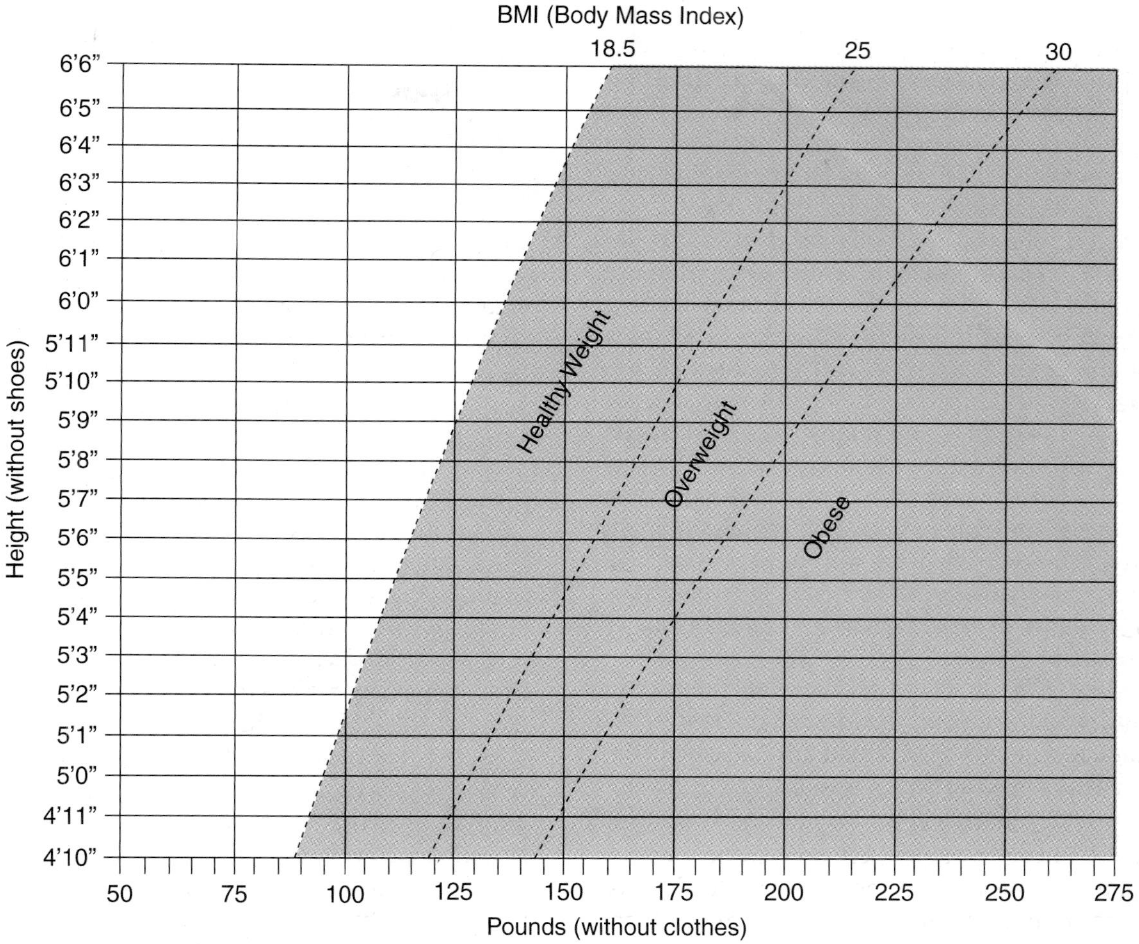

FIGURE 8-1. BODY MASS INDEX (BMI).

Source: Report of the Dietary Guidelines Advisory Committee on the Dietary Guidelines for Americans 2000

your lifestyle rather than a behavior you adopt from time to time.

HOW IS FAT STORED AND WHERE DO YOU FIND IT?

Fat is found in all of the body's cells. Some essential fat is necessary for cushioning organs, regulating temperature, and storing energy for future needs. Nonessential fat gradually accumulates when your food intake exceeds your energy demands. A special type of cell, the adipose cell, stores fat. The **adipose cell** stores triglyceride (a liquid form of fat), which moves in and out of the cell according to energy needs. The greater the amount of triglyceride contained in the adipose cells, the greater the amount of total body weight that is composed of fat.

adipose cell: a type of cell that stores triglyceride, a liquid form of fat

About half of the body's fat is located under the skin (**subcutaneous fat**). The fat distribution in adults tends to follow particular patterns that are largely inherited. In general, people tend to have large stores of fat in the abdominal area; women tend to store more fat in their hips and thighs than men. A useful estimate of overweight, obesity, and body fat distribution involves measurement of waist circumference (Figure 8-2). It appears that the location of fat on the body is significant. If the majority of fat is found around the waist, you are more likely to develop health problems than if most of your fat is in your hips and thighs. This is true even if your BMI falls within the normal range. Males with a waist measurement of more than 40 inches or females with a waist measurement of greater than 35 inches may have a higher disease risk than people with smaller waist measurements because of where the majority of their fat is found.

The term cellulite is often used in magazines and advertisements to identify a type of fat that appears to be dimpled and usually is deposited in the buttocks, upper thighs, and upper arms. Cellulite is a nonmedical term for the ordinary adipose tissue that is found in these sites. Losing weight and exercising will reduce all body fat, including cellulite.

WHAT DETERMINES HOW MUCH FAT YOU HAVE?

Two factors determine the amount of fat found in the body: (1) the number of adipose cells and (2) the size of the adipose cell. The number of adipose cells increases before birth and continues to rise until puberty. Children who become obese at an early age are believed to have too many fat cells (hyperplasia). Adolescents who become overweight seem to develop a greater number of fat cells than those of normal weight. It is thought that by early adulthood the number of fat cells becomes fixed. However, some recent evidence suggests that fat cell number may increase under certain conditions during adulthood.

In addition to cell number, cell size is a factor in obesity. The size of the adipose cell depends on the amount of fat stored within it. Fat cell size increases (hypertrophies) until early adulthood. In the mature adult, fat cell size fluctuates as a function of caloric balance. If more calories are consumed than are needed, the excess is converted to fat and stored in the adipose cells. Under this condition, adipose cells swell with fat. When the energy from fat is needed to fuel activities, the fat cells lose stored fat and shrink in size.

Contrary to popular belief, a fat baby does not necessarily become a fat child or fat young adult. However, after the age of two, a child begins to adopt the eating behaviors and activity patterns of his or her family members. If this child is still too fat by the time he or she starts school, then it is more likely that he or she will become a fat adolescent and adult. In

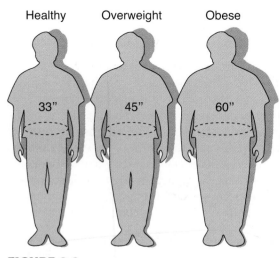

FIGURE 8-2.

Source: Report of the Dietary Guidelines Advisory Committee on the Dietary Guidelines for Americans 2000

subcutaneous fat: the fat that is found directly under the skin

fact the chances of this happening are
times greater in the obese child than in
dren of normal body weight.

In children who become obese at an
age, weight increases are primarily due
creases in the number of fat cells. In ac
weight loss or gain is primarily a functi
the changes in fat cell size, not cell num
Thus obese adults tend to exhibit a great
of adipose cell hypertrophy.

WHAT IS BODY COMPOSITIC

Body composition refers to both the fa
the nonfat components of the body. The
tion of total body weight that is compos
fat tissue is referred to as the percentage
fat. **Lean body weight** is made up by €. ₋₎
type of body tissue that is not fat (i.e., bone,
muscle, tendon, ligament, connective tissue,
nerves, skin, hair, etc.). Generally, the goal is
to maximize the percentage of total body
weight that is composed of lean tissue, and
minimize the percentage of total body weight
composed of fat. Assessment of body composition is perhaps a bit more difficult than
simply stepping on a scale and measuring
actual body weight in pounds. **However,
body weight as determined by a scale does
not take into account how much of the
weight is lean tissue and how much of the
weight is fat.** Body composition measurements are more accurate in attempting to determine precisely how much weight a person
may gain or lose.

In the traditional college student age range,
the average female has between 20 and 25 percent of her total body weight made up of fat.
The average male has between 15 and 20 percent body fat. However, persons who engage
in strenuous physical activities on a regular
basis tend to have a lower percentage body fat.
Male endurance athletes may get their fat percentage as low as 8 to 12 percent, and female
endurance athletes may reach 12 to 18 percent

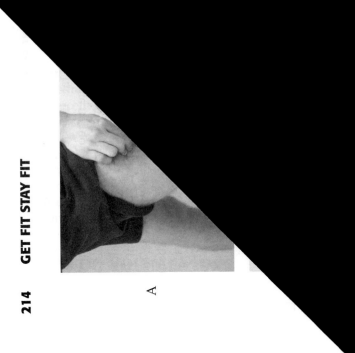

A

involves placing a subject in a specially
designed underwater tank to determine
body density.
2. Measurement of electrical impedance pre-
dicts the percentage body fat by assessing
resistance to the flow of electrical current
through the body between selected points.
3. Measurement of skinfold thickness is the
simplest and most commonly used
method.

▶ Measuring Skinfold Thickness

The third technique is based on the idea that
about 50 percent of the fat in the body is subcutaneous (under the skin). By measuring the
thickness of this layer of fat, the total percentage of body fat can be estimated. Skinfolds are
measured at various body sites using skinfold

> **body composition:** the fat and nonfat
> components of the body
>
> **lean body weight:** the portion of the
> total body weight that is composed of
> nonfat or lean tissue

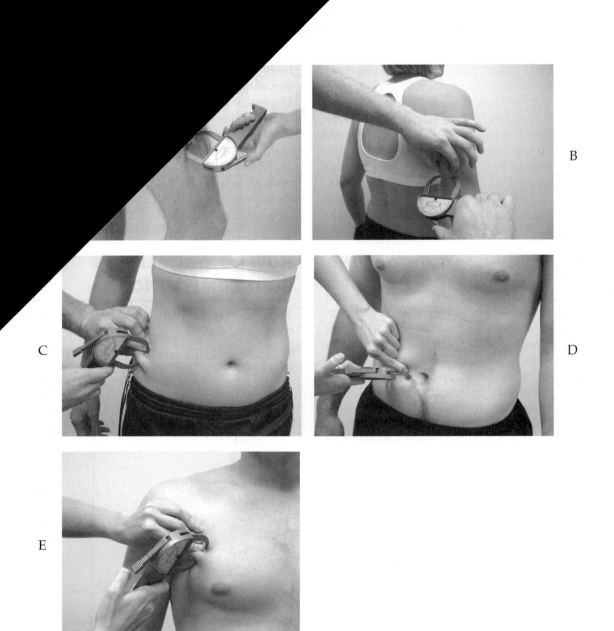

FIGURE 8-3. SKINFOLD MEASUREMENT SITES.
A, *Thigh (males & females);* **B,** *Tricep (females only);* **C,** *Suprailiac (females only);* **D,** *Abdominal (males only);* **E,** *Chest (males only).*

calipers (see Figure 8-3). Men and women tend to develop fat deposits in different body areas; skinfold measurements must be taken at these specified places. A number of different methods for calculating percent body fat using skinfold measurements have been developed. The technique proposed by Jackson and Pollack will be used in Lab Activity 8-2 to determine body fat composition. Although skinfold measurement is a less accurate method than underwater weighing and about same as electrical impedence, almost every can learn to perform this technique. Furth more, the calipers are less costly and tir consuming to use than the other equipmen

When taking a series of skinfold measu ments over time to determine changes, i important that the same person take measurements all the time. Due to the pot tial error that is always possible with cali measures, having the same person take peated measurements will minimize err and give a more accurate indication of solute changes in body composition.

Once you have calculated the percentage your total body weight that is made up of tissue, you may determine that you have much fat. It would be helpful to determine how much weight you have to lose to achieve a normal percent body fat. A worksheet is provided in Lab Activity 8-2 to help you calculate your desired body weight.

HOW DO YOU ACHIEVE CALORIC BALANCE?

It is important to reemphasize that fat in the form of triglyceride moves in and out of the adipose cell according to energy demands. If you have been able to maintain your weight, you are in a state of **caloric balance.** That is, the number of **calories*** that you consume in food equals the number that you use or expend. If you are trying to gain weight, then you need to consume more calories than you expend. The extra calories will be stored, and you will gain weight (*positive caloric balance*). Conversely, if you want to lose weight, you need to expend more energy than you are

*A calorie is simply a measure of the energy value of a foodstuff. A calorie by defintion is the amount of energy necessary to raise the temperature of 1 gram of water 1°C. However, this unit is too small to be easy to use, so the term kilocalorie is more appropriate. A **kilocalorie** is equal to 1,000 caolories. Thus subsequent mention to a specific number of calories in this text refers to kilocalories, which will be denoted as kcal or calories.

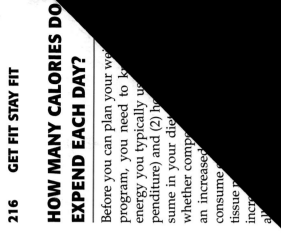

HOW MANY CALORIES DO EXPEND EACH DAY?

Before you can plan your we program, you need to k energy you typically us penditure) and (2) h sume in your die whether comp an increased consume tissue incr

percentage or total body weight that is composed of fat is highly related to the level of physical activity. Persons who have an excess of fat tend to be sedentary and therefore are in a positive calorie situation. In behavioral terms, the number of calories in food ingested and the number of calories expended can be modified. You can eat less and exercise more. However, for many who do not overeat, gradual weight gain often occurs as a result of decreased activity and muscle mass reduction that occurs with aging. The caloric expenditure of physical activities and resting metabolism declines with aging. It will become necessary to decrease caloric intake by about 2.5 percent for every 10 years over the age of 25. Thus, as you age, it becomes increasingly important to either increase exercise levels or decrease caloric intake to avoid gaining body fat.

caloric balance: the number of calories consumed equals the number of calories expended

calories: a measure of the energy value of a foodstuff

kilocalorie: 1,000 calories

YOU

ght modification
...ow (1) how much
...e each day (caloric ex-
...w much energy you con-
... each day. Physical activity,
...titive or recreational, results in
... need for energy. The goal is to
...enough nutritious foods to meet basic
...eeds plus an additional amount to meet
...eased energy needs for the activity. Gener-
...ly, people who participate in physical activity
need more energy supplied by the three food-
stuffs but not additional vitamins or minerals.
As they increase their activity, people usually
increase their food intake, which meets nutritional needs.

If a physically active person's daily energy
intake does not match the energy expenditure,
body weight loss will occur. For individuals
who want to maintain or alter their weight,
some estimation of caloric expenditure and
intake is necessary.

To estimate caloric expenditure, you must
calculate both your **basal metabolic rate** (BMR)
and the total energy required for all activities
you are involved in throughout the course of
a day. It is first necessary to determine the
number of calories (energy) needed to support your basal metabolism. This is the minimal level of energy required to sustain the
body's vital functions such as respiration,
circulation, and maintenance of body temperature. The BMR is the rate at which calories
are spent for these maintenance activities. Fit
List 8-1 describes various factors that influence BMR. Lab Activity 8-3 will help you
determine your BMR.

Once BMR has been determined, Lab Activity 8-4 will help you calculate energy requirements of all activities done in a 24-hour
period. There is a wide variation in energy
output for different types of activity and thus

FIT LIST 8-1

Factors Influencing BMR

Age: In general, the younger the person, the
higher the BMR.

Body surface area: The greater the amount of
body surface area, the higher the BMR.

Gender: Men generally have a higher
metabolic rate than women.

Diet: There is a dramatic and sustained
reduction in BMR that occurs with very-low-
calorie dieting.

Exercise: Consistent exercise tends to
increase the BMR during the activity and for
a period of time after the activity ceases.

there is some difficulty in achieving accuracy
in this exercise. It is determined by the type,
intensity, and duration of a physical activity.
Body size is also a factor; heavier people expend more energy in an activity than lighter
ones. Specific energy expenditures may be determined by consulting charts that predict energy used in an activity based on (1) the time
spent in each activity in minutes and (2) the
metabolic costs of each activity in kilocalories
per minute per pound (kcal/min/lb) of body
weight. If you were to carefully calculate energy costs of all daily activities such as sitting,
walking, and studying, you can estimate the
amount of energy used in a day. By determining your caloric needs for BMR and daily

basal metabolic rate: the rate at
which calories are spent for carrying on
the body's vital functions and maintenance activities

activities, you can calculate your total daily caloric expenditure.

HOW MANY CALORIES DO YOU EAT EACH DAY?

Once you have some idea of how many calories you expend each day, you need to determine how many calories you are consuming. A physically active person needs a sufficient number of calories from food to maintain body weight and composition. Determining caloric intake requires consulting food composition tables such as the ones in Appendix A. Appendix A indicates the nutritive value of commonly used foods. This chart identifies specific foods and indicates the number of calories per specified serving size. For example, if you consult Appendix A, you will see that 1 ounce of cheddar cheese provides 115 calories. Maintaining a daily food intake log like that in Lab Activity 8-5 can determine not only your caloric intake but also your eating patterns and habits. Factors unrelated to nutrition often influence what kinds of foods are selected and how much is eaten. These factors include your mood and social environment at mealtimes. From this table you may calculate your daily caloric intake.

ASSESSING YOUR CALORIC BALANCE

If the daily logs for estimating caloric intake and caloric expenditure have been accurately kept, it will be relatively easy to compare the total caloric values to determine whether you are in caloric balance. It is not easy to maintain caloric balance on a daily basis. One reason is that schedules never seem to be the same from one day to the next. Eating meals may be inconsistent, as are times spent engaged in physical activity. Estimations of caloric intake range from between 1,000 to 5,000 calories per day.

Estimations of caloric expenditure range from between 2,200 and 4,400 calories per day. Energy demands will be higher for those who are physically active and considerably higher for endurance-type athletes, who may require 7,000 calories or more per day. If you desire to lose weight, you must modify your behaviors so that you are burning more calories for energy than you are taking in. If you want to gain weight, you must consume more calories than you expend. The Worksheet for Estimating Caloric Balance (page 249) will indicate whether you are in a state of positive or negative caloric balance based on your estimation of caloric intake and expenditure.

SET POINT THEORY OF WEIGHT CONTROL

If you completed the Lab Activities and kept track of your weight, you may have noticed that although your caloric balance fluctuated from day to day, your weight did not go up or down. **Set point theory** is intended to explain why it is so difficult to lose or gain weight. It is hypothesized that the body tends to maintain a certain level of body fat. This theory maintains that the body has a "set point" or some mechanism for maintaining a specific body weight. It operates like a thermostat that is set to control a house's temperature. When the temperature in the house drops below the set point, the furnace turns on. When the temperature warms to the setting, the furnace shuts off. For people, it may be that the body's fat level is set at a particular point, and attempts to reduce this level are met with resistance by the body.

body maintains weight

set point theory: a mechanism for maintaining body weight at a specific level

It is unclear how this set point is controlled. It may be that the fat cells tend to maintain a certain degree of fat stored within them and resist efforts to reduce their size. Exercise in combination with caloric restriction appears to be the only way to reduce the set point. In any case, the set point theory is just that, a theory that may explain why so many people are unsuccessful at keeping off the fat lost through dieting.

WHAT CAN YOU DO TO LOSE BODY FAT?

There are many fat reduction techniques available; some are based on sound scientific and nutritional principles, and others are dangerous or a waste of money. Losing body fat boils down to creating a situation of negative caloric balance. First, food intake may be decreased by dieting. Second, caloric expenditure may be increased by increasing the amount of physical activity. Finally, a combination of approaches can be attempted.

LOSING BODY FAT BY DIETING

Fat loss through dieting alone is difficult. Much of what we choose to eat is influenced not by hunger but by other factors such as customs, advertising, our moods, and the attractiveness and availability of the food supply. Pizza can be delivered to your door with a phone call. Food has meaning to us; we associate sweet, "rich" desserts with rewards for good performances or just to make us feel better. Furthermore, dieting is viewed as the deprivation and punishment one must endure for overindulgence. Every so often, we literally starve ourselves, lose a few pounds, and then promptly return to our old eating habits and regain the body fat that was lost. The behavior is repeated without achieving lasting weight control. Thus periodic dieting

is ineffective. At best, long-term weight control by dieting alone is successful only 20 percent of the time.

Obviously, in any weight-loss program the goal is to lose fat, not lean tissue. Unfortunately, many popular diets, the so-called starvation diets, recommend reduction of caloric intake to dangerous levels. It is recommended that the minimum caloric intake for a female not go below 1,000 to 1,200 calories per day and for a male not below 1,200 to 1,500 calories per day. A minimum level of 1,200 calories may be needed to avoid entering a starvation metabolism. It should also be added that it is difficult to maintain adequate nutrition when caloric intake is at this level for long periods of time. Low calorie eating plans require careful planning to avoid nutritional deficits.

Starvation diets that restrict caloric intake below these recommended levels may actually reduce metabolic rate, thus making losing fat more difficult. The body's metabolic rate goes into "low gear" and conserves calories. The ideal situation is to keep the metabolic rate at normal or raise it to burn more calories. The initial weight loss that occurs with severe caloric restriction for the first few days of the diet may be encouraging. However, the majority of this weight loss is not due to the loss of much fat but results from loss of water weight (dehydration). More moderate reductions of total calories are recommended to lose body fat.

LOSING BODY FAT BY EXERCISING

Clearly, dieting alone is not the answer to long-term weight control. However, the weight lost through exercise involves primarily loss of fat tissue (estimates are as high as 90 percent) and almost no loss of lean tissue. Establishing new behaviors that include daily physical activity takes a great deal of motivation. For most of us, exercise habits were establishe early in life. Physical activity in adolescenc can prevent the formation of excess adipos tissue and results in an increase in lean bod weight. At any age, physical activity, whe combined with caloric reduction, can lead t substantial losses of body fat while preserv ing lean tissue. Keep in mind that physical ac tivity in the sedentary college student ma result in increases in muscle tissue, which i more dense and has greater weight than fe tissue. Thus, for anyone, initial attempts e weight loss through increased activity level may be frustrating. You weigh yourself an see no change or even an increase in weigh Instead of relying on scales, which provide n information about changes in body composi tion, every few weeks you should measure skinfold thickness to determine fat loss.

It must be emphasized that the increase in muscle mass will eventually produce an in crease in metabolism which in the long term helps to burn fat stores.

▶ Moderate Intensity Aerobic Activity

To maximize weight loss during exercise you can turn to the FITT principle discussed in Chapter 4. For weight loss you should exercise using an aerobic activity at intensity of 60 per cent to 70 percent of your maximum aerobic capacity or maximum heart rate. Certainly you want to expend calories during the activity. While exercising at an intensity above 70 per cent of your maximum heart rate over an ex tended period of time may allow you to burn more calories, less of those calories will be from fat. If the body can't use your fat stores it begins to utilize lean muscle stores. For the most effective weight loss we want the calories to come from fat stores, not from lean muscle stores. Increasing the time of the exercise will help to expend additional calories. Therefore, slowing down and exercising longer is a quicker and more effective route to losing weight.

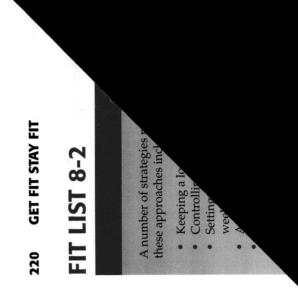

FIT LIST 8-2

A number of strategies these approaches inc

- Keeping a lo
- Controllir
- Setting
  wee

People trying to exercise solely for the pur pose of losing fat are not likely to stick with an exercise program for a long time. However, it is essential to realize that physical exercise not only will result in weight reduction from losing body fat but also may enhance car diorespiratory endurance, improve strength, and increase flexibility. For this reason, exer cise has some distinct advantages over dieting in any weight-loss program.

LOSING BODY FAT BY DIETING AND EXERCISING

Undoubtedly the most efficient method of decreasing the percentage of body fat is through some combination of diet and exer cise. A moderate caloric restriction combined with a moderate increase in caloric expendi ture will result in a negative caloric balance. This method is relatively fast and easy com pared with either of the others, especially if it focuses on changing eating habits and activity

spot reducing: a useless attempt to re duce fat stored in a specific area

... may be involved in a behavior modification approach to weight loss. Some of ... ude the following:

- ... g of the times, settings, reasons, and feelings associated with your eating
- ... g negative emotions such as boredom, loneliness, anger, and frustration while eating
- ... realistic, long-term goals (for example, loss of a pound per week instead of 5 pounds per ... k)
- ... voiding the total deprivation of enjoyable foods (occasionally reward yourself with a small treat)
- ... Eating slowly and realizing that the sacrifices you are making are what *you* feel are important for *your* health and happiness
- Putting more physical activity into your daily routine (taking stairs instead of elevators, or parking in the distant part of a parking lot, for example)
- Rewarding yourself when you reach your goals (with new clothes, sporting equipment, a vacation trip)
- Sharing your commitment to weight loss with your family and friends (then they can support your efforts)
- Keeping careful records of daily food consumption and weight change
- Being prepared to deal with occasional plateaus and setbacks in your quest for weight loss
- Cutting back consumption of "junk foods" and trying to adjust cooking habits (see the Health Links in Chapter 7).

From Payne W, Hahn D: *Understanding your health,* St Louis, 2000, McGraw-Hill.

levels. You don't have to starve and run 6 miles a day. If caloric intake is reduced by 200 to 300 calories per day and if caloric expenditure is increased by 200 to 300 calories per day, over a 7-day period this will result in a loss of approximately 3,500 calories, or 1 pound of body fat.

In any weight-loss program, the maximum weight loss should be 1 to 2 pounds per week. The rate of weight loss depends on how much body fat the person has at the start of the period of caloric restriction. In general, the greater the amount of body fat, the more rapidly one loses while on a calorie-reduced diet. This explains why some people lose 4 pounds or more the first week on a low-calorie diet. They had maintained their excess weight on relatively high calorie levels, and the reduction creates a major need for energy from fat stores.

A slower rate of weight loss indicates that the person is making minor lifestyle changes, particularly in regard to eating and physical activity behaviors, that they can maintain over time. The adoption of new behaviors and attitudes takes time. Fit List 8-2 lists suggestions for weight-loss strategies to help keep one motivated in weight control efforts.

EMPHASIZING THE LONG-HAUL APPROACH TO MINIMIZING BODY FAT

In any program for losing body fat, the "long haul" must be emphasized. It generally took a long time to accumulate that extra body fat, and it will take time to lose it safely. This fact is frustrating to the impatient individual who wants results fast. Many of these people starve themselves to lose body fat, shed some pounds, then return to their former eating habits and experience weight gain, the so-called "yo-yo" effect. This behavior makes subsequent efforts to lose body fat even more difficult, since the body tends to protect its existing fat stores.

WEIGHT-LOSS GIMMICKS AND FADS

Even educated people will resort to almost anything in a desperate effort to lose weight. Each year (especially before the summer months), Americans spend billions of dollars trying to find any method that promises they will lose weight quickly and without much effort. People are willing to spend money and time on diet programs, creams, gadgets, books, and equipment that claim to "melt pounds fast." Claims are made for rubberized suits that are supposed to "sweat" off pounds, mechanical devices to shake, vibrate, or roll off the fat; and creams and powders to remove "cellulite." Many people resort to the use of diet pills. Advertisements display physically attractive people who are reported to have lost dozens of pounds while using a device or diet plan. Most weight-loss gimmicks are based on unsound nutritional information and have no basis in scientific fact. Although people may lose weight at first, they become bored with the technique and lose interest. Any weight that was lost is regained.

What about the numerous diet plans? It seems that a new diet plan appears in a book that makes the best-seller list monthly. It is not easy to determine whether or not a diet plan is reliable and safe to follow. Table 8-1 reviews some of the more popular weight-loss plans. You will continue to see or hear about unreliable methods as long as people are unable to make the lifestyle changes needed to maintain control over their body weight.

SETTING REALISTIC GOALS FOR WEIGHT LOSS

Once you have decided to change your lifestyle to decrease your percent body fat, you must set some weight-loss goals. First, determine a desirable weight that is realistic in terms of your age, height, and bone structure. Goals must be reasonable and attainable. If you set too high a goal, you may become dissatisfied with any degree of weight loss that does not meet the goal. Ultimately, your goal should be to reach the standards for at least achieving the "good" body fat percentages for your age group as shown in Table 8-2. The second important goal is to determine a reasonable and safe rate of weight loss; it may be as low as ½ pound per week or as high as 2 pounds, depending on how much weight you have to lose. You may lose weight faster at first, but the rate slows and eventually averages out to become close to the goal rate within a few weeks.

WHAT IF YOU WANT TO INCREASE LEAN BODY MASS?

As a society we seem to be preoccupied with losing weight. However, there are people who would like to gain weight. The aim of a weight-gaining program should be to increase lean body mass—that is, muscle, as opposed to body fat. Muscle mass should be increased only by muscle work combined with an increase in food consumption. It cannot be increased by the intake of any special food or vitamin. Unfortunately, as was indicated in Chapter 7, muscle mass and weight may also be increased in an unsafe manner through the use of steroids or growth hormones.

The recommended rate of weight gain is a maximum of 1 to 2 pounds per week. This can be achieved through positive caloric balance. One pound of fat represents the equivalent of 3,500 calories. Lean body tissue, which contains less fat, more protein, and more water

TABLE 8-1
OVERVIEW OF DIET PLANS

Type of Diet	Advantages	Disadvantages	Examples
High-Protein, Low-Carbohydrate Diets			
Usually include all the meat, fish, poultry, and eggs you can eat	Rapid initial weight loss because of diuretic effect	Too low in carbohydrates	Dr. Stillman's Quick Weight Loss Diet
Occasionally permit milk and cheese in limited amounts	Very little hunger	Deficient in many nutrients—vitamin C, vitamin A (unless eggs are included), calcium, and several trace elements	Calories Don't Count by Dr. Taller
Prohibits fruits, vegetables, and any bread or cereal products		High in saturated fat, cholesterol, and total fat	Dr. Atkin's Diet Revolution
		Will result in ketosis because the major energy sources are protein and fat—both dietary and body. Extreme diets of this type could cause death	Scarsdale Diet
			Air Force Diet
			Mastering the Zone Diet
		Impossible to adhere to these diets long enough to lose any appreciable amount of weight	Carbohydrate Addict's Lifespan Program
		Dangerous for people with kidney disease	South Beach Diet
		Weight loss, which is largely water, is rapidly regained	Protein Power
		Diet does not develop a new and useful set of eating habits	Schwarzbein Principle
		Expensive	Sugar Busters
		Unpalatable after first few days	
		Difficult for dieter to eat out	
Low-Calorie, High-Protein Supplement Diets			
Usually a premeasured powder to be reconstituted with water or a prepared liquid formula	Rapid initial weight loss	Usually prescribed at dangerously low kilocalorie intake of 300 to 500 kcal	Metracal Diet
	Easy to prepare—already measured	Will result in ketosis	Cambridge Diet
	Palatable for first few days	Do not retrain dieters in acceptable eating habits	Liquid Protein Diet
			Last Chance Diet
			Diet Divas

From Guthrie HA: Introductory nutrition, St. Louis, 1989, Mosby.   *Continued*

TABLE 8-1
OVERVIEW OF DIET PLANS—CONT

Type of Diet	Advantages	Disadvantages	Examples
Low-Calorie, High-Protein Supplement Diets—cont'd	Usually fortified to provide recommended amounts of micronutrients Must be labeled if >50% protein	Overpriced; initially, users are often urged to buy several large cans of different flavors of the diet food (which is usually non-fat dried milk) Low in fiber and bulk—constipating in short amount of time Frequently cause loss of potassium with resultant weakness and heart arrhythmias Often contain poor quality protein	Oxford Diet
Restricted-Calorie, Balanced Food Plans	Sufficiently low in kilocalories to permit steady weight loss Nutritionally balanced Palatable Include readily available foods Reasonable in cost Can be adapted from family meals Permit eating out and social eating Promote a new set of eating habits	Do not appeal to people who want a "unique" diet Do not produce immediate and large weight losses	Weight Watchers Diet Prudent Diet (American Heart Association) The I Love New York UCLA Diet Time-calorie Displacement (TCD) Overeaters Anonymous The Beyond Diet Take Off Pounds Sensibly (TOPS) Fit or Fat Target Diet Ediet

Continued

TABLE 8-1
OVERVIEW OF DIET PLANS—CONT

Type of Diet	Advantages	Disadvantages	Examples
Fasting/Starvation Diet	Rapid inital loss	Nutrient deficient Danger of ketosis >60% loss is muscle <40% loss is fat Low long-term success rates	ZIP Diet 5-day Miracle Diet 3-day Diet
High-Carbohydrate Diet	Emphasizes grains, fruits, vegetables High in bulk Low in cholesterol	Limits milk, meat Nutritionally very inadequate for calcium, iron, and protein	Low Fat Diet New Beverly Hills Diet Quick Weight Loss Diet Pritikin Diet Carbohydrate Cravers Hilton Head Metabolism Diet
High-Fiber, Low-Calorie Diets	High satiety value Provide bulk	Irritating to the lower colon Decrease absorption of trace elements, especially iron Nutritionally deficient Low in protein	High Fiber Diet Volumetrics Pritikin Diet F Diet Zen Macrobiotic Diet Rice Diet Eat More, Weigh Less Heart Smart Diet

Continued

TABLE 8-1
OVERVIEW OF DIET PLANS—CONT

Type of Diet	Advantages	Disadvantages	Examples
Protein-Sparing Modified Fats <50% protein: 400 kcal	Safe under supervision High-quality protein Minimize loss of lean body mass	Decreases BMR Monotonous Expensive	Optifast Medifast Cambridge Diet Last Chance Diet Slimfast Ultrafast
Premeasured Food Plans	Provides the prescribed portion sizes—little chance of too small or too large a portion Total food programs Some provide adequate calories (1,200) Nutritionally balanced or supplemented	Expensive Do not retrain dieters in acceptable eating habits Precludes eating out or social eating Often low in bulk Monotonous Low long-term success rates	Nutri-System Carnation Plan Jenny Craig Herbalife Genesis
Limited Food Choice Diets	Reduce the number of food choices made by the users Limited opportunity to make mistakes Almost certainly low in calories after the first few days	Deficient in many nutrients, depending on the foods allowed Monotonous—difficult to adhere to Eating out and eating socially are difficult Do not retrain dieters in acceptable eating habits Low long-term success rates No scientific basis for these diets	Mayo Clinic Diet Cabbage Soup Diet Banana and milk Diet Grapefruit and cottage cheese Diet Kempner rice Diet Lecithin, vinegar, kelp, vitamin B_6 Diet Beverly Hills Diet Fit for Life Low Sodium Diet Healthy Soy Diet

TABLE 8-2
PERCENT FAT BASED ON SKINFOLDS

Rating	9%–17% Men				Rating	17%–25% Women			
	Ages 20–29	Ages 30–39	Ages 40–49	Ages 50+		Ages 20–29	Ages 30–39	Ages 40–49	Ages 50+
Dangerously Low	<5	<5	<5	<5	Dangerously Low				
Excellent	5–8.9	5–10.9	5–11.9	5–12.9	Excellent	12–16.9	12–17.9	12–19.9	12–20.9
GOOD	9–12.9	11–13.9	12–15.9	13–16.9	GOOD	17–20.9	18–21.9	20–23.9	21–24.9
Fair	13–16.9	14–17.9	16–20.9	17–21.9	Fair	21–23.9	22–24.9	24–27.9	25–30.9
Poor	17–19.9	18–22.9	21–25.9	22–27.9	Poor	24–27.9	25–29.9	28–31.9	31–35.9
Very Poor	>19.9	>22.9	>25.9	>27.9	Very Poor	>27.9	>29.9	>31.9	>35.9

than fat tissue, represents approximately 2,500 calories. Therefore to gain 1 pound of muscle, a weekly excess of approximately 2,500 calories is needed. Adding 500 to 1,000 calories daily to the usual diet will provide the energy needs of gaining 1 to 2 pounds per week and fuel the increased energy expenditure of the muscle training program. Weight training must be part of the program; otherwise, the excess energy intake will be converted to fat. Safe Tip 8-1 offers suggestions for an individual concerned about a safe weight-gaining program. For recommendations regarding weight training, refer to Chapter 5.

Athletes in training for competition require very-high-calorie diets. They often believe that more protein is needed to build bigger muscles. Actually, a relatively small amount of additional protein is needed for the muscles developed in a training program. Most Americans consume about twice the amount of protein needed; therefore, protein is obtained by eating natural food sources rather than by consuming protein supplements. Furthermore, protein supplements may have undesirable effects on the body.

One should monitor body weight weekly to ensure a gradual weight gain. Having the same person measuring skinfold thickness regularly will detect any increases in body fat. An increase in the skinfold thickness indicates a need for a reduction in caloric intake or an increase in training, or both, until it is demonstrated that the percentage of body fat is not increasing.

WHAT IS DISORDERED EATING?

To this point we have been discussing the problems with and the consequences of being overweight and of obesity. Clearly diet and eating patterns that result in overweight and obesity are the most common forms of disordered eating. Obesity represents an extreme in the eating continuum. Unfortunately for many people in our society, weight loss has

SAFE TIP 8-1

Guidelines for Gaining Weight

- Set a reasonable goal. An exercise program should begin in advance of the competing season. Rapid weight gain indicates increase in fat, not muscle.
- Follow an exercise program prescribed by a fitness professional and designed to develop the desired muscles (see Chapter 3).
- Determine the usual caloric intake, then estimate the additional calories needed daily to gain lean weight.
- For a young individual, an additional 500 to 1,000 calories per day may be needed to gain lean weight. Therefore it is important to plan both the composition and the timing of meals and snacks. The diet should be based on the food groups (see Chapter 7), with additional calories obtained from larger portions of foods rich in complex carbohydrates. It is recommended that the diet contain less than 25% of calories from fat. The fat component of the diet should be low in saturated fats and cholesterol.

become an obsession that poses a threat to health and well-being. The media bombard the public with an ideal body image that is super-model thin. This creates social and internal pressures, especially for young women, to become overly concerned with the relationship of body image to self-image. Pursuing an ideal body image, even one that is unrealistic and unhealthy, becomes an attainable goal. A person who believes that a thinner body is the key to becoming more satisfied with oneself is susceptible to adopting bizarre behaviors in an attempt to find happiness. Some people adopt such extreme dieting behavior that they literally starve themselves to death. The next sections describe some of the more common eating disorders associated

FIT LIST 8-3

Identifying Behaviors Associated with Disordered Eating

Reports or observation of the following signs or behaviors should arouse concern:

- Repeated expression of concerns about being or feeling fat even when weight is below average.
- Expressions of fear about being or becoming obese that do not diminish as weight loss continues.
- Refusal to maintain even a minimal normal weight consistent with the individual's sport, age, and height.
- Consumption of huge amounts of food not consistent with the person's weight.
- A pattern of eating substantial amounts of food, followed promptly by trips to the bathroom and resumption of eating shortly thereafter.
- Periods of severe calorie restriction or repeated days of fasting.
- Evidence of purposeless, excessive physical activity.
- Depressed mood and expression of self-deprecating thoughts after eating.
- Apparent preoccupation with the eating behavior of other people, such as friends, relatives, or teammates.
- Known or reported family history of eating disorders or family dysfunction.

with self-image problems. Also, Fit List 8-3 provides some clues to identifying those with dangerous weight-control behaviors.

BULIMIA NERVOSA

Bulimia nervosa, believed to be one of the more common eating disorders, involves recurrent episodes of binge-type eating ("pigging out") followed by purging (vomiting and laxative abuse). Usually the binge consists of foods high in calories from fat or sugar, such as bags of cookies, doughnuts, and chips. A typical binge involves the consumption of 1,000 calories or more during a 1- to 2-hour time period. These binges may occur once a month or, in severe cases, several times a day. To avoid gaining weight from the positive caloric situation, the person follows the binge with purging through vomiting, laxatives, or fasting. People who engage in such behavior tend to binge and purge in secret; in particular, the purging behavior is hidden from friends and family members.

Bulimia is most common in college-aged women who are about average in weight or not excessively overfat. Reports of bulimic behavior in young men involve the consumption of large quantities of beer and foods such as pizza followed by vomiting.

Although many people with bulimia are extroverts and socially active, they tend to have problems with interpersonal relationships. They suffer from low self-esteem and feel isolated because of their behavior. Bulimics believe that this behavior is disgusting and beyond their control. They become depressed and anxious, which in turn leads to more binging and purging episodes. In severe cases, bulimics become so obsessed with obtaining enough food and laxatives that they have little money for other needs. Sometimes they are arrested in the act of shoplifting these items from stores.

If untreated, the purging episodes can damage the body. The depressed bulimic may decide that suicide is the only solution to this abnormal behavior. If you know someone who seems to be able to eat huge amounts of food, is not physically active, yet is not gaining weight, you may suspect this disorder. It often helps to discuss the possibility of bulimia with them and

bulimia nervosa: an eating disorder involving recurrent episodes of binge-type eating followed by purging

to encourage them to obtain counseling. Treatment should focus on the causes of the behavior, including reasons for the low self-esteem and how to build supportive relationships. Individuals benefit from counseling that teaches how to cope with stress in a more constructive manner than binging and purging. Success is often measured in reducing the behavior rather than totally eliminating it. Thus it is essential to be realistic about changing bulimic behaviors; habits take time to change.

ANOREXIA NERVOSA

Anorexia nervosa is a psychological disease in which a person develops an aversion to food and a distorted body image. Over a period of time, the person loses a considerable amount of body weight so that health and life are threatened. Recently, anorexia nervosa has become a more widespread problem, although not as widespread as bulimia. About 90 percent of people with anorexia nervosa are female, and the disorder usually begins around puberty. It is very obvious that these individuals are anorexic. They are so thin that they appear to have a terminal disease such as cancer. The subcutaneous fat layer is nearly absent, so veins can be seen on arms and legs. The typical feminine shape that is due to body fat deposits is absent. Extreme physical activity behaviors are also characteristic of the illness; the anorexic may jog or work out tirelessly. The normal female hormonal cycle depends on a certain minimal level of body fat; most of these women fail to menstruate.

In certain players of sports, as well as in dancers, anorexic behaviors may be apparent, particularly for those individuals who think a thin appearance is important. These sports include gymnastics, wrestling, dancing, ballet, cheerleading, track, and, to some degree, tennis. This has been called *anorexia athletica*. These athletes seem to associate a slender appearance with the ability to perform successfully and appear more attractive.

In many instances the condition begins as an attempt to reduce body fat through caloric reduction and increased exercise. Instead of being satisfied with reaching a healthy goal weight, these individuals become obsessed with the ability to control body weight and continue the effort. They may fast, but often they eat small, precisely measured quantities of food that do not supply enough calories to fuel the high energy demands of their physical activity and maintain a reasonable amount of body fat. Reports of a combination of anorexia nervosa and bulimic behaviors are not uncommon. This is often called *bulimia nervosa*. An estimated 20 percent of those affected with this psychological disease die from the effects of severe malnutrition or the chemical imbalances created by purging.

Individuals with anorexia nervosa cannot be convinced that they are "too thin." Their body image is so distorted that even while looking at themselves in a mirror, they think they could lose some more weight. Therefore treating the condition is beyond the abilities of a health or physical educator. Simply referring the person to a health clinic is not effective unless specialists are on staff who are qualified to deal with these cases. Anorexics should be referred to a licensed psychologist or a medical doctor who specializes in treating such cases. In severe cases, long-term hospitalization is necessary. The key to treatment is getting patients to realize that they can gain control over their lives in ways that do not involve dieting. Unfortunately, many of those who do survive do not fully recover but remain underweight and fearful of any future weight gain.

> **anorexia nervosa:** a psychological disease in which a person develops an aversion to food and a distorted body image

FEMALE ATHLETE TRIAD SYNDROME

Female athlete triad syndrome is a potentially fatal problem that involves a combination of an eating disorder (either bulimia or anorexia), amenorrhea, and osteoporosis (diminished bone density). It occurs primarily in female athletes. The incidence of this syndrome is uncertain; however, some studies have suggested that eating disorders in female athletes may be as high as 62 percent in certain sports, with amenorrhea being common in at least 60 percent. However, the major risk of this syndrome is that the bone lost in osteoporosis may not be regained.

SUMMARY

- Body composition analysis indicates the percentage of total body weight composed of fat tissue versus the percentage composed of lean tissue.
- The size and number of adipose cells determine percent body fat, which can be measured by measuring the thickness of the subcutaneous fat with a skinfold caliper at specific areas.
- Changes in percent body fat are caused almost entirely by a change in caloric balance, which is a function of the number of calories taken in and the number of calories expended.
- Caloric expenditure may be calculated by maintaining accurate records of the number of calories expended for metabolic needs and in activities performed during the course of a day. Caloric intake measurement requires recording the number of calories consumed.
- Body fat can be lost either by increasing caloric expenditure through exercise or by decreasing caloric intake through reducing food intake. Most effective is a combination of moderate caloric restriction and a moderate increase in physical exercise during the course of each day.
- Fat loss should be accomplished gradually over a long period.
- Weight gain should be accomplished by increasing caloric intake and engaging in a weight-training program to increase lean body mass.
- Bulimia nervosa is an eating disorder that involves periodic binging and subsequent purging.
- Anorexia nervosa is a form of mental illness in which a person reduces food intake and increases energy expenditure to the extent that the loss of body fat threatens health and life.

SUGGESTED READINGS

Agatston, A. 2003. *The South Beach Diet: The delicious, doctor-designed, foolproof plan for healthy weight loss.* Emmaus, PA: Rodale Press.

Atkins, R. 2002. *Dr. Atkins new diet revolution.* New York: Harper Collins Publishers.

Barnes, D. E. 2004. Eating well and controlling your weight. In *Action plan for diabetes,* edited by D. E. Barnes. Champaign, IL: Human Kinetics.

Beals, K. A. 2004. *Disordered eating among athletes: A comprehensive guide for health professionals.* Champaign, IL: Human Kinetics.

Brownell, K., and C. Fairburn. 2002. *Eating disorders and obesity: A comprehensive handbook.* New York: Guilford Press.

Brownell, K., and K. Horgen. 2003. *Food fight: The inside story of America's obesity crisis—and what we can do about it.* New York: McGraw-Hill.

Byrne, S., and N. McLean. 2001. Eating disorders in athletes: A review of the literature. *Journal of Science and Medicine in Sport* 4(2):145–59.

Claude-Pierre, P. 1999. *The secret language of eating disorders.* New York: Vintage Books.

Coleman, E. 2002. The ACSM weight-loss position stand. *Sports Medicine Digest* 24(3):29, 31.

Cruise, J. 2005. *The 3-hour diet: How low-carb diets make you fat and timing makes you thin.* New York: Harper Collins.

Fulton, J. E., M. T. McGuire, C. J. Caspersen, and W. H. Dietz. 2001. Interventions for weight loss and weight gain prevention among youth: Current issues. *Sports Medicine* 31(3):153–65.

Jakicic, J. M., K. Clark, E. Coleman, and J. E. Donnelly. 2001. Appropriate intervention strategies for weight loss and prevention of weight regain for adults. *Medicine and Science in Sports and Exercise* 33(12):2145–56.

Karinch, M., ed. 2002. *Diets designed for athletes.* Champaign, IL: Human Kinetics.

Karinch, M. 2002. Gaining or cutting weight. In *Diets designed for athletes,* edited by M. Karinch. Champaign, IL: Human Kinetics.

Kruskall, L. J., L. J. Hohnson, and S. L. Meacham. 2002. Eating disorders and disordered eating—Are they the same? *ACSM's Health and Fitness Journal* 6(3):6–12.

Lebrun, C. M., and J. S. Rumball. 2002. Female athlete triad. *Sports Medicine and Arthroscopy Review* 10(1):23–32.

Litt, A. 2004. Lessons on losing weight. In *Fuel for young athletes,* edited by A. Litt. Champaign, IL: Human Kinetics.

Loucks, A. B. 2004. Energy balance and body composition in sports and exercise. *Journal of Sports Sciences* 22(1):1–14.

McArdle, W., F. Katch, and V. Katch. 2001. *Exercise physiology, energy, nutrition and human performance.* Baltimore: Lippincott Williams, & Wilkins.

McGraw, P. 2003. *The ultimate weight solution: The 7 keys to weight loss freedom.* New York: Simon and Schuster Adult Publishing.

McQuillan, S., E. Khosrova, and E. Saltzman. 1998. *The complete idiot's guide to losing weight.* Indianapolis: Macmillan.

Miller, W. C. 2001. Effective diet and exercise treatments for overweight and recommendations for intervention. *Sports Medicine* 31(10):717–24.

Nelson, C. 2003. In female athlete "triad," amenorrhea not necessary for poor bone quality: Is "disordered eating" the culprit? *Sports Medicine Digest* 25(6):61, 63–66, 70–71.

Schmitz, K. H. 2001. Effects on obesity of exercise- and diet-induced weight loss. *Clinical Journal of Sports Medicine* 11(2):130.

Schnirring, L. 2001. Body fat testing: Evaluating the options. *Physician and Sports Medicine* 29(5):13–14, 16.

Schultz, S. 2001. Disordered eating. In *Sports medicine handbook,* edited by S. J. Shultz et al. Indianapolis: National Federation of State High School Associations.

Sharkey, B. J. 2002. Weight-control programs. In *Fitness and health,* 5th ed., edited by B. J. Sharkey. Champaign, IL: Human Kinetics.

Swain, D. P., and B. C. Leutholz. 2002. Exercise prescription for weight loss. In *Exercise prescription: A case study approach to the ACSM guidelines,* edited by D. P. Swain and B. C. Leutholtz. Champaign, IL: Human Kinetics.

Thompson, J. 2003. *Handbook of eating disorders and obesity.* Hoboken, NJ: John Wiley & Sons.

Tribole, E. 2004. Losing and maintaining weight. In *Eating on the run,* edited by E. Tribole. 3rd ed., Champaign, IL: Human Kinetics

Van Marken Lichtenbelt, W. D., and F. Hartgens. 2004. Body composition changes in bodybuilders: A method comparison. *Medicine and Science in Sports and Exercise* 36(3):490–97.

Weyers, A. M., et al. 2002. Comparison of methods for assessing body composition changes during weight loss. *Medicine and Science in Sports and Exercise* 34(3):497–502.

Wong, S. L., P. T. Katzmarzyk, and M. Z. Nichaman. 2004. Cardiorespiratory fitness is associated with lower abdominal fat independent of body mass index. *Medicine and Science in Sports and Exercise* 36(2):286–91.

SUGGESTED WEB SITES

Food and Nutrition Center

Provides information on nutrition and safe dieting from WebMD.
http://my.webmd.com/nutrition

iVillage.com's Better Health's Diet & Nutrition Center

Get the latest dieting news and research, expert advice, interactive health assessment tools, scheduled chats, message boards and more.
www.betterhealth.com/diet

National Association of Anorexia Nervosa and Associated Disorders (ANAD)

This is the oldest nonprofit organization helping victims of eating disorders and their families.
http://members.aol.com/anad20/index.html

National Eating Disorders Organization

Get answers to any questions about eating disorders and their prevention. If you have (or know someone who has) an eating disorder, NEDO has information that may help.
www.laureate.com/nedointro.html

Weight Loss Support Groups

This is a comprehensive directory and list of weight support groups that can help you lose weight.
www.weightdirectory.com/support.htm

Weight Loss Tips

This site presents tips from *Prevention Magazine.*
www.healthyideas.com/report/980610/

CHAPTER 9

Practicing **Safe Fitness**

Objectives

After completing this chapter, you should be able to do the following:

- Realize that participation in physical activity sometimes creates situations in which injuries may occur.
- Discuss the principles and guidelines of injury prevention.
- Describe fractures, contusions, ligament sprains, muscle strains, muscle soreness, tendinitis, and bursitis.
- Identify the causes of low back pain and describe how such pain can best be avoided.
- Describe the RICE approach to the initial treatment of injuries.
- Identify exercises that may be dangerous or contraindicated.
- Discuss the precautions that should be exercised when working out in either a hot or a cold environment.

HOW CAN YOU PREVENT INJURIES?

Certainly, you don't participate in physical activities with the idea that you are going to be injured. Ironically, the nature of participation in any type of physical activity increases the possibility that injury will occur. Fitness programs will hopefully make you more fit and should ultimately reduce the possibility of injury. The overload demands placed on the body during exercise enable it to handle added stresses and strains that occur during physical activity. Thus the first step in practicing "safe fitness" and in preventing injuries associated with physical activity involves designing a well-planned fitness program based on the principles of overload, progression, consistency, individuality, and safety.

If you are involved in some physical activity and realize that a specific part of your body is causing discomfort or pain that affects your performance, it is strongly recommended that this problem be evaluated immediately. Injuries should be evaluated by persons experienced in dealing with sport-related injuries, such as physicians, physical therapists, or athletic trainers. The sooner an injury is diagnosed and

KEY TERMS

low back pain	*heat-related illness*
RICE	*hypothermia*

treatment begun, the less chance there is that continued activity will make the problem worse. The popular quote "No pain, no gain" holds no credibility with regard to an activity program.

Pain indicates that something is wrong. You should stop activity immediately and determine what is producing the pain. There is a great difference between overloading the system while you are working hard during exercise and pushing yourself to exercise when you are hurt. When you are dealing with injuries, common sense is of prime importance. Injuries are to a large extent preventable, and paying attention to some simple guidelines can make exercise safer and more enjoyable.

Perhaps the biggest mistake that people make when beginning a physical activity program is starting at a level that is too advanced and then trying to progress too quickly. If you are physically inactive, you must begin at a much lower level and gradually increase your level of activity. Some people stop exercising for a variety of reasons, and when they start exercising again, there is a tendency to try to begin where they left off. They do too much, too fast, too soon. Safe Tip 9-1 provides you with some tips for practicing "safe fitness."

WHAT TYPES OF INJURIES MIGHT OCCUR IN AN EXERCISE PROGRAM?

Several different types of injuries typically occur through participation in physical activity. These injuries are briefly identified here.

Fractures—Cracks or breaks in bones that usually require some type of immobilization in a cast.

Contusions—A bruise of the skin, fat, or muscle tissue.

SAFE TIP 9-1

Injury Prevention

- Always warm up properly before engaging in any activity.
- Do not neglect the cool-down period after exercise.
- Make certain that muscles are stretched sufficiently. Use full range-of-motion static stretching during an active warm-up period and vigorous stretching during the cool-down period.
- Avoid passive overstretching to reduce the possibility of injury to the ligaments or joint capsule.
- Avoid any movements, exercises, or activities that produce compression or impingement of joint motion.
- Begin at a low intensity and progress within your individual limits to higher intensities. Do not try to do too much too soon.
- Avoid holding your breath and straining too hard during intense activity.
- Choose a level of intensity that is compatible with your abilities in terms of strength, power, and endurance.
- Select the appropriate clothing for exercising in hot or cold environments.
- Make sure you are acclimated to the environment in which you are exercising, regardless of whether it is extremely hot or cold.
- Select and use high-quality equipment when engaging in any physical activity. Breakdown of cheap or low-quality equipment may prove to be more expensive in the long run should injury occur.
- Listen to what your body is telling you. If you experience pain during activity, stop immediately.
- Do not engage in any activity that you think may have the potential to result in injury.

Sprains—Damage to a ligament, which connects bone to bone, thus providing a support to a joint.

Strains—Separation or tearing of muscle fibers.

Muscle soreness—Delayed onset pain in muscle following physical activities that you are not accustomed to.

Tendinitis—Inflammation of a tendon, which connects muscle to bone.

Bursitis—Inflammation of a bursa, which is a membrane that functions to reduce friction between bone and muscle, ligament and bone, muscle and ligament, etc.

A detailed discussion of the many injuries, both acute and chronic, that can occur with participation in physical activity is beyond the scope of this text. However, a few injuries seem to occur frequently with physical activity. Table 9-1 provides a brief description of the causes and signs of the more common injuries.

LOW BACK PAIN

There is no question that **low back pain** is one of the most common, annoying, and disabling ailments known. Many causes and cures for low back pain have been proposed. However, so many different things can cause pain in the

> **low back pain:** pain in the lower back caused by muscle imbalances, muscle strain, ligament sprain, or disk degeneration

lower back that no single incriminating cause or absolute cure can be identified.

▶Causes of Low Back Pain

Of all the causes of low back pain, none is more common than imbalances between the strength and flexibility of the various muscle groups associated with the lower back. In most cases, the abdominal muscles are weak and stretched out, the spinal muscles are tight and inflexible, and the hamstring muscles are also tight. Therefore an exercise program that attempts to increase the strength and the tone of the abdominal muscles, improve the flexibility of the spinal muscles in the lower back, and stretch the tight hamstring muscles may alleviate many complaints of low back pain. Health Link 9-1 details some of the causes.

▶Prevention of Low Back Pain

Some knowledge of the source of low back pain is important to treat the injury, but it is more important to understand how low back pain can be avoided. To prevent low back pain, the practice of avoiding unnecessary stresses and strains should be integrated into your daily life. The back is subjected to these stresses and strains when one is standing, lying, sitting, lifting, and exercising. Care should be taken to avoid postures and positions that can cause injury. Figure 9-1 shows examples of safe postures.

Exercises for Treating Low Back Pain. The specific exercises used to treat low back pain will vary depending upon the specific conditions causing the pain. In general, back pain

HEALTH LINK 9-1

Causes of Low Back Pain

Low back pain may result from the following associated problems:

1. Disk degeneration and rupture (herniation).
2. A sprain of the intervertebral ligaments in the lumbosacral region of the spine.
3. A sprain of the ligaments in the sacroiliac region.
4. Muscle imblances—weak abdominal muscles/tight low back muscles/tight hamstrings.

TABLE 9-1 SUMMARY OF COMMON INJURIES ASSOCIATED WITH PHYSICAL ACTIVITY	
Injury	**Cause/Signs and Symptoms**
Achilles tendinitis	A chronic tendinitis of the "heel cord" or muscle tendon located on the back of the lower leg just above the heel. It may result from any activity that involves forcefully pushing off of the foot and ankle, such as running and jumping. This inflammation involves swelling, warmth, tenderness to touch, and pain during walking and especially running.
Ankle sprains	Stretching or tearing of one or several ligaments that provide stability to the ankle joint. Ligaments on the outside or lateral side of the ankle are more commonly injured by rolling the sole of the foot downward and to the inside. Pain is intense immediately after injury followed by considerable swelling, tenderness, loss of joint motion, and some discoloration over a 24- to 48-hour period.
Athlete's foot	A fungal infection that most often occurs between the toes or on the sole of the foot and that causes itching, redness, and pain. If the skin breaks down, a bacterial infection is possible. It may be prevented by keeping the area dry; using powder; and wearing clean, dry socks that do not hold moisture. It is best treated using over-the-counter medications (e.g., Micatin) that contain the active ingredient miconazole.
Blisters	Friction blisters can occur anywhere on the skin where there is friction or repetitive rubbing, but they most often occur on the hands or feet. The blister takes on a reddish color, becoming raised and filling with fluid. It can be quite painful, and if it occurs on the foot it may be disabling. Taking measures to reduce friction, such as wearing gloves, breaking in new footwear, and wearing appropriately fitting socks, is helpful in preventing blisters.
Groin pull	A muscle strain that occurs in the muscles located on the inside of the upper thigh just below the pubic area resulting either from an overstretch of the muscle or from a contraction of the muscle that meets excessive resistance. Pain will be produced by flexing the hip and leg across the body or by stretching the muscles in a groin stretch position.
Hamstring pull	A muscle strain of the muscles of the back of the upper thigh that most often occurs while sprinting. In most cases, severe pain is caused simply by walking or in any movement that involves knee flexion or extension of the hamstring muscle. Some swelling, tenderness to touch, and possibly some discoloration extending down the back of the leg may occur in severe strains.
Patellofemoral knee pain	Nonspecific pain occurring around the knee, in particular the front part of the knee, or kneecap (patella). Pain can result from many causes, including improper movement of the kneecap in knee flexion and extension; tendinitis of tendon just below the kneecap caused by repetitive jumping; bursitis (swelling) either above or below the kneecap; osteoarthritis (joint surface degeneration) between the kneecap and thigh bone. This may possibly involve inflammation with swelling, tenderness, warmth, and pain with movement.

TABLE 9-1
SUMMARY OF COMMON INJURIES ASSOCIATED WITH PHYSICAL ACTIVITY—CON'T

Injury	Cause/Signs and Symptoms
Plantar fascitis or arch pain	Chronic inflammation and irritation of the broad ligament that runs from the heel to the base of the toes, forming part of the long arch on the bottom of the foot. It most often occurs in runners or walkers. It is frequently caused by wearing shoes that do not have adequate arch support. At first, pain is localized at the attachment on the heel; it then tends to move more onto the arch. It is most painful when you first get out of bed and then in the evening when you have been on your feet for long periods.
Quadriceps contusion, "charlie horse"	A deep bruise of the muscles in the front part of the thigh caused by a forceful impact or by some object that results in severe pain, swelling, discoloration, and difficulty flexing the knee or extending the hip. Small calcium deposits may develop in the muscle without adequate rest and protection from additional trauma.
Racquetball or golfer's elbow	Similar to tennis elbow, except the pain is located on the medial or inside surface of the arm just above the elbow at the attachment of the wrist and finger flexor muscles. It occurs in those activities that involve repeated forceful flexion of the wrist, such as hitting a forehand stroke in racquetball. Golfers also develop this inflammation in the trailing arm from too much wrist flexion in a golf swing.
Shin splints	A "catch-all" term used to refer to any pain that occurs in the front part of the lower leg or shin, most often caused by excessive running on hard surfaces. Pain is usually caused by muscle strains of those muscles that move the ankle and foot at their attachment points in the skin. It is usually worse during activity. In more severe cases it may be caused by stress fractures of the long bones in the lower leg, with the pain being worse after activity is stopped.
Shoulder impingement	Chronic irritation and inflammation of muscle tendons and a bursa underneath the tip of the shoulder, which results from repeated forceful overhead motions of the shoulder such as in swimming, throwing, spiking a volleyball, or a tennis serve. Pain is felt when the arm is extended across the body above shoulder level.
Sunburn	An extremely common problem for anyone who exercises outside. Overexposure to the sun can ultimately cause certain types of skin cancer. It is critical to protect yourself from the sun by applying sunscreens and paying attention to the SPF (sun protection factor). Wearing a hat and other protective clothing to cover the skin can further help to minimize overexposure to ultraviolet light.
Tennis elbow	Chronic irritation and inflammation of the lateral or outside surface of the arm just above the elbow at the attachment of the muscles that extend the wrist and fingers. It results from any activity that requires forceful extension of the wrist. This typically occurs in tennis players who are using faulty techniques hitting backhand ground strokes. Pain is felt above the elbow after forcefully extending the wrist against resistance or applying pressure over the muscle attachment above the elbow.

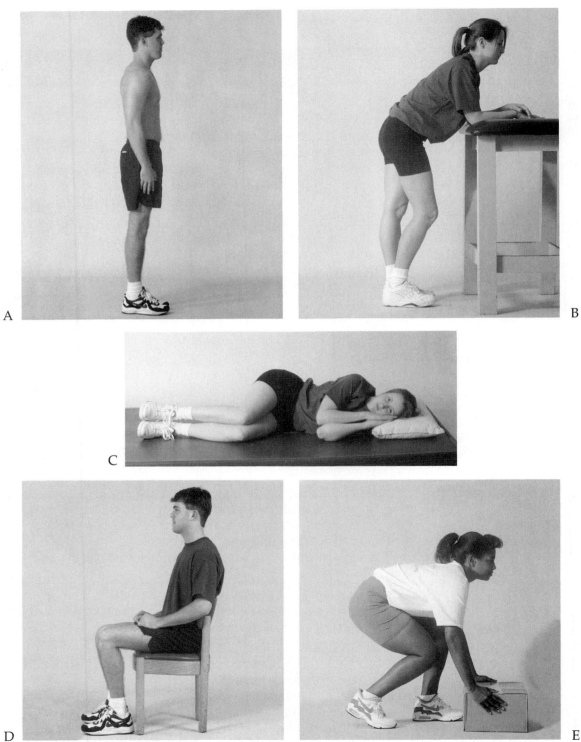

FIGURE 9-1. EXAMPLES OF SAFE POSTURES

A, Ideal standing posture. B, Correct leaning posture. C, Correct sleeping position.
D, Ideal sitting position. E, Correct lifting position.

may be caused by tightness or a lack of fl
bility in a number of different muscle gr
related to movement of the low back. Fl
bility exercises for muscle groups that
need to be stretched in treating low back
were discussed and illustrated previousl
Chapter 6 (see Figures 6-10 through 6-
Strengthening exercises can involve ei
flexion or extension exercises. Flexion e
cises are used to strengthen the abdom
muscles and to stretch the low back mus
(see Figures 5-33, 5-36, and 5-37). Exten:
exercises are used to strengthen back ex
sors and to stretch the abdominal mus
(see Figures 5-39B and 5-42). Core stabil
tion exercises discussed previously in Cl
ter 5 are widely used to treat low back
(see Figure 5-42).

TREATMENT AND MANAGEMENT OF INJURIES

Initial first-aid and management techniques for most fitness injuries associated with physical activity are fairly simple and straightforward. Regardless of which type of injury we are talking about, there is one problem they all have in common—swelling. Swelling is most likely during the first 72 hours after an injury. Once swelling has occurred, the healing process is significantly retarded. The injured area cannot return to normal until all the swelling is gone. Therefore everything that is done in terms of first-aid management of any of these conditions should be directed toward controlling the swelling. If the swelling can be controlled initially in the acute state of injury, it is likely that the time required for rehabilitation will be significantly reduced.

To control and severely limit the amount of swelling, the RICE principle can be applied. **RICE** stands for Rest, Ice, Compression, and Elevation (Figure 9-2). Each factor plays a critical role in limiting swelling, and all four methods should be used simultaneously.

WHAT EXERCISES SHO BE AVOIDED?

Throughout this text, an eff
recommend specific exe
fective and safe. Ove
have recommende

approximately 72 hours before a rehabilitation program is begun.

Ice—Ice should be applied to the injured area in a plastic bag to slow bleeding and for decreasing pain.

Compression—The purpose of compression is to reduce the amount of space available for swelling by applying pressure around the injured area using an elastic wrap (such as an Ace bandage).

Elevation—The injured part, particularly an extremity, should be elevated to eliminate the effects of gravity on blood pooling in the extremities.

The goal of rehabilitation should be to return the person to the usual physical activities as quickly and as safely as possible. Long-term rehabilitation programs require the supervision of a trained professional if they are going to be safe and effective. An injury that is not given proper rehabilitation may continue to cause many problems with increasing age.

RICE: initial first-aid technique for treating injuries including rest, ice, compression, and elevation

...rt has been made to ...rcises that are both ef-... the years, other sources ...d and widely used a number of exercises that place abnormal stresses, strains, or compression forces on particular muscles or joints. Such exercises potentially predispose these structures to injury. Appropriate stretching, strengthening, conditioning, and in some cases corrective exercises are described in detail within individual chapters. Figures 9-3 through 9-14 identify a series of exercises that for one

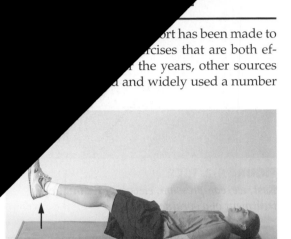

FIGURE 9-3. STRAIGHT-LEG LIFTS.
Used for strengthening abdominal muscles and hip flexors. Tends to tilt the pelvis forward, thus causing hyperextension of the lower back, which compresses the intervertebral disks. Alternative safe exercises: See Figures 5-33, 5-36 to 5-38.

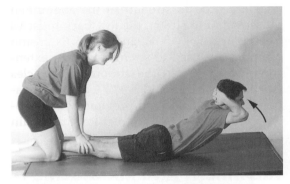

FIGURE 9-4. BACK HYPEREXTENSIONS.
Used to strengthen lower back muscles and stretch abdominal muscles. Causes compression of intervertebral disks with possible disk herniation or spinal nerve impingement. Alternative safe exercise: See Figure 5-42.

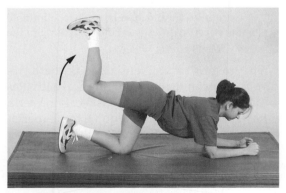

FIGURE 9-5. DONKEY KICKS.
Used to develop extensor muscles of the lower back. Involves a ballistic backward and upward kick with the leg and an extension of the neck. Causes compression of intervertebral disks and possible disk herniation or spinal nerve impingement. Alternative safe exercise: See Figure 5-39B.

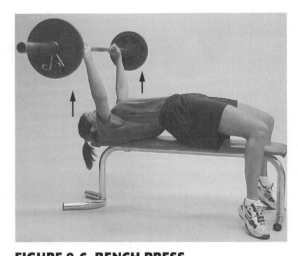

FIGURE 9-6. BENCH PRESS.
Used for strengthening pectoral and triceps muscles. This lift, when done with the feet on the floor and an arched back, hyperextends the lower back. Alternative safe exercise: See Figure 5-5.

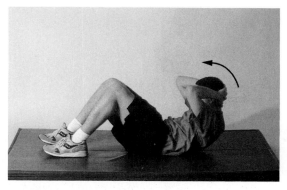

FIGURE 9-7. SIT-UPS WITH HANDS BE-HIND NECK.
Used for strengthening abdominal muscles. Pulls head and neck into hyperflexed position, stretching the intervertebral joint ligaments of the cervical spine. Alternative safe exercise: See Figure 5-33.

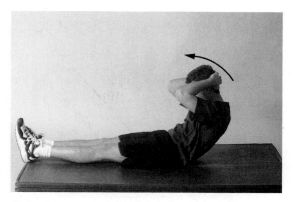

FIGURE 9-8. STRAIGHT-LEG SIT-UPS.
Causes a forward tilt of the pelvis, placing the lower back in a hyperextended position, thus adding unnecessary compression forces. Alternative safe exercise: See Figure 5-33.

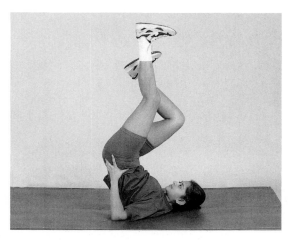

FIGURE 9-9. UP-RIGHT BICYCLING.
Used for strengthening abdominal muscles. Places the cervical and upper thoracic regions of the spine in a hyperflexed position, creating increased compression forces on intervertebral disks and stretching intervertebral ligaments. Alternative safe exercise: See Figure 5-38.

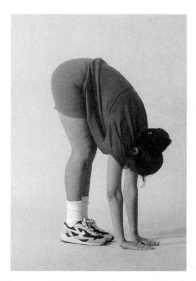

FIGURE 9-10. STANDING TOE-TOUCHES.
Used to stretch the hamstring muscles. Causes hyperextension of the knees and also pressure in the lower back, especially if the hamstring muscles are tight. Alternative safe exercises: See Figures 6-10 and 6-15.

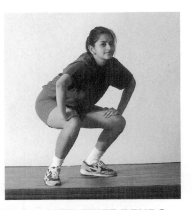

FIGURE 9-11. DEEP KNEE BENDS.
Used for strengthening hip and knee extensors. Places extreme compressive forces on the knee joint, stressing ligaments, joint capsule, and cartilage (menisci). Alternative safe exercise: See Figure 5-40.

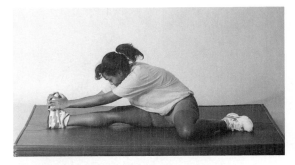

FIGURE 9-12. HURDLERS' STRETCH.
Used for stretching the quadriceps muscle and hamstring muscles. Rotation of the tibia with compression of the knee joint causes stress to the medial ligaments and compression of the medial cartilage. Alternative safe exercises: See Figures 6-12 and 6-15.

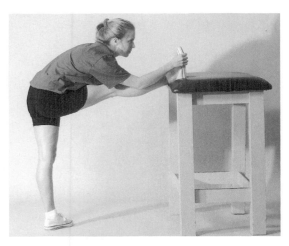

FIGURE 9-13. BAR STRETCH.
Used for stretching hamstring muscles. Hyperextends the knee, placing stress on the posterior joint capsule and ligaments. Also stretches and may irritate the sciatic nerve, which innervates most of the muscles in the posterior leg. Alternative safe exercise: See Figure 6-15.

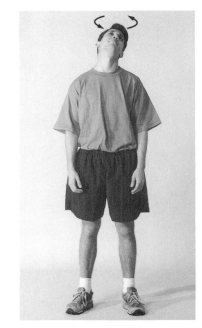

FIGURE 9-14. NECK CIRCLES.
Used for range of motion in the cervical spine. Requires hyperextension of the cervical spine, which causes unnecessary compression of the cervical intervertebral disks. Alternative safe exercise: Stretching should be done statically in all directions.

reason or another are *not* recommended as being safe and may potentially result in injury.

WHAT PRECAUTIONS SHOULD YOU TAKE WHEN EXERCISING IN HOT OR COLD ENVIRONMENTS?

EXERCISING IN THE HEAT

Regardless of your level of physical conditioning, extreme caution must be taken when exercising in extreme environmental climates. Prolonged exposure to extreme heat can result in heat stress. Heat stress is certainly preventable, but each year many people will suffer illness or perhaps death from some heat-related cause. People who exercise in the heat are particularly vulnerable to heat stress. Body temperature must be maintained within a normal range. Maintaining a normal temperature in a hot environment depends on the ability of the body to eliminate heat. It should be obvious that heat-related problems have the greatest chance of occurring on those days when the sun is bright and the temperature and relative humidity are high. But it is certainly true that various forms of heat stress, including heat cramps, heat exhaustion, or heatstroke, can occur whenever the body's ability to dissipate heat is impaired.

▶ Heat Cramps

Heat cramps are extremely painful muscle spasms that most commonly occur in the calf and abdomen, although any muscle can be involved. Heat cramps may be prevented by adequate replacement of water. The immediate treatment for heat cramps is ingestion of large quantities of a sports drink or water and mild stretching with ice massage of the muscle in spasm. Ingestion of salt tablets is not recommended. Various sport drinks have been rec-

ommended and appear to be more effective than water in preventing heat cramps.

▶ Heat Exhaustion

Like heat cramps, heat exhaustion results from inadequate replacement of fluids lost through sweating. Clinically, the victim of heat exhaustion will collapse and manifest profuse sweating, pale skin, mildly elevated temperature, dizziness, rapid breathing, and rapid pulse. Immediate treatment of heat exhaustion requires ingestion of large quantities of sport drinks or water. If possible, the person should be placed in a cool environment, although it is more essential to replace fluids.

▶ Heatstroke

Unlike heat cramps and heat exhaustion, heatstroke is a serious, life-threatening emergency. The specific cause of heatstroke is unknown; however, there is a breakdown of the sweating mechanism, and the body loses the ability to sweat. It is characterized by sudden collapse with loss of consciousness; red, relatively dry skin; and most important, a very high body temperature. Heatstroke can occur suddenly and without warning. Usually, the victim will not experience signs of heat cramps or heat exhaustion. Every first-aid effort should be directed to lowering body temperature. It is imperative that the victim be transported to a hospital as quickly as possible. The possibility of death from heatstroke can be significantly reduced if body temperature is lowered to normal within 45 minutes.

▶ Prevention of Heat-Related Illness

To a large extent **heat-related illness** can be prevented by simply paying attention to the following recommendations.

heat-related illness: exercising in a hot environment may cause heat cramps, heat exhaustion, or heatstroke

Acclimatization. It is most important to acclimate yourself to the existing heat and humidity conditions. This is the process of gradually preparing your body to be able to work in heat by slowly exposing the system to the stresses of a hot, humid environment. Heat dramatically reduces performance capabilities, and abrupt exposure to these conditions can predispose a person to heat-related illness. Acclimatization to heat generally occurs rapidly, usually within 5 to 7 days of gradually increasing periods of exercise in the heat. It is enhanced by being in good physical condition and by adequate fluid replacement.

Replacing Fluids. During hot weather it is essential to continually replace fluids lost through evaporation by drinking large quantities of fluid, regardless of whether you are thirsty. There is little question that adequate replacement of fluids is the best defense against heat stress. The most recent research has indicated that sport drinks are recommended as the most effective fluid replacement during exercise. Fluids should be replenished as often and in as great a quantity as necessary during exercise. (See Chapter 7.)

Clothing. When exercising in the heat, wear as little clothing as possible to allow maximal evaporation. Light-colored, 100 percent cotton material allows maximal evaporation. Caution should be used when wearing a hat because about 40 percent of all heat lost from the body is lost through the head. Thus a hat tends to interfere with keeping cool. The use of sunscreens and sunglasses is also recommended to reduce the long-term effects of exposure to the sun.

Exercise Your Common Sense When Exercising. If possible, do not exercise during the hottest parts of the day—between 11:00 AM and 4:00 PM. The temperature is usually highest at about 4:00 PM. Try to avoid exercising on surfaces such as asphalt, concrete, or Astroturf, which tend to absorb and hold heat. If you experience any of the heat-related problems, stop the activity immediately, get into a cool environment, and drink large quantities of cool water. Common sense is the best prevention for heat stress.

EXERCISING IN THE COLD

Although being able to dissipate heat is a problem in hot, humid weather, conserving heat becomes a major concern when exercising in cold weather. It is essential to consider the environmental factors that may combine to significantly lower body temperature or produce **hypothermia.** These major factors are temperature, dampness, and wind, which collectively can be a real problem. Most cases of hypothermia occur when the temperature is in the 50 to 60°F range and when it is also damp and windy. Hypothermia results when the body's temperature drops below 35°C (95°F). Essentially it is a breakdown in the body's ability to produce heat. Initially there is shivering followed by loss of coordination and difficulty speaking. As the body's temperature continues to drop, shivering stops, the muscles stiffen, and the person becomes unconscious. People who have hypothermia should be taken to the hospital for treatment, and all efforts should be directed toward elevating body temperature. Safe Tip 9-2 provides recommendations that may help reduce the chances of hypothermia.

PHYSICAL ACTIVITY DURING PREGNANCY

In the past, pregnancy was considered to be an abnormal condition. Today it is recognized as an altered physical state in which the woman's body undergoes a variety of changes to support the development of an unborn baby. The internal environment is very protective of the unborn baby. The developing baby is surrounded by the amniotic fluid, which acts as a shock absorber, dispersing the force of any direct blow to the mother's abdomen.

hypothermia: exercising in cold can cause a lowered body temperature

SAFE TIP 9-2

Hypothermia Prevention

- Use common sense, and be aware of the environmental conditions that predispose to hypothermia.
- Wear a hat to reduce loss of body heat through the head.
- Dress in layers of clothing, which can be removed layer by layer to prevent sweating. Remember that dampness is one of the more critical factors. If possible, wear materials such as Gortex, which allow moisture to escape from the body while keeping out moisture from the environment.
- Wear sufficiently protective clothing on the feet, hands, ears, and neck to prevent frostbite.
- Gradually acclimate yourself to exercising in the cold. Acclimatization to exercising in the cold is just as important as acclimatization when exercising in a hot, humid environment.

The type of exercise recommended will depend on the condition of the woman when her pregnancy begins and the health of the pregnancy. The pregnant woman should avoid becoming overheated. When the woman's body temperature rises, the unborn baby's environment also heats up. This temperature increase has been linked to birth defects, especially if it occurs during the first 3 months of pregnancy.

The key to being able to exercise during pregnancy is to become fit before getting pregnant. It is advisable to curtail contact sports and sports that involve severe exertion, especially in highly competitive situations.

The following are suggested activities that can be done during pregnancy:

- Swimming seems to be suitable throughout the pregnancy. It is self-limiting, and the individual may perform at her own speed. Water is good for relaxation of muscles and provides a soothing effect. Pregnancy-induced changes in body composition make the female more buoyant, and swimming remains easy as pregnancy advances. Swimming may be started during pregnancy even though the woman had not been swimming before.
- Bicycling is another non-weight-bearing activity. A stationary bike may be preferable to standard cycling because of weight and balance changes during pregnancy. Also, it is possible to control climate indoors so that the expectant mother does not become overheated.
- Walking is an excellent activity during pregnancy, even though it is weight-bearing. Walking keeps the muscles of the trunk, pelvis, and legs in good tone during pregnancy. Like swimming and cycling, it offers aerobic benefits as well.
- Running is an activity of questionable value for the pregnant female. It is likely that few problems would develop during the first two trimesters of pregnancy. However, during the last trimester, running should be done with extra caution because of expected increases in body weight.
- Aerobic exercise, like running, should be avoided during the third trimester, especially because it involves a considerable amount of bouncing.

The American College of Obstetrics and Gynecology has developed guidelines for pregnant women to follow when exercising. Fit List 9-1 summarizes guidelines designed to ensure the safety, health, and fitness of the pregnant woman and her developing baby.

SUMMARY

- Listen to what your body is telling you. The "No pain, no gain" mentality will likely worsen an existing injury. The best way to prevent injury is to pay close attention to the basic principles of training and conditioning.

FIT LIST 9-1

Guidelines for Exercise During Pregnancy

- Consult your physician before starting an exercise program.
- It is better to modify your prepregnancy exercise program than to start a new one.
- Do not exercise to exhaustion.
- Avoid any activities that involve bouncing, jarring, or twisting motions.
- Avoid any activities that require rapid stops and starts.
- Do not perform any activity that puts the abdomen in jeopardy.
- Be aware that your body's center of gravity changes during pregnancy; it may be harder to keep your balance during some exercises.
- Do not exercise while lying on your back, particularly after the fourth month.
- Do not exercise during hot, humid weather.
- Drink plenty of fluids before, after, and sometimes during the workout.
- During your workout, make sure your temperature stays below 100°F and your heart rate does not exceed 140 beats per minute.

Modified from Alexander L. L., LaRosa J. H.: New dimensions in women's health, Boston, 1994, Jones & Bartlett; and Agostini R., Medical and orthopedic issues of active and athletic women, Philadelphia, 1994, Hanley & Belfus.

- Low back pain can have many causes, but the most common are herniated disks, lumbosacral strains, sacroiliac sprains, excessive tightness of the hamstrings, and weak abdominal muscles.
- Low back pain can be prevented by paying attention to standing, lying, sitting, and lifting posture to prevent the lower back from being placed in potentially injurious positions.

- All injuries should be initially managed using rest, ice, compression, and elevation (RICE) to control swelling and thus reduce the time required for rehabilitation.
- It is important to understand the dangers involved in exercising in extreme environmental conditions.

SUGGESTED READINGS

Artal, R., and M. O'Toole. 2003. Guidelines of the American College of Obstetricians and Gynecologists for exercise during pregnancy and the postpartum period. *British Journal of Sports Medicine* 37(1):6–12.

Binkley, H. M., J. Beckett, and D. J. Casa. 2002. National Athletic Trainers' Association Position Statement: Exertional heat illness. *Journal of Athletic Training* 37(3):329–43.

Boyle, D. 1999. *The sports medicine handbook for parents and coaches.* Washington, DC: Georgetown University Press.

Brown, W. 2002. The benefits of physical activity during pregnancy. *Journal of Science and Medicine in Sport* 5(1):37–45.

Brukner, P., and K. Khan. 2002. Principles of injury prevention. In *Clinical sports medicine,* 2nd rev. ed., edited by P. Brukner. New York: McGraw-Hill.

Burruss, P. et al. 1998. Winter sports: Risks during cold exposure. *Sports Science Exchange-Roundtable* 9(4):1–6.

Carpenter, D. M., and B. W. Nelson. 1999. Low back strengthening for the prevention and treatment of low back pain. *Medicine and Science in Sports and Exercise* 31(1):18–24.

Casa, D. 1999. Exercise in the heat II. Critical concepts in rehydration, exertional heat illnesses, and maximizing athletic performance. *Journal of Athletic Training* 34(3):253–62.

Clapp, J. F. 2000. Exercise during pregnancy: A clinical update. *Clinics in Sports Medicine* 19(2):273–86.

Clapp, J. 2002. *Exercising through your pregnancy.* Omaha, NE: Addicus Books.

Gallaspie, J., and D. May. 2001. *Signs and symptoms of athletic injuries.* St. Louis: McGraw-Hill.

Galloway, S. D. R. et al. 1997. Exercise in the heat: Factors limiting exercise capacity and methods for improving heat tolerance. *Sports Exercise and Injury* 3(1):19–24.

2003. Heat illness symptoms and treatments. *JOPERD—The Journal of Physical Education, Recreation & Dance* 74(7):12–13.

2001. Heat-related illness. In *Sports medicine handbook,* edited by S. J. Shulz, Indianapolis: National Federation of State High School Associations.

Hinch, D. E., and M. W. Radomski. 2003. Exercise in the cold. *WellnessOptions* 4(11):43–44.

McGill, S. 2002. *Low back disorders: Evidence-based prevention and rehabilitation.* Champaign, IL: Human Kinetics.

Mellion, M. (ed.). 2002. *Sports medicine secrets.* Philadelphia: Lippincott, Williams & Wilkins.

Micheli, L., and M. Jenkins. 2001. *The sports medicine bible for the young athlete.* New York: Harper Perennial.

Moran, D. S. 2001. Potential applications of heat and cold stress indices to sporting events. *Sports Medicine* 31(13):909–17.

Pfeiffer, R., and B. Magnus. 2004. *Concepts of athletic training.* Boston: Jones & Bartlett.

Porterfield, J., C. Derosa, and M. Bilbas. 1998. *Mechanical low back pain: Perspectives in functional anatomy.* Philadelphia: W. B. Saunders.

Prentice, W. 2006. *Arnheim's principles of athletic training.* New York: McGraw-Hill.

Prentice, W. 2005. *Essentials of athletic injury management.* New York: McGraw-Hill.

Prentice, W. 2004. *Rehabilitation techniques in sports medicine and athletic training.* New York: McGraw-Hill.

Rucker, K. S. 2001. *Low back pain: A symptom-based approach to diagnosis and treatment.* Burlington, MA: Butterworth-Heinemann.

Rush, S. 2001. Winter exercise. *ACSM's Health and Fitness Journal* 5(6):23–25.

Rush, S. 2002. Sports medicine approach to low back pain. *ACSM's Health and Fitness Journal* 6(2):22–24.

Shirreffs, S. M., L. E. Armstrong, and S. N. Cheuvront. 2004. Fluid and electrolyte needs for preparation and recovery from training and competition. *Journal of Sports Sciences* 22(1):57–63.

Vad, V., and H. Hinzmann. 2004. Back Rx: *A 15-minute-a-day yoga-and-pilates-based program to end low-back pain.* New York: Gotham.

Suggested Web Sites

American Orthopaedic Society for Sports Medicine

This site has a directory of doctors, publications, links to other sites, an ask the doctor section, and the *Sports Medicine Journal.*
www.sportsmed.org

Common Sports Injuries

This site presents background information and Quick Time movies on injuries such as ankle sprain, pulled hamstring, and others.
www.southflorida.digitalcity.com/DCSports

ESPN.com: Training Room

This site has articles about fitness and conditioning, sports injuries, and sports nutrition.
http://espn.go.com/trainingroom

Gatorade Sport Science Institute

This site provides a wide range of information on exercise and nutrition.
www.gssiweb.com

Hughston Sports Medicine Hospital

This is the nation's first hospital specifically designed to treat patients suffering from activity related injuries and disorders. It is in Columbus, Georgia.
www.mindspring.com/~hughston/~

National Athletic Trainers' Association

Provides links to injury information, news about the organization, research and education, the *Journal of Athletic Training,* and other related topics.
www.nata.org

Spine-Health, your back pain and neck pain resource

This site presents in-depth information on back pain and neck pain, sciatica, scoliosis, herniated disc, degenerative disc disease, spinal stenosis.
www.spine-health.com/

Sports Science, Sport Medicine & Physical Education

Sports Science Directory on SPORTQuest provides links to sport science/medicine and related topics.
www.sportquest.com/sportscience.html

Sportsmedicine.com

The sports medicine network offers information on education, organizations, and topics about sports medicine, plus a chat room, mail list, and message board to connect people interested in sports medicine.
www.sportsmedicine.com

The Female Athlete

This site presents information about typical women's sports health issues like knee injuries, osteoporosis, and strength training.
www.sportsmed.org/d/answers/jan97.htm

WebMD/Lycos-Article-Recommendations for Exercise in Pregnancy

Provides recommendations for Exercise in Pregnancy. Prenatal exercise is a crucial part of staying healthy while you're pregnant.
http://webmd.lycos.com/content/article

Becoming a Wise **Consumer**

Objectives

After completing this chapter, you should be able to do the following:

- Describe what is necessary to be a careful consumer of health and fitness products.
- Discuss the various types of exercise equipment that may be used in a health and fitness program.
- Explain how clothing should be selected for exercising in hot or cold environments.
- Identify special considerations for selecting a health or fitness club.
- Discuss what you should look for in health and fitness books and magazines.

ARE YOU A WISE CONSUMER OF FITNESS PRODUCTS?

To say that the emphasis on health and fitness in American society has increased significantly during the past decade is a gross understatement. The consumer of health and fitness products has become the target of an unprecedented media advertising blitz. The stereotypical image of the healthy and fit body appears in countless magazines at newsstands, on television, in infomercials, in newspaper ads, and on the Internet. Advertising includes everything from health foods and vitamins to exercise equipment, fitness centers, and weight-loss centers.

Further evidence of the magnitude of the interest in fitness and exercise is seen in the expenditures for sporting goods and exercise equipment. These expenditures have reached an all-time high. The sale of sporting goods has become big business. Sales of about $23 billion were recorded in the early 2000s. The athletic shoe business alone has become a $2.5 billion-a-year business. Recent sales figures show that close to $5 billion is being spent on athletic clothing annually. Sales of home exercise equipment have skyrocketed to about $3 billion today as individuals seek the convenience of being able to work out at home. Stationary bicycles, rowing machines, treadmills, stair climbers, and weight systems are the most popular items. Sales of diet and exercise books continue to rise. Corporate fitness programs and commercial health clubs have

KEY TERM

consumerism

267

attracted a record number of members. The list goes on and on. There is little doubt that a significant amount of misinformation is being disseminated in an effort to merchandise a lucrative health and fitness industry.

Marketing and advertising experts are extremely sensitive to the vulnerability of American consumers when it comes to buying products that promise to make them look and feel better. How can the consumer separate fact from hype when considering advertisements for health and fitness products? It is essential for consumers to educate themselves by taking a critical look at a product or service to be purchased. For example, if you are going to buy a new automobile, perhaps you begin by looking at advertisements. You may wish to consult an independent consumer magazine to look at performance specifications, maintenance records, and so on. Then you go to the dealers to find who can offer the best price along with a reputation for good service. Chances are that you will buy your new car from that dealer.

The point is that most people shop around and are careful when making a choice about a large purchase such as an automobile. They take the time necessary to learn everything they can about the product. The wise consumer will take a similar approach when buying health and fitness products. You should realize that it is easy to be "taken in" by advertisements that project an image that seems to be in demand by consumers. Practicing **consumerism** means that wise consumers will take the time to analyze the entire product and to decide if the outlay of money is necessary to reap the benefits they desire.

consumerism: taking the time to analyze the entire product and to decide if the outlay of money is necessary to reap the desired benefits

WHAT DO YOU NEED TO CONSIDER WHEN BUYING FITNESS EQUIPMENT?

The extent and variety of fitness and exercise equipment available to the consumer are at times mind-boggling. Prices of equipment can range from between $5 for a jump rope or Frisbee to $60,000 for certain computer-driven isokinetic devices. One of the most important facts that the consumer of health and fitness products and services must understand is that it is certainly not necessary to purchase expensive exercise equipment to see good results. You will achieve many of the same physiological benefits from using a $5 jump rope, an exercise mat, or dumbells that result from running on a $10,000 treadmill. The following discussion identifies some of the more popular pieces of exercise equipment.

FREE WEIGHTS VS. WEIGHT MACHINES

Various types of weight training equipment can be used with progressive resistive exercise including free weights (barbells and dumbbells) or weight machines (such as Cybex, Eagle, DP, Soloflex, Body Master, and Free Motion Fitness) (Figure 10-1). Dumbbells and barbells require the use of iron plates of varying weights that can be easily changed by adding or subtracting equal amounts of weight to both sides of the bar. Most of the weight machines have a stack of weights that are lifted through a series of levers or pulleys. The stack of weights slides up and down on a pair of bars that restrict the movement to only one plane. Weight can be increased or decreased simply by changing the position of a weight key.

There are advantages and disadvantages to both the free weights and weight machines. The machines are relatively safe to use in

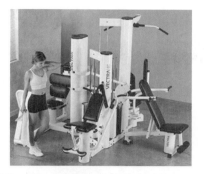

FIGURE 10-1. MULTISTATION EXERCISE MACHINE.
(Courtesy Vectra Fitness, 7901 South 190th St. Kent, WA 98032.)

comparison with free weights. For example, if you are doing a bench press with free weights, it is essential to have someone "spot" you (help you lift the weights back onto the support racks if you don't have enough strength to complete the lift); otherwise you may end up dropping the weight on your chest. With the weight machines you can easily and safely drop the weight without fear of injury. It is also a simple process to increase or decrease the weight by moving a single weight key with the weight machines, although changes can generally be made only in increments of 10 or 15 pounds. With free weights, iron plates must be added or removed from each side of the barbell.

A discussion of using free weights as compared to using exercise machines was included in Chapter 5 (pp. 101–103). Costs of purchasing free weights are substantially lower than the weight machines. Regardless of which type of equipment is used, the same principles of isotonic training may be applied.

STATIONARY EXERCISE BIKES

Many different exercise bikes are available to the consumer (Figure 10-2, *A*). Bicycle companies such as Schwinn or Ross, as well as Tunturi and Vitamaster, which specifically manufacture exercise equipment, are well-known name

brands. Exercise bikes priced below $150 tend to be somewhat unstable. Most good models range between $150 and $700. Computerized exercise bikes used in health clubs may cost between $1,500 and $3,500.

There are essentially two types of exercise bikes. When you pedal a "single-action" model, resistance is created from a device such as a flywheel. With the flywheel you can change the resistance with a twist of a knob. The "dual-action" models also let you pump the handlebars back with your arms. Most of these bikes use a fan to create resistance, which can be increased by pumping the arms and legs faster. The dual-action models allow you to rest your feet on coaster pedals and exercise only your arms. Obviously, those models that work both the upper and lower extremities require a higher energy expenditure. Most models have you sitting on a bicycle seat in a standard position. Some design variations allow you to sit in a recumbent position. This position exercises the hamstring muscles to a greater degree and is useful for individuals who have back problems or poor balance.

Training stands hook a resistance device to your regular bicycle, allowing you to convert it to a stationary bike at relatively low cost. Features that are important to look for include a comfortable padded seat and some type of monitor that tells you how far you have pedaled or the time. Models with pedal straps will work your legs on the upstroke in addition to the downstroke.

Individuals who are unable to use their lower extremities on a regular exercise bike can use an upper-extremity bicycle ergometer (Figure 10-2, *G*).

TREADMILLS

An exercise treadmill is a belt stretched between two rollers (Figure 10-2, *B*). The belt may be driven manually in the least expensive models or by a motor in more expensive ones. Sears, Tunturi, Vitamaster, Voit, DP, Precor, and

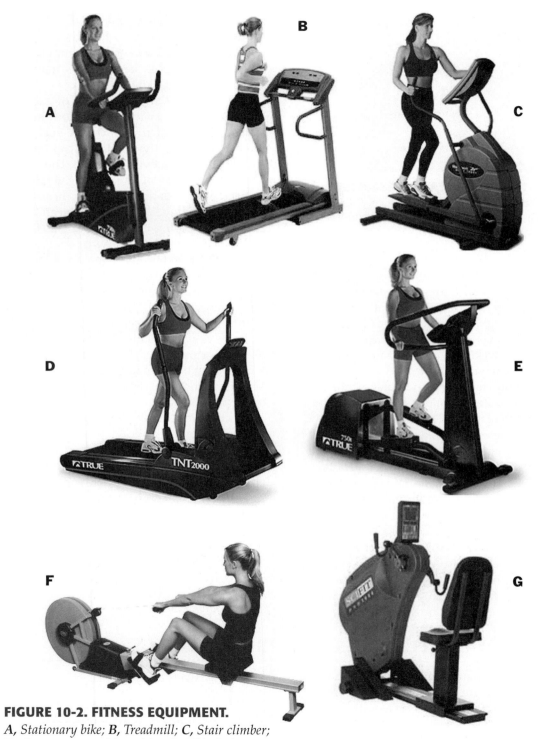

FIGURE 10-2. FITNESS EQUIPMENT.
*A, Stationary bike; B, Treadmill; C, Stair climber;
D, Cross-country ski machine; E, Elliptical exerciser; F, Rowing machine; G, Upper-extremity ergometer.*

Proform are among the more common brands of treadmills manufactured for home use. Costs range from $400 to $1,000. More expensive machines have a bigger motor, a wider belt, and a faster top speed (up to about 5 mph). It is difficult to find a good motor-driven treadmill for under $500. Treadmills subjected to high use in health clubs cost between $1,000 and $12,000. Most of the more expensive motor-driven treadmills allow you to adjust both the speed of the belt and the incline angle to alter intensity.

Machine motors vary in both type and size. The type of motor can be either AC or DC. AC motors run at full speed, all the time relying on a transmission-like pulley system to regulate speed. This means most models start up at full speed and can be somewhat dangerous when getting on. Treadmill motors that are DC can be run at different speeds, thus start-up is not much of a problem. All models come with some type of speed control. Motor size varies from 1/2 horsepower to more than 1 horsepower. Bigger motors can handle heavier loads and higher speeds. A running gait requires that the treadmill is able to go at least 5 mph.

STAIR CLIMBERS

Stair climbers have become one of the more popular types of exercise machines (Figure 10-2, C). They are essentially a set of levers attached to some resistance device. Your legs pump the levers as if you are climbing stairs. Models vary in how they apply resistance, using either a flywheel, a hydraulic piston, a drive train, or wind resistance. In some models, the stairs are linked. As one goes down, the other automatically goes up. Dual-action models allow you to work both the arms and the legs simultaneously. The more expensive models have a series of stairs that rotate as if you were climbing the wrong direction on an escalator. Monitors on many models display information such as time, steps per minute, and energy expenditure. Some may be pro-

grammed to vary both the speed and the amount of resistance during the course of a workout. Sears, Tunturi, DP, and Precor are brand names of the typical home models. Stairmaster makes most of the more expensive units for commercial use. Stair-climbing machines cost between $200 and $3,000. Most of the home models are around $500. Programmable units cost a minimum of $800.

SKI MACHINES

A ski machine offers many of the aerobic benefits of cross-country skiing without having to worry about the snow. These machines have two flat boards, one for each foot, that slide back and forth in a groove on rollers. The arms are also involved, using either telescoping poles or a rope and pulley instead of the ski poles. The design of these machines allows you to simultaneously exercise both the upper and lower extremities. (Figure 10-2, D).

Ski machines have either dependent or independent leg motion. With a dependent machine, the leg boards are connected. As one goes forward, the other goes backward. On independent machines, the leg boards slide independently, making them somewhat more difficult to master but also affording you a better workout. Resistance on the ski machine comes from either an electromagnetic flywheel or from a belt wrapped around a flywheel that provides friction. Some models do not have variable resistance. More expensive models may also incline, increasing the stress on the quadriceps muscles in the front of the thigh. Most machines have some type of monitor that can show heart rate, resistance, speed, calories expended, etc. Most of these machines can be folded and require little space for storage.

There are several manufacturers of ski machines, including NordicTrack, Precor, Proform, DP, Vitamaster, and Tunturi. Ski machines range in price from $300 to as high as $2,000 for health club models.

ELLIPTICAL EXERCISERS

Elliptical machines provide a new mode of cardiovascular exercise that makes use of a no-impact, elliptical-shaped stride (Figure 10-2, *E*). When using the machine, you stand upright while striding in a forward or reverse motion and holding handrails. An electronically adjustable ramp allows you to raise or lower ramp incline, adjust resistance, and use both forward and reverse motion. These options let exercisers simulate no-impact versions of their favorite exercise activities, such as walking, running, cycling, cross-country skiing, and stairclimbing. Lower ramp levels can simulate cross-country skiing or the walking or running options of a treadmill. Higher ramp levels can produce a safe, comfortable cycling or stair-climbing motion. Elliptical machines are manufactured by Vision Fitness, Life Fitness, Star Trac, Precor, NordicTrack, ICON Health and Fitness, Inc., Guthy-Renker, and Quantum Television. They range in price from $200 for home models to $3,500 for more sophisticated commercial models.

ROWING MACHINES

Rowing machines are designed to mimic the action of rowing a boat or sculling. Most brands have some type of movable handles, which are similar to oars, and a sliding seat. Exercise involves pressing against stationary footplates with the legs while sliding backward on the seat and simultaneously pulling on the handles to create a rowing motion. Rowing machines are similar to stair climbers in terms of their resistance mechanisms, which may include a flywheel, a hydraulic piston, or wind resistance. (Figure 10-2, *F*).

Sears, DP, and Tunturi are the most common home models of rowing machines. Costs range between $200 and $800 for home models. Rowing machines for health clubs range between $1,000 and $3,000.

PASSIVE EXERCISE DEVICES AND TECHNIQUES

Unfortunately, many consumers of health and fitness products are lured into thinking that there is some easy way to achieve physical fitness with little or no physical effort. The marketing of a variety of devices such as rubberized suits that let you sit around and sweat off weight, electrical devices that make muscles contract, and mechanical devices that shake, vibrate, or roll fat off can seem to be very appealing shortcuts to getting fit. There are, however, no shortcuts.

▶ Passive Motion Machines

These machines have only been introduced into the health and fitness market in recent years. Passive motion machines are designed to exercise individual body parts by moving them for you with no effort on your part. You are simply required to lie or sit still while the machine does all the work. For example, one machine is designed to flex and extend your trunk and lower back, while another may flex and extend your hip and your knee. Manufacturers claim that these machines will help improve muscular endurance since a particular body part is moving repeatedly, improve flexibility by using slow continuous movement, and burn off fat while reducing cellulite in the exercised areas. All of these claims are totally ludicrous. The only potential benefit offered to healthy individuals by these machines may be relaxation. However, similar passive exercise devices, referred to as constant passive motion (CPM) machines, are widely and effectively used in rehabilitation for postsurgical patients to minimize development of scar tissue.

▶ Motor-Driven Exercise Bikes

Stationary exercise bikes or rowing machines that are motor driven may have some value in increasing circulation, particularly around joints. However, they are totally ineffective in elevating heart rate and thus stressing the cardiovascular system.

▶Vibrating Belts and Rolling Machines

Vibrating belts placed around the trunk or the extremities that shake fat and muscle tissue or rolling machines that use movable wooden rollers to compress fat and muscle tissue in a rolling fashion have been promoted to break up fat tissue, thus making it easier to burn off. They also falsely claim to increase muscle tone and improve posture. The truth is that they do not "break up" fat, but they may damage connective tissue around joints and within a muscle. The rollers may also cause bruising of the skin and fat from repeated compression. Use of these machines should definitely be avoided by people with low back pain and by pregnant women.

▶Massage

Massage can be an extremely effective therapeutic technique. It is most typically used for stimulating circulation, for inducing relaxation, and for loosening up muscles. However, as in the case of rolling machines, it will not selectively rub fat away from a specific spot.

▶Rubberized or Inflatable Suits

Rubberized inflatable suits are also called sauna shorts or sauna sleeves. Promoters claim that the pressure created by the garment will help to break down fat tissue by squeezing it and that the rubber garment will help you "sweat off" fat. Once again these claims are ridiculous. Fat cannot be "squeezed off." Furthermore, sweating does not burn off a significant amount of fat.

Wearing rubberized suits may help you lose body weight fairly quickly, but the weight loss represents the water weight of perspiration rather than loss of fat tissue. Elevation of body core temperature by wearing rubberized suits may predispose an individual to various forms of heat stress and can potentially be very dangerous for individuals with high blood pressure.

▶Electrical Stimulating Devices

In general, electrical stimulating devices use low-amperage electrical current of sufficient intensity to cause involuntary muscle contraction. The technique involves connecting the electrodes to specific areas of the body and generating a weak electrical current to contract the muscles. (Promoters claim that the muscle contraction requires energy, thus calories will be used from stored fat to supply energy.) Once again, there is no credibility to the value of this technique for weight loss or fitness.

Electrical stimulating currents are routinely used by qualified rehabilitation specialists for treating many different musculoskeletal and neurological problems. When appropriate treatment limits are selected, electrical currents can be effectively used for pain control and muscle reeducation after injury, as well as to decrease muscle spasm and to reduce muscle atrophy. The indiscriminant use of electrical currents by untrained individuals is strongly discouraged and in many states is against the law.

SPAS, STEAM BATHS, SAUNAS

In the health and fitness industry, the use of spas (hot tubs), steam baths, and saunas is widespread. Most health and fitness clubs offer the use of at least one form of these to their members. Hot tubs and whirlpool baths are increasingly being installed in private homes. Of all their therapeutic benefits, perhaps none is more important than the relaxation factor. Relaxation seems to be the primary reason why so many people are interested in using them. However, claims that sitting in either water or air at high temperatures will cause fat loss are again totally unfounded. Whatever weight is lost is due to a loss of water. Water loss should be immediately replaced through proper rehydration from beverages.

Saunas are likely to produce the greatest amount of body water loss because the air is hot and extremely dry. Thus significant amounts of water will be lost through the rapid evaporation of sweat. Temperatures in a sauna should not be higher than 180°F. You should limit yourself to no more than 15 minutes in the sauna at that temperature.

Steam baths, which should be no higher than 120°F., have a much lower temperature than saunas. However, the humidity in a steam bath is 100 percent. Thus individuals will appear to be sweating more heavily in a steam bath. Under humid conditions, sweat cannot evaporate to dissipate body heat, and body temperature rises rapidly. It is necessary to limit time in a steam bath to no longer than 10 minutes.

Spas or hot tubs involve full-body immersion in a whirlpool at a temperature that should be no higher than 100°F. for no longer than 10 minutes.

Certain precautions should be taken when using any of these units:

1. If you have a heart condition or skin infection or are pregnant, you should avoid their use.
2. Do not use any of these without cooling down after exercise.
3. Wash off all oils or lotions before use.
4. Never drink alcohol before use.
5. If you feel faint for any reason, get out immediately.
6. Always have someone with you when using any of these.

TANNING BEDS

For years, having a deep, golden-brown tan was associated with being fit and healthy. During the past decade, artificial tanning beds have become very popular in the health and fitness club industry. These tanning salons, beds, and booths usually consist of an array of long tubes that produce ultraviolet light. The lights are positioned in some type of frame that allows for exposure of the entire body.

We now know beyond any doubt that prolonged or continuous exposure to ultraviolet light rays predisposes an individual to the development of skin cancer. Manufacturers of artificial tanning devices claim the ultraviolet light produced by tanning devices is safe. The Food and Drug Administration (FDA) has warned the public that sunlamps and tanning beds are dangerous. Besides the risk of skin cancer, long-term exposure to a form of ultraviolet light (UVA) causes premature aging of the skin with wrinkling and sagging. Production of UVA tanning beds is largely unregulated. Furthermore, there is generally no standard of training for people who operate these machines. Their knowledge of the tanning process and the danger of exposure to ultraviolet radiation may be limited at best. Therefore, extreme caution should be exercised whenever you are exposed to ultraviolet radiation, either from sunlight or from artificial sources.

HOW SHOULD YOU CHOOSE APPROPRIATE CLOTHING AND SHOES FOR EXERCISE?

CLOTHING FOR EXERCISING IN HOT, HUMID WEATHER

Guidelines for selecting clothing for exercising in hot, humid weather are relatively simple and straightforward. Clothing chosen should allow for maximal dissipation of body heat through evaporation of sweat while minimizing the heat gained from the environment. By far the most effective means of heat loss involves the process of evaporation. If sweat remains on the skin, it will not produce heat loss. Thus the material worn must be lightweight and dry very quickly by permitting sweat to evaporate. The body area that has the greatest number of sweat glands is the upper back, and shoulders. Consequently a tank top will allow for greatest exposure for evaporation. Radiation of heat from the sun or other hot surfaces such as pavement will cause the body to gain heat. Clothing should be a light color to reflect as much radiant heat energy as possible.

Wearing a hat will help block some of the radiant heat energy from the sun. However, it is critical that the hat be made of some type of mesh fabric to allow heat to be dissipated from the head. About 40 percent of the heat lost from the body is from the head.

It should be reemphasized that making certain you are well hydrated is the best way to minimize heat-related problems.

CLOTHING FOR EXERCISING IN COLD WEATHER

In situations where the weather is cold, the goal of wearing clothing is to create a "semi-tropical microclimate" for the body and to prevent chilling. The clothing should not restrict movement and should be as lightweight as possible. The material should permit free passage of sweat and body heat. Otherwise, sweat would accumulate on the skin or in the clothing and provide a chilling effect when activity ceases. This dampness, in combination with cold and wind, plays a critical role in the development of hypothermia. Individuals should routinely dress in thin layers of clothing that can be easily added or removed when the temperature increases or decreases. Constant adjustment of these layers will reduce sweating and the likelihood that clothing will become damp or wet.

Before exercise, during activity breaks, and after exercise, a warm-up suit or sweat clothes should be worn to prevent chilling. Activity in cold, wet, or windy weather poses some problem because such weather reduces the insulating value of the clothing. Consequently, the individual may be unable to achieve a level of metabolic heat production sufficient to keep pace with body heat loss. In cold weather, a hat should be worn to minimize excessive heat loss from the head. It is also a good idea to wear gloves to minimize the effects of cold and wind on the hands and fingers.

SHOE SELECTION

The athletic and fitness shoe manufacturing industry has become extremely sophisticated and offers a number of options when it comes to purchasing shoes for different activities. Terms like forefoot varus support or rearfoot valgus wedge are confusing to a person who simply wants to buy a pair of good running, aerobic, or court shoes. Most people are simply interested in finding a shoe that is designed for a specific activity that will last for a long time, and that will provide good support and comfort. Figure 10-3 shows the major parts of a shoe. For the average individual, the following guidelines can help you select the most appropriate shoe to fit your needs.

▶ Toe Box

There should be plenty of room for your toes in the fitness shoe. Most experts recommend a 1/2- to 3/4-inch distance between toes and the front of the shoe. A few fitness shoes are made in varying widths. If you have a very wide or narrow foot, most shoe salespersons can recommend a specific shoe for your foot. The best way to make sure there is adequate room in the toe box is to have your foot measured and then try on the shoe. If the shoe feels too tight or there are areas of friction or pressure when trying the shoe in a store, it is like that there will be some continuing problems with the shoe fitting properly when you begin exercising.

▶ Sole

The sole should possess two qualities. First, it must provide a shock-absorptive function; second, it must be durable. Most shoes have

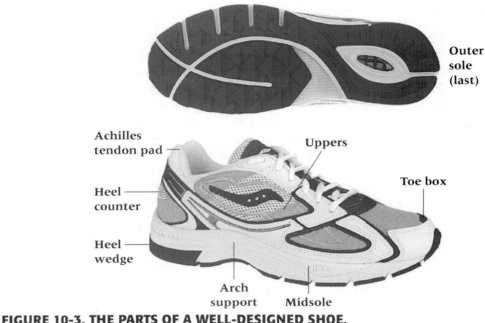

Outer
sole
(last)

Achilles
tendon pad

Uppers

Toe box

Heel
counter

Heel
wedge

Arch
support   Midsole

FIGURE 10-3. THE PARTS OF A WELL-DESIGNED SHOE.

three layers on the sole: a thick spongy layer, which absorbs the force of the foot strike under the heel; a midsole, which cushions the midfoot and toes; and a hard rubber layer, which comes in contact with the ground. The average runner's feet strike the ground 1,500 to 1,700 times per mile. Thus it is essential that the force of the heel strike be absorbed by the spongy layer to prevent overuse-type injuries from occurring in the ankles and knees. "Heel wedges" are sometimes inserted on either the inside or the outside surface of the sole underneath the heel counter to accommodate and correct for various structural deformities of the foot that may alter normal biomechanics of the running gait. A flared heel may be appropriate for running shoes but is not recommended in aerobic or court shoes. The sole must provide good traction and must be made of a tough material that is resistant to wear. Most of the better-known brands of shoes tend to have well-designed, long-lasting soles.

▶ Heel Counters

The heel counter is the portion of the shoe that prevents the foot from rolling from side to side at heel strike. The heel counter should be firm but well fitted (snug) to minimize movement of the heel up and down or side to side. A good heel counter may prevent ankle sprains and painful blisters.

▶ Shoe Uppers

The upper part of the shoe is made of some combination of nylon and leather. The uppers should be lightweight, capable of quick drying, and well ventilated. The uppers should have some type of extra support in the saddle area, and there should also be some extra padding in the area of the Achilles tendon just above the heel counter. While running shoes are designed for straight ahead motion, court shoes and aerobic shoes have to absorb lateral motions and thus the uppers should be reinforced appropriately.

►Arch Support

The arch support should be made of some durable yet soft supportive material and should smoothly join with the insole. The support should not have any rough seams or ridges inside the shoe, which may cause blisters.

►Price

Unfortunately, for many people price is the primary consideration in buying running shoes. Running shoes and court shoes range from $40 to $160 per pair. Aerobic shoes tend to be less expensive, in the $30 to $80 range. When buying fitness shoes, remember that in many fitness activities, shoes are important for performance and prevention of injury. Thus it is worth a little extra investment to buy a quality pair of shoes.

WHAT DO YOU LOOK FOR WHEN SHOPPING FOR A HEALTH CLUB?

It's easy to get caught up in a desire to join a health club. You walk in the front door and may immediately be greeted by an attractive, energetic receptionist who quickly introduces you to an attractive, energetic "fitness consultant," which is the term frequently used in fitness centers to label the salesperson. You may be escorted into a large exercise room with plush carpeting on the floor, mirrors on every wall, chrome-plated exercise equipment, and high-energy music coming from the stereo system. Your eyes tend to ignore the overweight gentleman or the frail lady working on machines in the corner and go straight to the Adonis or Aphrodite working out in the center of the room. It is easy to think, "Hey, this place is beautiful, and if it can make me feel comfortable and look like that at the same time, I want to join—NOW." Unfortunately, in this situation the consumer has already decided to purchase the hype without investigating the facts.

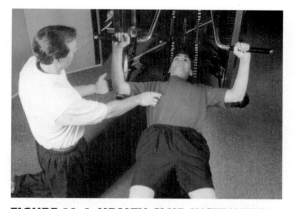

FIGURE 10-4. HEALTH CLUB INSTRUCTION. *Well-qualified instructors are an important factor to consider when selecting a health club.*

Certainly it is possible to find health clubs that offer good-quality instruction and guidance (Figure 10-4) in addition to an aesthetically pleasing environment in which to work out. The guidelines described here are important for those individuals who are considering joining a health or fitness club.

TYPES OF FACILITIES

Familiarize yourself with the many different types of facilities available, including spas, gyms, YMCA/YWCAs, and facilities at universities or high schools. Many times local schools or colleges will offer excellent facilities for public use at little or no cost. You can most often find a listing of facilities in the telephone book. It is important to contact all the available sources to get the most detailed information.

LOCATION OF FACILITY

Certainly the location of the facility is an important factor in deciding whether to join.

- Is it close or easily accessible to your home or apartment?

- Will you be stopping to exercise on your way to or from work or school?
- What is the traffic like near the facility at the times of day you are most likely to go?

EQUIPMENT AVAILABLE

Check the type of equipment available.

- Do they have weight equipment (free weights, exercise machines)?
- Is there a pool, whirlpool, sauna, steam room, running track, racquetball court, and aerobic exercise room?
- Is there sufficient available locker space, with showers and changing areas?
- Do they have the type of equipment necessary for your fitness program?

PROGRAMS OFFERED

Check the type and quality of programs offered, such as individualized and supervised weight training, aerobic exercise classes, spinning classes, kick-boxing classes, jogging classes, yoga, weight-control programs, and cardiac rehabilitation programs. Do any of these cost extra?

HOURS OF OPERATION

- What are the hours of operation of the facility?
- Are they open 7 days per week?
- Is it a co-ed facility?
- Can both males and females work out there 7 days a week?
- What are the most crowded times?

QUALIFICATIONS OF PERSONNEL

You must be careful to consider the qualifications of the instructors. Many health and fitness clubs employ attractive, fit individuals whose primary function is to sell memberships to the club. Ask the salesperson the following questions:

- What is the background of the personnel who will be supervising your program?
- Do they have a background in physical education, exercise physiology, athletic training, or physical therapy?
- Are they certified by the American College of Sports Medicine as Exercise Leaders, Health/Fitness Instructors, or Exercise Specialists?
- Are they certified as aerobics instructors by the Aerobics and Fitness Association of America (AFAA), American Council on Exercise (ACE), Cooper Institute for Aerobics Research, or Exercise Safety Association (ESA)?
- Are they certified as personal trainers by the National Academy of Sport Medicine (NASM), the Aerobics and Fitness Association of America (AFAA), American Council on Exercise (ACE), Cooper Institute for Aerobics Research, Exercise Safety Association (ESA), International Fitness Institute, or the National Strength and Conditioning Association (NSCA)?

TYPES OF MEMBERSHIP CONTRACTS

Health and fitness clubs tend to offer a wide range of membership contract options, ranging from pay-by-the-visit to lifetime memberships. It is a good idea to avoid long-term contracts, especially in the beginning. Health clubs sell a lot of memberships because people tend to get caught up by the aesthetics of the facility and are manipulated by some very good salespeople. The firm commitment to consistently use the facility three to four times per week that is made in the sales office tends to become less important for most people over time. If all the people who bought memberships in a club were to show up at one time, it is likely that you would not be able to get in the door. If you do decide to join, check on various payment options that best suit your budget. Also check on additional fees that you may have to pay for extras, such as reserving racquetball courts or enrolling in aerobics classes.

TRIAL PERIODS

Before signing a contract, it is a good idea to spend several sessions working out at the club, talking with the instructors and with other club members. Current members can answer specific questions about the quality of the facility as well as identify its deficiencies. If there is some objection to doing this on the part of the management, then you should exercise extreme caution about signing a contract.

BE KNOWLEDGEABLE ABOUT FITNESS

It is probably wise to avoid the clubs or organizations that advertise programs, classes, equipment, or techniques that claim to result in "overnight" strength gains, weight loss, or improvements in appearance. You must realize that reaching your fitness goals requires selecting an activity you enjoy. The activity should not overload the body but progress within your individual limitations. Furthermore, by being consistent in your training program, you will accomplish your goals safely by paying attention to the basic principles outlined within this text.

WHAT TO LOOK FOR IN FITNESS MAGAZINES, BOOKS, AND VIDEOS

As with the various types of exercise equipment, consumer demand for literature and other media dealing with health and fitness issues makes publication in this area an extremely lucrative enterprise.

It is difficult, if not totally impossible, to pick up a popular magazine that does not contain at least one article about health and fitness. It is reasonable to assume that the majority of people in the United States obtain most of their health and fitness information while standing in line at the grocery store. This is certainly not to say that grocery store sources of health and fitness information are unreliable, but there is a tremendous amount of misinformation relative to health and fitness issues routinely spread through the popular media. Often, the articles in magazines are written by individuals with little or no health or fitness expertise who may interview fitness experts. Occasionally, you will find experts writing the articles. The same is true for so-called experts who appear on television or radio talk shows. These people have charming personalities but often lack reliable credentials.

A trip to the local bookstore, public library, or Internet booksellers, to locate books dealing with health, wellness, fitness, exercise, sports, diet, and nutrition can be overwhelming. Many excellent, accurate books are available. These books are written by health and fitness experts. Unfortunately, the majority of the best-selling books, and certainly the best-marketed ones, are written by celebrities who look fit and attractive. Some of these books contain excellent information. Others include some facts along with misinformation and border on being dangerous.

For anyone who has ventured into a video store, it is easy to see that celebrities also like to star or be featured in exercise videos or DVDs. Again the available choices can be overwhelming. Many consumers choose to purchase exercise videos or DVDs as an alternative to joining a health club. The convenience of having someone lead you through a workout at home certainly appeals to some people who have neither the time nor the motivation to leave home to participate in an exercise program. As is the case with books and magazines, the consumer must make informed choices when it comes to purchasing exercise videos or DVDs. Remember, they don't always do exactly what the infomercials tell you they can do.

How do you know whether information presented in the popular media is reliable? Simply by being an informed consumer. The information presented in this text is accurate and up-to-date. The knowledge you have obtained from this text should make you a more informed consumer.

THE BOTTOM LINE FOR THE CONSUMER

Regardless of the type of exercise equipment, the aesthetics of a health club, or the claims of nutritional products, the bottom line is that the responsibility for getting fit and healthy ultimately lies with you. Remember, a commitment to a fitness program is first and foremost a commitment to yourself. Being cautious, asking a number of questions, and being well informed will help you make the best choice possible. Basing your physical activity program on the facts rather than on marketing techniques is the way to get fit. If you find that joining a health club or buying expensive exercise equipment in some way motivates you to adhere to your program, then by all means, do so. But never neglect the basic principles.

SUMMARY

- Be a conscientious and well-informed consumer when selecting products related to health and fitness.
- Don't be afraid to ask questions and fully investigate a health and fitness club before joining.
- There is an incredible amount and diversity of exercise equipment available to the consumer.
- Deciding what type of equipment is best for you to use or purchase should be based primarily on individual interests

and the goals of your physical activity program.
- Remember, there is no shortcut to fitness. Passive exercise devices are essentially useless when it comes to improvement in fitness levels.
- Spas, saunas, and steam baths should be used for relaxation and are not effective in reducing your percent body fat.
- The use of tanning beds and tanning booths is generally not recommended.
- Select appropriate clothing for exercising in either hot or cold environments to prevent heat stress or hypothermia.
- Selecting and purchasing a quality fitness shoe can reduce the likelihood of injury.
- Fitness books, magazine articles, and videos should be critically analyzed by the informed and educated consumer of health and fitness products.

SUGGESTED READINGS

2004. Athletic shoes: The facts about fit. Forget the fancy gear and gadgets. All you really need for a great run or powerwalk is the right pair of shoes. *Active Woman Canada* 2(3):40–43.

Burfoot, A. 2004. Treadmill nation: They help you lose weight, lower your race times, and stay fit wherever you are. Is it any wonder millions of Americans are running on treadmills? Here, the 20 best ways to make the most of your time inside. *Runner's World* 39(1):56–60.

Burke, E. 1996. *Complete home fitness handbook.* Champaign, IL: Human Kinetics.

Consumer Reports. 2006. *Consumer Reports 2006 buying guide.* New York: Consumer Reports.

2004. Creating together: Equipment, supplies and people provide the tools for successful programs. *IDEA Health & Fitness Source* 22(1):53–57.

Dickey, C. 2004. Tools for the trade: Books, looks, and stuff. *ACSM's Health & Fitness Journal* 8(2):32–33. 2004.

Editors of on Health and Consumer Report. 2005. *Consumer Reports diet, health, and fitness guide.* New York: Time Incorporated Home Entertainment.

Faigenbaum, A. D. 2000. Weight machines. In *Strength and power for young athletes,* edited by A. D. Faigenbaum. Champaign, IL: Human Kinetics.

Fall 2002: Shoe buyer's guide. 2002. *Runner's World* (September), 48–49ff.

Forness, L. 2001. *Don't get duped: A consumer's guide to health and fitness.* Boston: Prometheus Books.

Gledhill, K. 2001. *Fitness and exercise sourcebook: Basic consumer health information about the fundamentals of fitness and exercise* (Health Reference Series). Detroit, MI: Omnigraphics.

Goldstein, D., and J. Flory. 1996. *Online consumer guide to healthcare and wellness: The best online sites, resources and services in: Health and fitness, diet and weight loss, alternative medicine, family health, stress management, disease and medical conditions, emergency care.* New York: McGraw-Hill.

Gormley, B. 2005. Understanding strength training equipment: Add some muscle to your strength equipment purchasing decisions. *Fitness Business Canada* 6(1):22–24.

Grantham, W., R. Patten, and T. York. 1998. *Health fitness management: A comprehensive resource for managing and operating programs and facilities.* Champaign, IL: Human Kinetics.

Grisanti, S. 2002. *Industry of illusions: Health and fitness industry scams, frauds, fakes, and personal trainers exposed.* Rye, NY: Rivercat.

Hamilton, A. 2004. Rowers: Having looked at home-use bikes, treadmills and elliptical cross-trainers, it's time to consider rowers. Now you might think that a humble rowing machine, bereft of electronic gizmos, won't really cut the mustard when it comes to serious aerobic training, but you'd be wrong! *Ultra-FIT* 14(1):56–58.

Herbert, D. L. 1998. New standards for health and fitness facilities from the American Heart Association (AHA) and the American College of Sports Medicine (ACSM). *Exercise Standards and Malpractice Reporter* 12(3):46–47.

Holt, S. 2001. Mechanics of machines: Selecting the right piece of equipment. When choosing strength equipment, make sure the machine's mechanics replicate the members' body mechanics. *Fitness Management* 17(8):56–58, 60–61.

2005. Home gym guide 2005. *Ultra-fit Australia* 84:78–88, 90–100, 102.

Industry books, catalogs/literature. 2002. *Fitness Management* 18(7):60.

Jung, A. P., and D. C. Nieman. 2000. An evaluation of home exercise equipment claims: Too good to be true. *ACSM's Health and Fitness Journal* 4(5):14–16, 30–31.

Kreighbaum, E., and M. A. Smith (eds.). 1996. *Sports and fitness equipment design.* Champaign, IL: Human Kinetics.

Manning, S. 2000. Anatomy of a shoe. *Runner's World* (November/December), 34–35.

Napolitano, F. 1999. The American College of Sports Medicine health/fitness facility standards, what they mean and how to apply them to your facility: Part 1. *American College of Sports Medicine Health and Fitness Journal* 3(1):39–49.

Peterson, J. 1997. American *College of Sports Medicine health/fitness facility standards and guidelines.* Champaign, IL: Human Kinetics.

Porcari, J. P., et al. 2002. Effects of electrical muscle stimulation on body composition, muscle strength, and physical appearance. *Journal of Strength and Conditioning Research* 16(2):165–72.

Skinner, T., and M. Cardona. 2004. *Sneaker Book: 50 Years of Sports Shoe Design.* Atglen, PA: Schiffer Publishing, Ltd.

Strength training equipment and accessories: Product information provided by the manufacturers. 2002. *Fitness Management* 18(7):62, 64–68.

Teare, T. 2001. Shoe review 2001: Shape's top 26 picks for running, walking and more. *Shape* 20(8):60, 62, 64, 66.

2004. What's new: The latest products & services from industry suppliers. *Fitness Business Canada* 5(4):8.

SUGGESTED WEB SITES

Exercise Equipment At Beyond Moseying

This site features exercise equipment, fitness machines, athletic equipment, gym apparatus, treadmills, ellipticals, versaclimbers, homegyms, bikes, steppers and body building equipment.
www.fitnessstore.net

Fitness Brokers

This site specializes in genuine Nautilus exercise equipment.
www.fitnessbrokers.com

Fitness Factory Outlet

This is a source for aerobic, strength training, and fitness equipment. It includes fitness tips, exercise charts, and the lowest prices on the highest quality health and fitness products available.
www.fitnessfactory.com

Healthrider

Find great treadmill deals, check your fitness age, buy equipment like treadmills, and check the weekly fitness special. Enjoy relaxation therapy, massage chairs, hydrotherapy, and spas.
www.healthrider.com

Nellies Exercise Fitness Equipment

This site presents a complete line of treadmills, home gyms, bikes, pulse and heart monitors. We carry free weights and strength training and more.
www.nellies.com

NordicTrack Exercise Equipment Site

This site features the leading manufacturer of high-quality treadmill, cycle, skier, strength training, and other fitness equipment products. Purchase conveniently online.
www.nordictrack.com

Precor USA

This is the industry leader in high quality fitness equipment.
www.precor.com

4Sneakers

This is a shopping directory of sneakers and athletic shoes.
www.4sneakers.com

EPILOGUE

NOW DO YOU SEE WHY YOU SHOULD CARE ABOUT GETTING FIT?

Throughout this text, I have tried to emphasize the value of establishing lifelong patterns of healthy living and physical activity. I have tried to provide you with facts and principles that establish the basis for motivating you to incorporate some form of physical activity into your daily life. The text has also identified the exercises, activities, resources, and assessment instruments that can be used in developing an individualized, well-rounded physical activity program. Although there are many different approaches that will ultimately lead to being physically fit, following certain principles and guidelines makes the pursuit of a healthy lifestyle safer and more effective. How, where, or what you choose to do or use to get yourself fit and healthy is of little consequence as long as you pay attention to the basic principles that have been detailed in each of the chapters in this text.

APPENDIX

For more information on nutrition resources, including the nutrient content of fast foods, please visit our nutrition website at **www.mhhe.com/catalogs/sem/nutrition/nutrilinks.**

FOOD COMPOSITION TABLE

Food Name	Serving	KCAL Kc	PROT Gm	CARB Gm	FAT Gm	CHOL Mg	SAFA Gm	FIBD Gm
BABY FOODS								00.000
Baby-carrots	ounce	8	0.2	1.7	0	0	0	0.7
Baby-teething biscuits	item	43	1.2	8.4	0.5	0	-	0.1
Baby-mixed cereal/milk	ounce	32	1.3	4.5	1	0	-	0.25
Baby-oatmeal cereal/milk	ounce	33	1.4	4.3	1.2	0	-	0.7
Baby-rice cereal/milk	ounce	33	1.1	4.7	1	0	-	0.25
Baby-beef lasagna	ounce	22	1.2	2.8	0.6	-	-	0.1
Baby-beef stew	ounce	14	1.4	1.5	0.3	3.55	0.16	0.34
Baby-mixed vegetables	ounce	11	0.3	2.7	0.028	0	0	0.25
Baby-turkey & rice	ounce	14	0.5	2.1	0.4	2.84	0.12	0
Baby-veal & vegetables	ounce	20	1.7	1.7	0.8	-	-	0.1
Baby-apple blueberry	ounce	17	0.1	4.6	0.1	0	0	0.1
Baby-applesauce	ounce	12	0.1	3.1	0	0	0	0.7
Baby-peaches	ounce	20	0.1	5.4	0	0	0	0.7
Baby-pears	ounce	12	0.1	3.1	0	0	0	0.55
Baby-apple juice	fl oz	14	0	3.6	0	0	0	0.25
Baby-apple peach juice	fl oz	13	0	3.2	0	0	0	0.25
Baby-orange juice	fl oz	14	0.2	3.2	0.1	0	0	0.25
Baby-beef	ounce	30	3.9	0	1.5	-	0.73	0
Baby-chicken	ounce	37	3.9	0	2.2	-	0.58	0
Baby-egg yolks	serving	58	2.8	0.3	4.9	223	1.47	0
Baby-ham	ounce	32	3.9	0	1.6	-	0.55	0
Baby-lamb	ounce	29	4	0	1.3	0	0.66	0
Baby-liver	ounce	29	4.1	0.4	1.1	52	0.39	0
Baby-pork	ounce	35	4	0	2	-	0.68	0
Baby-turkey	ounce	32	4	0	1.7	-	0.54	0
Baby-beans-green	ounce	7	0.4	1.7	0	0	0	0.39
Baby-cookie-arrowroot	item	24	0.4	4.3	0.9	0	0.2	0.1
Baby-garden vegetables	ounce	11	0.7	1.9	0.1	0	0	0.7
Baby-peas	ounce	11	1	2.3	0.1	0	0	0.7
Baby-squash	ounce	7	0.2	1.6	0.1	0	0	0.7
Baby-sweet potatoes	ounce	16	0.3	3.7	0	0	0	0.7
Baby-pretzels	item	24	0.7	4.9	0.1	0	0	0
Baby-Zwieback	piece	30	0.7	5.2	0.7	1.46	0.28	0
Baby-cereal & egg yolks	ounce	15	0.5	2	0.5	18	0.17	0
Baby-apple betty	ounce	20	0.1	5.6	0	0	0	0.1
Baby-beef & egg noodles	ounce	15	0.6	2	0.5	-	-	0.1
Baby-beans-green-buttered	ounce	9	0.3	1.9	0.2	0	0	0.7
Baby-beets	ounce	10	0.4	2.2	0	0	0	0.4

FOOD COMPOSITION TABLE—cont'd

Food Name	Serving	KCAL Kc	PROT Gm	CARB Gm	FAT Gm	CHOL Mg	SAFA Gm	FIBD Gm
Baby-corn-creamed	ounce	16	0.4	4	0.1	0	0	0.9
Baby-peas-creamed	ounce	15	0.6	2.5	0.5	0	-	0.7
Baby-spinach-creamed	ounce	11	0.7	1.6	0.4	0	-	1.12
BEVERAGES								
Carn inst break-choc-env	item	130	7	23	1	-	-	-
Choc bev drink-no milk-dry	ounce	99.1	0.937	25.6	0.88	0	0.521	-
Beer-regular	fl oz	12.2	0.089	1.1	0	0	0	0.07
Whis/gin/rum/vod-80 proof	fl oz	64	0	0	0	0	0	0
Whis/gin/rum/vod-86 proof	fl oz	69.5	0	0.028	0	0	0	0
Whis/gin/rum/vod-90 proof	fl oz	72.9	0	0	0	0	0	0
Wine-dessert	fl oz	45.9	0.06	3.54	0	0	0	0
Wine-red-table	fl oz	21	0.059	0.502	0	0	0	0
Club soda	fl oz	0	0	0	0	0	0	0
Coffee-brewed	fl oz	0.592	0.03	0.118	0	0	0.001	0
Coffee-instant-prepared	cup	4.78	0.239	0.956	0	0	0.005	0
Tea-brewed	fl oz	0.296	0	0.089	0	0	0.001	0
Tea-instant-prep-unsweet	cup	2.37	0	0.474	0	0	0	0
Tea-instant-prep-sweetened	cup	88.1	0.259	22.1	0	0	0.008	0
Cordials/liqueur-54 proof	fl oz	97	-	11.5	0	0	0	0
Brandy-cognac-pony	item	73	-	-	0	0	0	0
Cider-fermented	fl oz	11.8	-	0.3	0	0	0	0
Whis/gin/rum vod-94 proof	fl oz	76.5	0	0	0	0	0	0
Whis/gin/rum vod-100 proof	fl oz	82	0	0	0	0	0	0
Champagne-domestic-glass	item	84	0.2	3	0	0	0	0
Wine-vermouth-dry-glass	item	105	0	1	0	0	0	0
Wine-vermouth-sweet-glass	item	167	0	12	0	0	0	0
Beer-light	fl oz	8.26	0.059	0.384	0	0	0	0
Hot cocoa-prep/milk-home	cup	218	9.1	25.8	9.05	33.3	5.61	3
Cream soda	fl oz	15.8	0	4.1	0	0	0	0
Perrier-mineral water	cup	0	0	0	0	0	0	0
Ovaltine-choc-prep/milk	cup	227	9.53	29.2	8.79	-	-	-
Coffee substitute-prepared	fl oz	1.52	0.03	0.303	0	0	0.002	0
Postum-inst grain bev-dry	ounce	103	1.93	24.1	0.028	0	0	0
Tang-inst drink-orange-dry	ounce	104	0	26.1	0	0	0	-
Wine-white-table	fl oz	20.1	0.03	0.236	0	0	0	0
Fruit punch drink-can	fl oz	14.6	0	3.69	0	0	0.001	0
Wine-cooler-white wine-7UP	serving	54.9	0.05	5.72	0	0	0	0
Water	cup	0	0	0	0	0	0	0
Lemon lime soda-7UP	fl oz	12.3	0	3.19	0	0	0	0
Tea-herb-brewed	fl oz	0.296	0	0.059	0	0	0.001	0
Gatorade-thirst quencher	fl oz	7.53	0	1.9	0	0	0	0
Tonic water-quinine soda	fl oz	10.4	0	2.68	0	0	0	0
Wine-rosé-table	fl oz	20.9	0.059	0.413	0	0	0	0
BREADS								
Bagel-egg	item	163	6.02	30.9	1.41	8	-	1.16
Bagel-water	item	163	6.02	30.9	1.41	0	0.2	1.16
Biscuits-prepared/mixed	item	104	1.63	13	5.05	1.4	3.31	0.504
Breadcrumbs-dry-grated	cup	390	13	73	5	0	1	3.65
Bread-cracked wheat	slice	65.5	2.32	12.5	0.868	0	0.1	1.33
Bread-french-enriched	slice	98	3.33	17.7	1.36	0	0.2	0.805

FOOD COMPOSITION TABLE—cont'd

Food Name	Serving	KCAL Kc	PROT Gm	CARB Gm	FAT Gm	CHOL Mg	SAFA Gm	FIBD Gm
Bread-raisin-enriched	slice	69.5	2.05	13.2	0.99	0	0.2	0.55
Bread-rye-American-light	slice	65.5	2.12	12	0.913	0	-	1.55
Bread-pumpernickel	slice	81.6	2.93	15.4	1.1	0	-	1.89
Bread-white-firm	slice	61.4	1.9	11.2	0.902	0	0.2	0.437
Bread-white-firm-toasted	slice	65	2	12	1	0	0.2	0.5
Bread-whole wheat-firm	slice	61.3	2.41	11.3	1.09	0	0.1	2.83
Bread-wheat-firm-toasted	slice	59	2.31	10.9	1.05	0	0.1	2.38
Crackers-graham-plain	item	27.5	0.5	5	0.5	0	0.1	0.224
Crackers-rye wafers	item	22.5	1	5	0	0	0	1.05
Crackers-saltines	item	12.5	0.25	2	0.25	0.75	0.1	0.072
Muffin-blueberry-home rec	item	110	3	17	4	21	1.1	0.85
Muffin-bran-home rec	item	112	2.96	16.7	5.08	21	1.2	2.52
Muffin-corn-home rec	item	125	3	19	4	21	1.2	0.95
Muffin-plain-home rec	item	120	3	17	4	21	1	0.85
Pancakes-buckwheat-mix	item	55	2	6	2	20	0.8	0.621
Pancakes-plain-home recipe	item	60	2	9	2	20	0.5	0.45
Pancakes-plain-mix	item	58.9	1.85	7.87	21.7	20	0.7	0.394
Roll-brown & serve-enr	item	85	2	14	2	0	0.4	0.988
Roll-hamburger/hotdog	item	114	3.43	20.1	2.09	0	0.5	1.01
Roll-hard-enriched	item	155	5	30	2	0	0.4	1.5
Roll-submarine/hoagie-enr	item	390	12	75	4	0	0.9	3.75
Waffles-enr-home recipe	item	245	6.93	25.7	12.6	45	2.3	1.05
Muffin-English-plain	item	133	4.43	25.7	1.09	0	-	1.29
Muffin-English-plain-toast	item	154	5.13	29.8	1.26	0	-	1.49
Bread-corn-home rec	slice	108	2.21	15.6	3.94	0	-	1.17
Crackers-cheese	item	5.38	0.091	0.52	0.327	-	0.09	0.025
Crackers-graham-sug/honey	item	30.1	0.519	5.4	0.732	0	0.1	0.119
French toast-home recipe	slice	153	5.67	17.2	6.73	-	-	2.02
Waffles-frozen	item	103	2.15	15.9	3.52	0	-	0.888
Bread-mixed grain	slice	64.3	2.49	11.7	0.93	0	-	1.58
Bread-whole wheat-home rec	slice	66.5	2.25	11.6	1.16	0	-	2.83
Bread-pita	item	105	3.95	20.6	0.57	0	-	0.608
Crackers-Rykrisp-natural	item	7.5	0.25	1.67	0.033	0	0	0.34
Crackers-animal	item	8.67	0.127	1.47	0.2	0	-	0.027
Crackers-cheddar snacks	item	7.22	0.144	1.11	0.261	-	-	0.056
Crackers-triscuits	item	21	0.4	3.1	0.75	0	-	0.155
Crackers-wheat thins	item	9	0.125	1.25	0.35	0	-	0.099
Roll-whole wheat-homemade	item	90	3.5	18.3	1	0	-	1.83
Croissant-roll-Sara Lee	item	109	2.3	11.2	6.1	-	-	0.56
Muffin-soy	item	119	3.9	16.7	4.4	0	-	0.835
Bread stick-vienna type	item	106	3.3	20.3	1.1	0	-	1.02
Crackers-Ritz	item	18	0.233	21.3	0.967	0	-	0.107
BREAKFAST CEREALS								
Cereal-corn grits-enriched	cup	145	3.39	31.5	0.484	0	0.073	0.6
Cereal-farina-cook-enr	cup	117	3.26	24.7	0.233	0	0.023	3.26
Cereal-wheat-rolled-cooked	cup	180	5	41	1	0	0.182	2.87
Cereal-wheat-wholemeal	cup	110	4	23	1	0	0.182	1.61
Cereal-frost flake-Kellogg	cup	133	1.75	31.7	0.07	0	0	0.77
Cereal-corn-shredded sugar	cup	95	2	22	0	0	0	1.54
Cereal-oats-puffed-sugar	cup	100	3	19	1	0	0.185	2.65

FOOD COMPOSITION TABLE—cont'd

Food Name	Serving	KCAL Kc	PROT Gm	CARB Gm	FAT Gm	CHOL Mg	SAFA Gm	FIBD Gm
Cereal-rice-puffed-plain	cup	56.3	0.882	12.6	0.07	0	0	0.1
Cereal-rice-puffed-sugar	serving	115	1	26	0	0	0	0.2
Cereal-wheat-flakes-sugar	cup	105	3	24	0	0	0	2.7
Cereal-wheat-puffed plain	cup	43.7	1.76	9.55	0.144	0	0	0.4
Cereal-wheat-puffed sugar	serving	138	5.59	30.2	0.456	0	-	2.11
Cereal-wheat-shred-biscuit	item	83	2.6	18.8	0.3	0	0	2.2
Cereal-wheat germ-toasted	cup	432	32.9	56.1	12.1	0	2.07	14.6
Cereal-cream/wheat-packet	item	132	2.5	28.9	0.4	0	0	2.02
Cereal-oatmeal-inst packet	item	104	4.4	18.1	1.7	0	0.289	1.62
Cereal-Ralston-cooked	cup	134	5.57	28.2	0.8	0	0	4.2
Cereal-All Bran	cup	212	12.2	63.4	1.53	0	-	25.5
Cereal-Alpha Bits	cup	111	2.2	24.6	0.6	0	-	0.3
Cereal-Bran Buds	cup	220	11.8	64.8	2.04	0	-	23.6
Cereal-Bran Chex	cup	156	5.05	39	1.37	0	-	7.9
Cereal-C.W. Post-plain	cup	432	8.7	69.4	15.2	0.184	11.3	2.2
Cereal-Cheerios	cup	88.8	3.42	15.7	1.45	0	0.27	0.863
Cereal-corn bran	cup	125	2.45	30.3	1.26	0	-	6.84
Cereal-Corn Chex	cup	111	2.02	24.9	0.114	0	0	0.5
Cereal-cornflakes-Kellogg	cup	88.3	1.84	19.5	0.068	0	0	0.454
Cereal-Cracklin Bran	cup	229	5.52	41.2	8.76	0	-	9.1
Cereal-Crispy rice	cup	112	1.82	25.2	0.114	0	0	1
Cereal-fortified oat flake	cup	177	8.98	34.8	0.72	0	0	1.2
Cereal-bran flakes-Kellogg	cup	127	4.91	30.5	0.741	0	0	5.5
Cereal-Frosted Mini Wheats	item	25.5	0.731	5.86	0.071	0	0	0.54
Cereal-granola-homemade	cup	594	15	67.3	33.2	0	5.84	12.8
Cereal-Grape Nuts	cup	407	13.3	93.5	0.456	0	0	5.47
Cereal-Grape Nuts Flakes	cup	116	3.48	26.6	0.358	0	0	2.08
Cereal-Heartland Natural	cup	499	11.6	78.5	17.7	0	-	5.4
Cereal-Honey Nut Cheerios	cup	125	3.63	26.5	0.759	0	0.132	1.3
Cereal-Honey Bran	cup	119	3.08	28.6	0.735	0	0	3.9
Cereal-Life-plain/cinnamon	cup	162	8.1	31.5	0.836	0	0	1.4
Cereal-Lucky Charms	cup	125	2.91	26.1	1.22	0	0.224	0.6
Cereal-granola-Nature Val	cup	503	11.5	75.5	19.6	0	13	4.2
Cereal-Nutri Grain-barley	cup	153	4.47	33.9	0.328	0	0	2.4
Cereal-Nutri Grain-corn	cup	160	3.36	35.4	0.966	0	-	2.6
Cereal-Nutri Grain-rye	cup	144	3.48	33.9	0.28	0	0	2.56
Cereal-Nutri Grain-wheat	cup	158	3.83	37.2	0.44	0	0	2.8
Cereal-100% bran	cup	178	8.25	48.1	3.3	0	0.587	19.5
Cereal-Product 19	cup	126	3.23	27.4	0.231	0	0	0.4
Cereal-Raisin Bran-Kellogg	cup	154	5.31	37.1	0.984	0	-	5.31
Cereal-Rice Chex	cup	99.5	1.34	22.5	0.101	0	0	0.151
Cereal-Rice Krispies	cup	112	1.93	24.8	0.199	0	0	0.1
Cereal-Special K	cup	83.1	4.2	16	0.085	0.028	0	0.17
Cereal-Sugar Corn Pops	cup	108	1.42	25.7	0.085	0	0	0.2
Cereal-Sugar Smacks	cup	141	2.65	33	0.72	0	0	0.531
Cereal-Team	cup	164	2.69	36	0.756	0	0	0.7
Cereal-Toasties	cup	87.8	1.84	19.5	0.045	0	0	0.386
Cereal-Total	cup	116	3.3	26	0.693	0	0.099	2.4
Cereal-Trix	cup	109	1.53	25.2	0.398	0	0	0.32
Cereal-Wheat Chex	cup	169	4.55	37.8	1.15	0	-	3.4

FOOD COMPOSITION TABLE—cont'd

Food Name	Serving	KCAL Kc	PROT Gm	CARB Gm	FAT Gm	CHOL Mg	SAFA Gm	FIBD Gm
Cereal-wheat germ-sugar	cup	426	24.6	68.7	9.04	0	1.57	5.7
Cereal-Wheaties	cup	101	2.8	23.1	0.5	0	0.07	2
Cereal-cream/wheat-reg-hot	cup	133	3.8	27.7	0.5	0	0	1.94
Cereal-cream/wheat instant	cup	153	4.4	31.6	0.6	0	0	2.21
Cereal-malt o meal-cook	cup	122	3.6	25.9	0.24	0	0	0.6
Cereal-Maypo-cook-hot	cup	170	5.8	31.8	2.4	0	-	1.2
Cereal-Roman Meal-cooked	cup	147	6.51	33	0.964	0	-	2.31
Cereal-Wheatena-cooked	cup	136	4.86	28.7	1.22	0	-	2.6
Cereal-whole wheat natural	cup	150	4.84	33.2	0.968	0	-	2.7
Cereal-oatmeal-raw	cup	311	13	54.2	5.1	0	0.9	4.6
COMBINATION FOODS								
Beef-Raviolios-canned	ounce	27.5	1.14	4.26	0.568	-	0.11	0.23
Salad-three-bean-Del Monte	ounce	22.4	0.71	5.06	0.056	0	0	1.52
Salad-tuna	cup	350	30	7	22	68	4.3	1.03
Beef-vegetable stew	cup	220	16	15	11	72	4.9	3.19
Beef potpie-home recipe	slice	515	21	39	30	44	7.9	3.9
Chili concarne/beans-can	cup	340	19	31	16	38	7.5	5
Chicken a la king-home rec	cup	470	27	12	34	186	12.9	1.2
Chicken chow mein-canned	cup	95	7	18	0	98	0	0.9
Chicken potpie-baked-home	slice	545	23	42	31	72	11	4.2
Macaroni & cheese-enr-can	cup	230	9	26	10	42	4.2	1.44
Macaroni & cheese-enr-home	cup	430	17	40	22	42	8.9	1.2
Pizza-cheese-baked	slice	140	7.68	20.5	3.21	9	1.54	1.59
Spaghetti/tom/che-home rec	cup	260	9	37	9	4	2	2.5
Spaghetti/tom/che-can	cup	190	6	39	2	4	0.5	2.5
Spaghetti/tom/meat-home	cup	330	19	39	12	75	3.3	2.73
Spaghetti/tom/meat-can	cup	260	12	29	10	39	2.2	2.75
Beans/pork/frankfurter-can	cup	365	17.3	39.6	16.9	15.4	6.05	12.8
Beans/pork/tom sauce-can	cup	248	13.1	49.1	2.61	17	0.999	13.8
Beans/pork/sweet sauce/can	cup	281	13.4	53.1	3.69	17.7	1.42	14
Salad-potato	cup	358	6.7	27.9	20.5	170	3.57	5.25
Vegetables-mixed-froz-boil	cup	107	5.21	23.8	0.273	0	0.056	6.92
Salad-fruit-can/juice	cup	125	1.27	32.5	0.075	0	0.01	1.64
Salad-coleslaw	tbsp	5.52	0.103	0.993	0.209	1	0.031	0.297
Taco	item	370	20.7	26.7	20.6	57	11.4	2.67
Pizza-pepperoni-baked	slice	181	10.1	19.9	6.96	14	2.24	1.48
Sand-bac/let/tom/mayo	item	282	6.8	28.8	15.6	-	-	2.88
Sandwich-club	item	590	35.6	41.7	20.8	-	-	4.17
Salad-macaroni	serving	50.7	0.7	5.3	3	-	-	0.29
Salad-carrot raisin-home	cup	306	3.8	55.8	11.6	-	-	16.7
Salad-mandarin orange gel	serving	22.7	0.4	5.7	0	0	0	0.57
Salad-chicken	cup	502	26	17.4	36.2	-	-	-
Chili with beans-canned	cup	286	14.6	30.4	14	43.4	6	6.93
Salad-green salad-tossed	serving	32	2.6	6.67	0.16	0	0.021	2.11
Meat loaf-celery/onions	serving	213	15.8	5.23	13.9	107	5.29	0.11
Salad-chef salad-ham/chees	serving	196	13.4	7.42	12.7	46	6.98	2.39
DAIRY PRODUCTS								
Cheese-blue	ounce	100	6.06	0.659	8.14	21	5.29	0
Cheese-camembert-wedge	item	114	7.52	0.18	9.22	27	5.8	0
Cheese-cheddar-shredded	cup	455	28.1	1.45	37.5	119	23.8	-

FOOD COMPOSITION TABLE—cont'd

Food Name	Serving	KCAL Kc	PROT Gm	CARB Gm	FAT Gm	CHOL Mg	SAFA Gm	FIBD Gm
Cheese-cottage-4% lar curd	cup	232	28.1	6.03	10.1	33.8	6.41	0
Cheese-cream	ounce	100	2.17	0.759	10	31.4	6.31	0
Cheese-mozzarella-skim milk	ounce	72	6.88	0.78	4.51	16	2.87	0
Cheese-parmesan-grated	cup	456	41.6	3.74	30	79	19.1	0
Cheese-provolone	ounce	100	7.25	0.61	7.55	20	4.84	0
Cheese-ricotta-skim milk	cup	340	28	12.6	19.5	76	12.1	0
Cheese-romano	ounce	110	9.02	1.03	7.64	29	4.85	0
Cheese-Swiss	ounce	107	8.06	0.96	7.78	26	5.04	0
Cheese-American-processed	ounce	106	6.28	0.45	8.86	27	5.58	0
Cheese-swiss-processed	ounce	95	7.01	0.6	7.09	24	4.55	0
Cheese food-American-proc	ounce	93	5.56	2.07	6.97	18	4.38	0
Cheese-spread-processed	ounce	82	4.65	2.48	6.02	16	3.78	0
Cream-half & half-fluid	cup	315	7.16	10.4	27.8	89	17.3	0
Cream-coffee-table-light	cup	469	6.48	8.78	46.3	159	28.9	0
Cream-whipping-heavy	cup	821	4.88	6.64	88.1	326	54.8	0
Cream-whip-pressurized	cup	154	1.92	7.49	13.3	46	8.3	0
Cream-sour-cultured	cup	493	7.27	9.82	48.2	102	30	0
Cream-whip-imit-froz	cup	239	0.94	17.3	19	0	16.3	0
Cream-whip-imit-pressurize	cup	184	0.69	11.3	15.6	0	13.2	0
Milk-whole-3.3% fat-fluid	cup	150	8.03	11.4	8.15	33	5.07	0
Milk-2% fat-lowfat-fluid	cup	121	8.12	11.7	4.68	18	2.92	0
Milk-2% milk solids added	cup	125	8.53	12.2	4.7	18	2.93	0
Milk-1% fat-lowfat-fluid	cup	102	8.03	11.7	2.59	10	1.61	0
Milk-buttermilk-fluid	cup	99	8.11	11.7	2.16	9	1.34	0
Milk-evaporated-whole can	cup	338	17.2	25.3	19.1	73.1	11.6	0
Milk-evaporated-skim can	cup	199	19.3	28.9	0.51	10.2	0.309	0
Milk-condensed-sweet can	cup	982	24.2	166	26.6	104	16.8	0
Milk-chocolate-whole	cup	208	7.92	25.9	8.48	30	5.26	0.15
Milk-eggnog-commercial	cup	342	9.68	34.4	19	149	11.3	0
Milkshake-chocolate-thick	item	356	9.15	63.5	8.1	32	5.04	0.75
Milkshake-vanilla-thick	item	350	12.1	55.6	9.48	37	5.9	0.2
Yogurt-fruit flavor-lowfat	cup	231	9.92	43.2	2.45	10	1.58	0.8
Yogurt-plain-low-fat	cup	144	11.9	16	3.52	14	2.27	0
Yogurt-plain-nonfat	cup	127	13	17.4	0.41	4	0.264	0
Yogurt-plain-whole	cup	139	7.88	10.6	7.38	29	4.76	0
Cheese-feta	ounce	75	4.03	1.16	6.03	25	4.24	0
Cheese-gouda	ounce	101	7.07	0.63	7.78	32	4.99	0
Cheese-limburger	ounce	93	5.68	0.14	7.72	26	4.75	0
Cheese-monterey	ounce	106	6.94	0.19	8.58	25.2	5.41	0
Cheese-roquefort	ounce	105	6.11	0.57	8.69	26	5.46	0
Cream-sour-half & half	tbsp	20	0.44	0.64	1.8	6	1.12	0
Cream-sour-imitation	ounce	59	0.68	1.88	5.53	0	5.04	0
Milk-whole-low sodium	cup	149	7.56	10.9	8.44	33	5.26	0
Milk-human-whole-mature	cup	171	2.53	17	10.8	34	4.94	0
DESSERTS								
Ice cream-van-hard-10% fat	cup	269	4.8	31.7	14.3	59	8.92	0
Ice cream-van-soft serve	cup	377	7.04	38.3	22.5	153	13.5	0
Ice milk-van-soft-2.6% fat	cup	223	8.03	38.4	4.62	13	2.88	0
Sherbet-orange 2% fat	cup	270	2.16	58.7	3.82	14	2.38	0
Custard-baked	cup	305	14	29	15	278	6.8	1.02

FOOD COMPOSITION TABLE—cont'd

Food Name	Serving	KCAL Kc	PROT Gm	CARB Gm	FAT Gm	CHOL Mg	SAFA Gm	FIBD Gm
Pudd-tapioca cream-home	cup	220	8	28	8	80	4.1	0.56
Pudd-choc-cooked-mix/milk	cup	320	9	59	8	32	4.3	0
Pudd-choc-inst-mix/milk	cup	325	8	63	7	28	3.6	0
Cake-angelfood-mix/prep	slice	142	4.2	31.5	0.122	0	-	0.037
Cupcake/chocolate icing	item	130	2	21	5	15	2	0.42
Cake-gingerbread-mix/prep	slice	175	2	32	4	1	1.1	1.83
Cake-yellow/icing-home rec	slice	268	2.9	40.3	11.4	36	3	0.552
Cake-fruit-dark-home rec	slice	56.9	0.72	8.96	2.3	6.75	0.48	0.313
Cake-sheet-no icing-home	slice	315	4	48	12	1	3.3	0.96
Cake-pound-home recipe	slice	160	2	16	10	68	54.9	0.08
Cake-sponge-home recipe	slice	188	4.82	35.7	3.14	162	1.1	0
Cookie-chocolate chip-mix	item	50	0.5	6.96	2.42	5.52	0.7	0.284
Cookie-choc chip-home rec	item	46.3	0.5	6.41	2.68	5.25	0.6	0.27
Cookie-macaroon	item	90	1	12.5	4.5	0	-	0.437
Cookie-oatmeal/raisin-mix	item	61.5	0.732	8.93	2.6	0	0.5	0.351
Cookie-sandwich-choc/van	item	50	0.5	7	2.25	0	0.55	0.15
Cookie-vanilla wafer	item	18.5	0.2	3	0.6	2.5	0.1	0.01
Danish pastry-plain	item	250	4.06	29.1	13.6	0	4.7	0.582
Doughnuts-cake-plain	item	104	1.28	12.2	5.77	10	1.2	0.325
Doughnuts-yeast-glazed	item	205	3	22	11.2	13	3	1.1
Pie-apple-home rec	slice	323	2.75	49.1	13.6	0	3.9	2.16
Pie-banana cream-home rec	slice	285	6	40	12	40	3.8	1.4
Pie-cherry-home rec	slice	350	4	52	15	0	4	1.08
Pie-custard-home rec	slice	285	8	30	14	-	4.8	2.08
Pie-lemon meringue-home	slice	300	3.86	47.3	11.2	-	3.7	1.44
Pie-mince-home rec	slice	365	3	56	16	0	4	1.96
Pie-peach-home rec	slice	345	3	52	14	0	3.5	1.82
Pie-pecan-home rec	slice	495	6	61	27	0	4	4.13
Pie-pumpkin-home rec	slice	275	5	32	15	0	5.4	3.51
Piecrust-mix/prep-baked	item	743	10	70.5	46.5	0	11.4	4.23
Granola bar	item	109	2.35	16	4.23	-	-	0.96
Cookie-sugar-mix	item	98.8	0.908	13.1	4.79	-	-	0.262
Cake-cheesecake-commercial	slice	257	4.61	24.3	16.3	-	-	1.79
Ice cream sundae-hot fudge	item	297	5.89	49.8	9.01	21.5	5.25	-
Turnover-apple	ounce	85.2	0.738	10.5	4.71	1.42	-	0.21
Cookie-peanut butter-mix	item	50	0.8	5.87	2.64	-	-	0.18
Pudd-rice/raisins	cup	387	9.5	70.8	8.2	-	-	1.42
Cake-strawberry shortcake	serving	344	4.8	61.2	8.9	-	-	2.14
Froz yogurt-fruit variety cup	216	7	41.8	2	-	-	-	-
Twinkie-Hostess	item	143	1.25	25.6	4.2	21	-	-
EGGS								
Egg-whole-raw-large	item	75	6.25	0.61	5.01	213	1.55	0
Egg-white-raw-large	item	17	3.52	0.34	0	0	0	0
Egg-yolk-raw-large	item	59	2.78	0.3	5.12	213	1.59	0
Egg-hard-large-no shell	item	77	6.29	0.56	5.3	213	1.63	0
Egg-poached-whole-large	item	74	6.22	0.61	4.99	212	1.54	0
Egg-substitute-liquid	cup	211	30.1	1.61	8.31	2.51	1.65	0
FATS/OILS								
Butter-regular-tablespoon	tbsp	100	0.119	0.008	11.4	30.7	7.07	0
Butter-whipped-tablespoon	tbsp	64.5	0.077	0.005	7.3	19.7	4.54	0

FOOD COMPOSITION TABLE—cont'd

Food Name	Serving	KCAL Kc	PROT Gm	CARB Gm	FAT Gm	CHOL Mg	SAFA Gm	FIBD Gm
Shortening-vegetable-soy	cup	1812	0	0	205	0	51.2	0
Margarine-diet Mazola	tbsp	50	0	0	5.7	0	1	0
Margarine-veg spray-Mazola	serving	6	0	0	0.72	0	0.08	0
Margarine-reg-hard-stick	item	812	1.02	1.02	91	0	17.9	0
Vegetable oil-corn	cup	1927	0	0	218	0	27.7	0
Vegetable oil-olive	cup	1909	0	0	216	0	29.2	0
Sal dress-blue cheese	tbsp	77.1	0.7	1.1	8	2.6	1.5	0.05
Sal dress-blue che-low cal	tbsp	10	0	1	1	4	0.5	0
Sal dress-French	tbsp	67	0.1	2.7	6.4	1.95	1.5	0.1
Sal dress-French-low cal	tbsp	21.9	0.033	3.5	0.9	0.978	0.13	0.09
Sal dress-Italian	tbsp	68.7	0	1.5	7.1	0	1	0.05
Sal dress-Italian-low cal	tbsp	15.8	0	0.7	1.5	1	0.2	0.09
Sal dress-mayonnaise type	tbsp	57.3	0.132	4.91	4.91	3.82	0.72	0
Sal dress-mayo-low cal	tbsp	20	0	2	2	2	0.4	0
Sal dress-Thousand Island	tbsp	58.9	0.14	2.4	5.6	4.9	0.9	0.6
Sal dress-Thous Isl-low cal	tbsp	24.3	0.1	2.5	1.6	2	0.2	0.3
Animal fat-cooking-chicken	tbsp	115	0	0	12.8	11	3.8	0
Margarine-corn-reg-hard	tsp	33.8	0	0	3.8	0	0.6	0
Margarine-corn-reg-soft	tsp	33.7	0	0	3.8	0	0.7	0
Mayonnaise-imitation-soy	tbsp	34.7	0.045	2.4	2.9	3.6	0.495	0
Sal dress-Russian-low cal	tbsp	23	0.082	4.5	0.652	1	0.1	0.2
Sal dress-Russian	tbsp	76	0.2	1.6	7.8	0	1.1	0
Sal dress-vinegar/oil-home	tbsp	70	0	0.39	7.81	0	1.42	0
Sandwich spread-commercial	tbsp	59.5	0.1	3.4	5.2	12	0.8	0.02
Mayonnaise-light-low-cal	tbsp	40	0	1	4	5	-	0
Miracle Whip-light-low cal	tbsp	45	0	2	4	5	-	0
Sal dress-Caesar	tbsp	70	0	1	7	-	-	0.04
Sal dress-ranch style	tbsp	54	0.4	0.6	5.7	-	-	0
FISH								
Fish-bluefish-baked/butter	item	246	40.6	0	8.1	108	1.83	0
Fish-clams-raw-meat only	serving	62.9	10.9	2.18	0.83	28.9	0.08	0
Fish-clam-can-solid/liquid	ounce	12.8	2.33	0.667	0.333	17.7	0.067	0
Fish-crab meat-king-can	cup	135	24	1	3.2	135	0.6	0
Fish-stick-bread-froz-cook	ounce	77.2	4.44	6.75	3.47	31.8	0.894	0.665
Fish-perch-breaded-fried	piece	195	16	6	11	32	2.7	0.05
Fish-oysters-raw-meat only	cup	171	17.5	9.7	6.14	136	1.56	0
Fish-salmon-pink-can	serving	118	16.8	0	5.14	46.8	1.3	0
Fish-sardines-can/oil	item	25	2.95	0	1.37	17	0.184	0
Fish-shad-bake/marg/bacon	serving	201	23.2	0	11.3	69.4	2.45	0
Fish-shrimp-meat-can	cup	154	29.5	1.32	2.51	221	0.477	0
Fish-shrimp-french fried	serving	206	18.2	9.75	10.4	150	1.77	0.48
Fish-tuna-can/oil-drained	serving	168	24.8	0	6.98	15.3	1.3	0
Fish-tuna-white can/water	serving	116	22.7	0	2.09	35.7	0.556	0
Fish-tuna-diet-low sodium	ounce	35.5	7.67	0.011	0.54	9.94	0.09	0
Fish-tuna-light-can/water	serving	111	25.1	0	0.525	15.3	0.136	0
Fish-anchovy-fillet can	item	8.4	1.16	0	0.388	3.4	0.088	0
Fish-cod-cooked-dry heat	piece	189	41.1	0	1.55	99	0.302	0
Fish-crab cake	item	93	12.1	0.288	4.51	90	0.89	0.03
Fish-crab-steamed pieces	cup	150	30	0	2.39	82.2	0.206	0
Fish-sole/flounder-baked	serving	148	30.7	0	1.94	86	0.461	0

FOOD COMPOSITION TABLE—cont'd

Food Name	Serving	KCAL Kc	PROT Gm	CARB Gm	FAT Gm	CHOL Mg	SAFA Gm	FIBD Gm
Fish-haddock-cook-dry heat	serving	95.2	20.6	0	0.79	62.9	0.142	0
Fish-mackerel-Atlantic-can	cup	296	44.1	0	12	150	3.53	0
Fish-rockfish-ckd-dry heat	serving	121	24	0	2.01	44	0.474	0
Fish-roe-raw-eggs	ounce	39.4	6.34	0.426	1.82	106	0.414	0
Fish-salmon-smoked	serving	117	18.3	0	4.32	23	0.929	0
Fish-scallops-steamed	ounce	31.8	6.59	0.511	0.398	15.1	-	0
Fish-swordfish-broil/marg	serving	174	28	0	6	4	-	0
Fish-trout-brook-cooked	serving	196	23.5	0.4	11.2	-	-	0
Fish-whitefish-bake/stuff	serving	215	15.2	5.8	14	-	-	0.58
Fish-white perch-fri-fillet	item	108	12.5	0	5.3	-	-	0
Fish-carp-cooked-dry heat	serving	138	19.4	0	6.1	71.4	1.18	0
Fish-catfish-fried-breaded	serving	195	15.4	6.83	11.3	68.9	2.79	0.8
Fish-flatfish-ckd-dry heat	serving	99.5	20.5	0	1.3	58	0.309	0
Fish-grouper-ckd-dry heat	serving	100	25.7	0	1.11	40	0.254	0
Fish-mackerel-ckd-dry heat	serving	223	20.3	0	15.1	63.8	3.55	0
Fish-ocean perch-ckd-dry	serving	103	20.3	0	1.78	45.9	0.266	0
Fish-perch-cooked-dry heat	serving	99.5	21.1	0	1	98	0.201	0
Fish-pollock-ckd-dry heat	serving	96.1	20	0	0.952	81.6	0.196	0
Fish-pompano-ckd-dry heat	serving	179	20.1	0	10.3	54.4	3.82	0
Fish-salmon-ckd-moist heat	serving	157	23.3	0	6.41	41.7	1.19	0
Fish-sea-bass-ckd-dry heat	serving	105	20.1	0	2.18	45.1	0.557	0
Fish-smelt-cooked-dry heat	serving	105	19.2	0	2.64	76.5	0.492	0
Fish-red snapper-ckd-dry	serving	109	22.4	0	1.46	40	0.31	0
Fish-surimi	serving	84.2	12.9	5.82	0.765	25.5	0.153	0
Fish-pollock-Atlantic-raw	serving	78.2	16.5	0	0.833	60.4	0.115	0
Fish-swordfish-cooked-dry	serving	132	21.6	0	4.37	42.5	1.2	0
Fish-trout-rainbow-ckd-dry	serving	128	22.4	0	3.66	62.1	0.707	0
Fish-tuna-yellowfin-raw	serving	91.8	19.9	0	0.81	38.3	0.2	0
Fish-whiting-ckd-dry heat	serving	98	20	0	1.43	71.4	0.269	0
Fish-crab-imitation-surimi	serving	86.7	10.2	8.69	1.11	17	0.221	0
Fish-crayfish-ckd-moist	serving	96.9	20.3	0	1.15	151	0.197	0
Fish-lobster-ckd-moist	ounce	27.8	5.82	0.364	0.168	20.4	0.03	0
Fish-shrimp-ckd-moist heat	serving	84.2	17.8	0	0.918	166	0.246	0
Fish-clams-breaded-fried	serving	172	12.1	8.78	8.78	51.9	2.28	0.32
Fish-clams-ckd-moist heat	serving	126	21.7	4.36	1.65	57	0.16	0
Fish-mussel-blue-ckd-moist	serving	147	20.2	6.28	3.81	47.6	0.723	0
Fish-oyster-Eastern-canned	cup	171	17.5	9.7	6.14	136	1.57	0
Fish-oyster-East-ckd-moist	serving	117	12	6.65	4.21	92.7	1.07	0
Fish-oysters-Pacific-raw	serving	68.9	8.03	4.21	1.96	42.5	0.434	0
Fish-squid-cooked-fried	serving	149	15.3	6.62	6.36	221	1.6	0.3
Fish-halibut-broiled-dry	serving	119	22.7	0	2.5	34.9	0.354	0
FROZEN DINNERS								
Fish divan-Lean Cuisine	item	270	31	16	10	85	-	-
Fettucini alfredo-Stouffer	item	270	8	19	18	-	-	-
Turkey pie-Stouffer	item	460	20	35	26	-	-	-
Meatballs/noodles-Stouffer	item	475	25	33	27	-	-	-
Beef/green peppers-Stouf	item	225	10	18	11	-	-	-
Lasagna-Stouffer	item	385	28	36	14	-	-	-
Chicken cacciatore-Stouf	item	310	25	29	11	-	-	-
Veal parmigiana-froz din	item	296	24	17	14	-	-	-

FOOD COMPOSITION TABLE—cont'd

Food Name	Serving	KCAL Kc	PROT Gm	CARB Gm	FAT Gm	CHOL Mg	SAFA Gm	FIBD Gm
Cabbage roll/tom sauc-Horm	ounce	23	1.1	3.2	0.7	3	0.281	-
Chicken kiev-Le Menu	item	500	21	35	30	-	-	-
Vegetable lasagna-Le Menu	item	400	15	30	24	-	-	-
Beef sirloin tips-Le Menu	item	400	29	27	19	-	-	-
Chicken parmigiana-Le Menu	item	390	26	28	19	-	-	-
Manicotti-cheese-Le Menu	item	310	18	29	13	-	-	-
Sole-light-Van de Kamps	item	293	16	17	18	-	-	-
Mexican dinner-Swanson	item	590	20	64	29	-	-	-
Beef dinner-Swanson	item	320	25	34	9	-	-	-
Turkey dinner-Swanson	item	340	20	42	10	-	-	-
Chicken dinner-Swanson	item	660	26	64	33	-	-	-
Egg roll-beef/shrimp/froz	item	27	0.9	3.5	1	-	-	0.12
Fish & chips-Van de Kamps	item	500	16	45	30	-	-	-
Meatloaf-froz din-Banquet	item	412	20.9	29	23.7	-	-	-
Ham-froz din-Banquet	item	369	16.8	47.7	12.2	-	-	-
Salisbury steak din-Banq	item	390	18.1	24	24.6	-	-	-
FRUITS								
Apples-raw-unpeeled	item	81	0.262	21.1	0.497	0	0.08	3.04
Apple-juice-canned/bottled	cup	116	0.15	29	0.28	0	0.047	0.52
Applesauce-can-sweetened	cup	194	0.459	50.8	0.47	0	0.077	3.06
Applesauce-can-unsweetened	cup	105	0.415	27.6	0.12	0	0.02	3.66
Apricot-raw-without pit	item	16.9	0.494	3.93	0.138	0	0.01	0.67
Apricots-dried-uncooked	cup	309	4.75	80.3	0.6	0	0.042	10.1
Apricots-dried-cooked-unsw	cup	213	3.24	54.8	0.4	0	0.028	19.5
Avocado-raw-California	item	306	3.65	12	30	0	4.48	6.13
Bananas-raw-peeled	item	105	1.17	26.7	0.547	0	0.211	1.82
Blackberries-raw	cup	74.9	1.04	18.4	0.562	0	0.07	8.93
Blueberries-raw	cup	81.2	0.972	20.5	0.551	0	0.07	3.34
Cherries-sweet-raw	item	4.9	0.082	1.13	0.065	0	0.015	0.1
Cranberry sauce-can-sweet	cup	418	0.554	108	0.416	0	0.06	3.2
Dates-natural-dried-chop	cup	490	3.51	131	0.801	0	0.05	15.5
Grapefruit-raw-pink & red	item	74	1.36	18.5	0.246	0	0.034	3.2
Grapefruit-raw-white	item	78	1.63	19.3	0.236	0	0.033	2.5
Grapefruit juice-raw	cup	96.3	1.24	22.7	0.247	0	0.035	0.5
Grapefruit juice-can-uns	cup	93.9	1.28	22.1	0.247	0	0.032	0.442
Grapefruit juice-can-sweet	cup	115	1.45	27.8	0.225	0	0.03	0
Grapefruit juice-froz-dilu	cup	101	1.36	24	0.321	0	0.047	0
Grape juice-can & bottle	cup	154	1.42	37.8	0.202	0	0.063	0
Grape juice-froz-diluted	cup	128	0.475	31.9	0.225	0	0.073	0
Grape drink-canned	cup	154	1.42	37.8	0.202	0	0.063	0
Lemons-raw-peeled	item	16.8	0.638	5.41	0.174	0	0.023	0.58
Lemon juice-raw	cup	61	0.927	21.1	0	0	0	0.732
Lemon juice-can & bottle	cup	51.2	0.976	15.8	0.708	0	0.093	0.732
Lemonade-froz-diluted	cup	105	0	28	0	0	0	0.56
Lime juice-raw	cup	66.4	1.08	22.2	0.246	0	0.027	0
Lime juice-can & bottle	cup	51.7	0.615	16.5	0.566	0	0.064	0
Melons-cantaloupe-raw	cup	56	1.41	13.4	0.448	0	0	1.28
Melons-honeydew-raw	cup	59.5	0.782	15.6	0.17	0	0	1.53
Oranges-raw-all varieties	item	61.6	1.23	15.4	0.157	0	0.02	3.14
Orange juice-raw	cup	111	1.74	25.8	0.496	0	0.06	1.98

FOOD COMPOSITION TABLE—cont'd

Food Name	Serving	KCAL Kc	PROT Gm	CARB Gm	FAT Gm	CHOL Mg	SAFA Gm	FIBD Gm
Orange juice-can	cup	104	1.47	24.5	0.349	0	0.045	0.26
Orange juice-froz-diluted	cup	112	1.69	26.8	0.149	0	0.017	0.498
Papayas-raw	cup	54.6	0.854	13.7	0.196	0	0.06	1.27
Peaches-raw-whole	item	37.4	0.609	9.66	0.078	0	0.009	1.39
Peaches-raw-sliced	cup	73.1	1.19	18.9	0.153	0	0.017	2.72
Peaches-can/water pack	cup	58.6	1.07	14.9	0.146	0	0.015	1.08
Peaches-dried-uncooked	cup	382	5.78	98.1	1.22	0	0.131	14
Peaches-dried-cooked-uns	cup	199	2.99	50.8	0.645	0	0.067	6.7
Peaches-froz-sliced-sweet	cup	235	1.58	60	0.33	0	0.035	5.99
Pears-raw-Bartlett-unpeeled	item	97.9	0.647	25.1	0.664	0	0.037	4.32
Pineapple-raw-diced	cup	76	0.605	19.2	0.667	0	0.05	1.88
Pineapple juice-can	cup	140	0.8	34.5	0.2	0	0.013	0.25
Plums-raw-prune type	item	20	0	6	0	0	0	0.588
Prunes-dried-uncooked	cup	385	4.2	101	0.837	0	0.066	11
Prune juice-can & bottle	cup	182	1.56	44.7	0.077	0	0.008	2.56
Raisins-seedless	cup	435	4.67	115	0.667	0	0.218	7.69
Raisins-seedless-packet	item	42	0.451	11.1	0.064	0	0.021	0.742
Raspberries-raw	cup	60.3	1.12	14.2	0.677	0	0.023	5.5
Rhubarb-raw-cooked-sugar	cup	380	1	97	0	0	0	5.4
Strawberries-raw-whole	cup	44.7	0.909	10.5	0.551	0	0.03	3.87
Tangerines-raw-peeled	item	37	0.53	9.4	0.16	0	0.018	1.68
Watermelon-raw	cup	51.2	0.992	11.5	0.688	0	-	0.64
Apples-raw-peeled-boiled	cup	90.6	0.45	23.3	0.61	0	0.099	4.1
Apple juice-frozen-diluted	cup	112	0.34	27.6	0.239	0	0.043	0.55
Apricots-can/juice	cup	119	1.56	30.6	0.09	0	0.007	2.81
Blackberries-frozen-unsw	cup	96.6	1.78	23.7	0.649	0	-	7.55
Blueberries-frozen-unsweet	cup	79.1	0.651	18.9	0.992	0	-	4.94
Boysenberries-frozen-unsw	cup	66	1.45	16.1	0.343	0	-	5.15
Figs-dried-uncooked	cup	507	6.07	130	2.33	0	0.466	18.5
Fruit cocktail-can/juice	cup	114	1.14	29.4	0.025	0	0.005	1.51
Kiwifruit-raw	item	46.4	0.752	11.3	0.334	0	0	2.58
Limes-raw	item	20.1	0.469	7.06	0.134	0	0.015	0.353
Melons-casaba-raw	cup	44.2	1.53	10.5	0.17	0	0	2
Nectarines-raw	item	66.6	1.28	16	0.626	0	-	2.18
Papaya nectar-can	cup	143	0.425	36.3	0.375	0	0.118	1.2
Pears-can/juice	cup	124	0.843	32.1	0.174	0	0.01	4.71
Pineapple-can/juice	cup	150	1.05	39.3	0.2	0	0.015	1.88
Pineapple juice-froz-dilu	cup	130	1	31.9	0.075	0	0.005	0.3
Pomegranates-raw	item	105	1.46	26.4	0.462	0	-	1.1
Strawberries-froz-unsweet	cup	52.2	0.641	13.6	0.164	0	0.009	3.9
Cranapple juice-can	cup	170	0.253	43.3	0	0	0	0
Fruit roll up-cherry	item	50	0	12	1	0	-	-
GRAINS								
Cornmeal-degerm-enr-cooked	cup	878	20.4	186	3.96	0	0.54	1.9
Macaroni-cooked-firm-hot	cup	183	6.2	36.9	0.871	0	0.124	2.08
Noodles-egg-enr-cooked	cup	200	7	37	2	50	-	3.52
Popcorn-popped-plain	cup	25	1	5	0	0	0	0.4
Popcorn-popped-sugar coat	cup	135	2	30	1	0	0.5	1.35
Pretzel-thin-stick	item	1.19	0.028	0.242	0.011	0	0	-
Rice-white-instant-hot	cup	162	3.4	35.1	0.264	0	0.073	1.32

FOOD COMPOSITION TABLE—cont'd

Food Name	Serving	KCAL Kc	PROT Gm	CARB Gm	FAT Gm	CHOL Mg	SAFA Gm	FIBD Gm
Rice-white-long grain-cook	cup	264	5.51	57.2	0.574	0	0.158	2.13
Rice-white-parboil-cooked	cup	199	4.01	43.3	0.473	0	0.128	0.875
Spaghetti-cooked-tender-hot	cup	155	5	32	1	0	-	2.24
Flour-wheat-enr-sifted	cup	419	11.9	87.7	1.12	0	0.178	3.11
Corn chips	ounce	155	1.7	16.9	9.14	0	1.5	1.66
Taco shells	item	49.8	0.967	7.24	2.15	0	-	0.88
Tortilla-corn	item	67.2	2.15	12.8	1.14	0	-	1.56
Rice-brown-Uncle Ben's	cup	220	5	46.4	1.82	0	0.462	2.48
Shake'n Bake	ounce	116	2.44	17.7	4.26	-	-	-
Bisquick mix-dry	cup	480	8	76	16	-	-	3.02
Tortilla chips-Doritos	ounce	139	2	18.6	6.6	0	1.43	1.85
Croutons-herb seasoned	cup	100	4.29	20	0	0	0	1.41
Tortilla-flour	item	95	2.5	17.3	1.8	0	-	0.778
Rice-Spanish-home recipe	cup	213	4.4	40.7	4.2	0	-	1.83
Stuffing-mix-dry form	cup	111	3.9	21.7	1.1	-	-	-
Stuffing-mix-prepared	cup	501	9.1	49.8	30.5	-	-	-
Rice cake-regular	item	35	0.7	7.6	0.28	0	-	0.158
Noodles-Ramen-oriental	cup	207	5.9	30.7	8.6	-	-	2.04
MEATS								
Bacon-pork-broiled/fried	slice	36.3	1.92	0.037	3.1	5.36	1.1	0
Roast beef-rib lean/fat	slice	308	18.3	0	25.5	73.1	10.8	0
Roast beef-rib-lean	slice	122	13.9	0	7.03	41.3	2.96	0
Steak-sirloin-lean/fat	item	238	23.3	0	15.3	76.5	6.38	0
Steak-sirloin-lean/broiled	item	116	17	0	4.89	49.8	2	0
Steak-round-lean/fat	slice	179	26.2	0	7.5	72	2.8	0
Corned beef hash-canned	cup	400	19	24	25	50	11.9	-
Lamb-chop-lean/fat-broiled	serving	307	18.8	0	25.2	84.2	10.8	0
Lamb-chop/rib-lean-broiled	serving	134	15.8	0	7.38	51.9	2.65	0
Lamb-leg-lean/fat-roasted	slice	219	21.7	0	14	79	5.85	0
Beef-liver-fried/marg	slice	184	22.7	6.67	6.8	410	2.4	0
Ham-reg-roasted-pork	cup	249	31.7	0	12.6	82.6	4.37	0
Ham-reg-lunch meat-11% fat	slice	52	4.98	0.88	3	16.2	0.962	0
Pork-chop-lean/fat-broiled	item	284	19.3	0	22.3	77	8.06	0
Pork-chop-lean/broiled	item	169	18.4	0	10.1	63	3.48	0
Pork-loin-lean/fat-roast	item	268	22.4	0	19.1	80	6.92	0
Pork-loin-lean-roasted	slice	173	20.5	0	9.42	65.5	3.25	0
Pork-tenderloin-lean-roast	ounce	47.1	8.18	0	1.37	26.3	0.471	0
Bologna-pork	slice	56.8	3.52	0.168	4.57	13.6	1.58	0
Braunschweiger-saus-pork	slice	64.6	2.43	0.56	5.78	28.1	1.96	0
Sausage-patty-pork-cooked	item	100	5.31	0.28	8.41	22.4	2.92	0
Deviled ham-canned	tbsp	45	2	0	4	10	1.5	0
Frankfurter-hot dog-no bun	item	183	6.43	1.46	16.6	28.5	6.13	0
Sausage-link-pork-cooked	item	48	2.55	0.13	4.05	10.8	1.41	0
Salami-dry or hard-park	slice	40.7	2.26	0.16	3.37	7.9	1.19	0
Salami-cooked-beef	slice	60.3	3.46	0.646	4.76	15	2.07	0
Italian sausage-pork-link	item	216	13.4	1.01	17.2	52	6.05	0
Canadian bacon-pork-grill	slice	43	5.64	0.315	1.96	13.5	0.66	0
Liverwurst/liver saus-pork	slice	59	2.54	0.4	5.14	28	1.91	0
Polish sausage-pork	item	740	32	3.71	65.2	159	23.4	0
Kielbasa-pork/beef	slice	80.6	3.45	0.56	7.06	17.4	2.58	0

FOOD COMPOSITION TABLE—cont'd

Food Name	Serving	KCAL Kc	PROT Gm	CARB Gm	FAT Gm	CHOL Mg	SAFA Gm	FIBD Gm
Knockwurst-pork/beef-link	item	209	8.08	1.2	18.9	39.4	6.94	0
Mortadella-pork/beef	slice	46.7	2.46	0.458	3.81	8.4	1.43	0
Bacon bits	tbsp	26.6	1.92	1.72	1.55	0	-	-
Spareribs-pork-braised	ounce	113	8.25	0	8.61	34.4	3.34	0
Steak-chicken fried	item	389	17.9	12.3	30	-	-	0
Pot roast-arm-beef-cooked	slice	231	33	0	9.98	101	3.79	0
Steak-rib-cooked	item	221	28	0	11.2	80	4.75	0
Hamburger-ground-reg-baked	serving	244	19.6	0	17.8	74	6.99	0
Hamburger-ground-reg-fried	serving	260	20.3	0	19.2	75.7	7.53	0
MISCELLANEOUS								
Pickle/hot dog relish	ounce	35	0	8	0	0	0	-
Pickle/hamburger relish	ounce	30	0	7	0	0	0	-
Baking powder-home use	tsp	3.87	0.003	0.936	0	0	0	-
Baking powder-low sodium	tsp	7.4	0.004	1.79	0	0	0	-
Gelatin-dry envelope	item	25	6	0	0	0	0	0
Gelatin dessert-prep	cup	140	4	34	0	0	0	0
Olives-green-pickled-can	item	3.75	0.1	0.1	0.5	0	0.05	0.104
Olives-mission-rice-can	item	5	0.1	0.1	0.667	0	0.067	0.09
Pickle-dill-cucumber-med	item	5	0	1	0	0	0	0.78
Pickle-fresh pack-cucumber	item	5	0	1.5	0	0	0	0.09
Pickle-sweet-gherkin-small	item	20	0	5	0	0	0	0.165
Pickle relish-sweet	tbsp	20	0	5	0	0	0	-
Popsickle	item	70	0	18	0	0	0	-
Vinegar-cider	tbsp	0	0	1	0	0	0	0
Yeast-baker-dry-act-packet	serving	20	3	3	0	0	0	2.21
Yeast-brewers-dry	tbsp	25	3	3	0	0	0	-
Baking soda	tsp	0	0	0	0	0	0	0
Jello-gel-sugar free-prep	cup	16	2	0	0	0	0	0
Gel-D Zerta-low-cal-prep	cup	16	4	0	0	0	0	0
Chewing gum-Wrigleys	item	10	0	2.3	-	0	0	-
Vinegar-distilled	cup	29	0	12	0	0	0	0
Chewing gum-candy coated	item	5	-	1.6	-	0	0	-
NUTS/SEEDS								
Nuts-almond-shelled-sliver	cup	677	22.9	23.5	60	0	5.69	10.7
Nuts-Brazil-dried-shelled	cup	918	20.1	17.9	92.7	0	22.6	10.8
Nuts-filbert-hazel-dri-chop	cup	727	15	17.6	72	0	5.29	9.77
Nuts-peanuts-oiled roasted	cup	837	37.9	27.3	71	0	9.85	12.8
Peanut-butter-smooth type	tbsp	94.1	3.94	3.32	8	0	1.53	0.96
Nuts-pecans-dried-halves	cup	720	8.37	19.7	73.1	0	5.85	7.02
Nuts-walnut-black-dri-chop	cup	759	30.4	15.1	70.7	0	4.54	8.08
Nuts-walnut-Persian/English	cup	770	17.2	22	74.2	0	6.7	5.76
Nuts-cashew-dry roasted	cup	786	21	44.8	63.5	0	12.5	10
Nuts-macadamia-dried	cup	941	11.1	18.4	98.8	0	14.8	12.4
Nuts-mixed-dry roasted	cup	814	23.7	34.7	70.5	0	9.45	11.6
Nuts-mixed-oiled roasted	cup	876	23.8	30.4	80	0	12.4	12.8
Nuts-peanuts-Spanish-dried	cup	828	37.7	23.6	71.9	0	9.98	11.7
Nuts-pecans-oil roasted	cup	754	7.65	17.7	78.3	0	6.27	8.47
Nuts-pistachio-dried	cup	739	26.3	31.8	61.9	0	7.84	13.8
Nuts-pistachio-dry roasted	cup	776	19.1	35.2	67.6	0	8.56	13.8
Seeds/pumpkin/squash-roast	cup	285	11.9	34.4	12.4	0	2.35	29.4

FOOD COMPOSITION TABLE—cont'd

Food Name	Serving	KCAL Kc	PROT Gm	CARB Gm	FAT Gm	CHOL Mg	SAFA Gm	FIBD Gm
Seeds-sesame-roasted-whole	ounce	161	4.82	7.31	13.6	0	1.91	5.32
Seeds-sunflower-oil roasted	cup	830	28.8	19.9	77.6	0	8.13	9.18
Peanut butter-low sodium	tbsp	95	5	2.5	8.5	0	1.36	1.7
Nuts-peanuts-oil-salted	cup	837	37.9	27.3	71	0	9.85	12.8
Peanut butter-chunk style	tbsp	94.8	3.87	3.48	8.04	0	1.54	1.06
Peanut butter-old fashion	tbsp	95	4.2	2.7	8.1	0	1.5	1.06
POULTRY PRODUCTS								
Chicken-breast-fried/flour	item	436	62.4	3.22	17.4	176	4.8	0.07
Chicken-drumstick-fried	item	120	13.2	0.8	6.72	44	1.79	0
Chicken-breast-fri/batter	item	728	69.6	25.2	36.9	238	9.86	-
Turkey-dark meat-no skin	cup	262	40	0	10.1	119	3.39	0
Turkey-light-no skin-roasted	cup	219	41.9	0	4.5	97	1.44	0
Turkey-light/dark-no skin	cup	238	41	0	6.95	107	2.29	0
Turkey-breast-no skin-roasted	item	826	184	0	4.5	508	1.47	0
Chicken-giblets-fri/flour	cup	402	47.2	6.31	19.5	647	5.5	-
Chicken-giblets-simmered	cup	228	37.5	1.37	6.92	570	2.16	0
Chicken-liver-simmered	cup	219	34.1	1.23	7.63	883	2.58	0
Chicken-breast-roasted	item	386	58.4	0	15.3	166	4.3	0
Chicken-breast-stewed	item	404	60.3	0	16.3	166	4.58	0
Chicken-breast-no skin-fried	item	322	57.5	0.88	8.1	156	2.22	0
Chicken-breast-no skin-roasted	item	284	53.4	0	6.14	146	1.74	0
Chicken-leg roasted	item	265	29.6	0	15.4	105	4.24	0
Chicken-leg-no skin-roasted	item	182	25.7	0	8.01	89	2.18	0
Chicken-leg-no skin-stewed	item	187	26.5	0	8.14	90	2.22	0
Chicken-thigh-fried/flour	item	162	16.6	1.97	9.29	60	2.54	0.04
Chicken-thigh-no skin-roasted	item	109	13.5	0	5.66	49	1.57	0
Chicken-wing-fried/flour	item	103	8.36	0.76	7.09	26	1.94	0
Chicken-wing-roasted	item	99	9.13	0	6.62	29	1.85	0
Chicken-wing-stewed	item	100	9.11	0	6.73	28	1.88	0
Duck-flesh & skin-roasted	item	2574	145	0	217	640	73.9	0
Duck-no skin-roasted	item	890	104	0	49.5	396	18.4	0
Chicken-frankfurter	item	116	5.82	3.06	8.76	45.5	2.49	0
Chicken-liver pate-can	tbsp	26	1.75	0.85	1.7	-	-	0.01
Chicken roll-light	slice	45	5.54	0.695	2.09	14.2	0.574	0
Chicken spread-canned	tbsp	25	2	0.7	1.52	-	-	-
Turk ham-cured thigh meat	slice	36.5	5.37	0.105	1.44	15.9	0.483	0
Turkey loaf-breast	serving	31.2	6.39	0	0.449	11.6	0.136	0
Turkey pastrami	slice	40	5.21	0.47	1.76	15.3	0.514	0
Turkey roll-light	ounce	41.7	5.31	0.15	2.05	12.2	0.574	0
SAUCES/DIPS								
Sauce-chili-bottled	tbsp	16	0.4	3.7	0	0	0	-
Sauce-Heinz 57	tbsp	15	0.4	2.7	0.2	0	0	-
Sauce-tartar-regular	tbsp	75	0	1	8	9	1.5	-
Dip-guacamole-Kraft	tbsp	25	0.5	1.5	2	0	-	-
Dip-French onion-Kraft	tbsp	30	0.5	1.5	2	0	-	-
Sauce-taco-canned	floz	11	0.4	2.2	0.7	0	-	-
Sauce-salsa/chilies-canned	fl oz	10	0.4	2	0.7	0	0	-
Sauce-picante-canned	fl oz	9	0.3	1.9	0.5	0	0	-
Tomato catsup	tbsp	15	0	4	0	0	0	-
Sauce-barbecue	cup	188	4.5	32	4.5	0	0.675	2.3

FOOD COMPOSITION TABLE—cont'd

Food Name	Serving	KCAL Kc	PROT Gm	CARB Gm	FAT Gm	CHOL Mg	SAFA Gm	FIBD Gm
Mustard-yellow-prepared	tsp	5	0.1	0.1	0.1	0	0	0.06
Sauce-bearnaise-mix/milk	cup	701	8.34	17.5	68.3	189	41.8	0.09
Sauce-cheese-mix/milk	cup	307	16	23.2	17.1	53	9.32	0.1
Sauce-curry-mix/milk	cup	269	10.7	25.7	14.7	35.4	6.04	0.9
Sauce-mushroom-mix/milk	cup	227	11.3	23.8	10.3	34	5.39	0.5
Sauce-sweet/sour-mix/prep	cup	294	0.751	72.7	0.063	0	0	-
Sauce-soy	tbsp	9.54	0.931	1.53	0.014	0	0.002	-
Gravy-beef-canned	cup	123	8.74	11.2	5.49	6.99	2.69	0.093
Gravy-chicken-canned	cup	188	4.59	12.9	13.6	4.76	3.36	-
Gravy-turkey-canned	cup	121	6.2	12.2	5.01	4.76	1.48	-
Sauce-marinara-canned	cup	170	4	25.5	8.38	0	1.2	-
Sauce-tomato-can-salt add	cup	73.5	3.26	17.6	0.417	0	0.059	3.68
Sauce-tomato-Spanish-can	cup	80.5	3.51	17.7	0.659	0	0.092	3.66
Sauce-spaghetti-canned	cup	271	4.53	39.7	11.9	0	1.7	-
Sauce-sour cream-mix/milk	cup	509	19.1	45.4	30.2	91	16.1	-
Sauce-Teriyaki-bottled	tbsp	15.1	1.07	2.87	0	0	0	-
Horseradish-prepared	tbsp	6	0.2	1.4	0	0	0	-
Sauce-Worcestershire	tbsp	12	0.3	2.7	0	0	0	-
Sauce-tabasco	tsp	0	0.1	0.1	0	0	0	0
Mustard-brown-prepared	cup	228	14.8	13.3	15.8	0	-	-
Sauce-tomato-can-low sod	cup	90	4	18	0	0	0	3.39
SOUPS								
Soup-cream/chick-can-milk	cup	191	7.46	15	11.5	27.3	4.64	0.5
Soup-cream/mushroom-milk	cup	203	6.05	15	13.6	19.8	5.13	-
Soup-tomato-can-milk	cup	161	6.1	22.3	6	17.4	2.9	0.8
Soup-bean/bacon-can-water	cup	173	7.89	22.8	5.94	2.53	1.52	3.2
Soup-beef broth-can-ready	cup	16.8	2.74	0.096	0.528	0	0.264	0
Soup-clam-Manhattan-water	cup	78.1	2.2	12.2	2.22	2.44	0.383	-
Soup-minestrone-can-water	cup	81.9	4.26	11.2	2.51	2.41	0.554	1.9
Soup-pea-split-can-water	cup	189	10.3	28	4.4	7.59	1.77	-
Soup-tomato-can-water	cup	85.4	2.05	16.6	1.92	0	0.366	0.9
Soup-vegetable beef-can	cup	78.4	5.61	10.2	1.91	4.9	0.858	0.98
Soup-vegetarian-can-water	cup	72	2.1	12	1.93	0	0.289	1.21
Soup-beef-broth-dehy-cubed	item	6.12	0.62	0.58	0.14	0.144	0.072	-
Soup-onion-dehy-packet	serving	115	4.52	20.9	2.33	1.95	0.538	2.2
Soup-cream/celery-can-milk	cup	164	5.68	14.5	9.7	32.2	3.94	0.77
Soup-cheese-can-milk	cup	230	9.46	16.2	14.6	47.7	9.11	-
Soup-chick broth-can/water	cup	39	4.93	0.93	1.39	0	0.39	0
Soup-chicken noodle-can	cup	74.7	4.05	9.35	2.46	7.23	0.65	1.45
Soup-clam-New England-milk	cup	163	9.47	16.6	6.6	22.3	2.95	-
Soup-cream/potato-can-water	cup	148	5.78	17.2	6.45	22.3	3.77	-
Soup-black bean-can-water	cup	116	5.63	19.8	1.51	0	0.395	-
Soup-beef-chunky-can	cup	170	11.7	19.6	5.14	14.4	2.55	-
Soup-chicken-chunky-can	cup	178	12.7	17.3	6.63	30.1	1.98	-
Soup-chicken/rice-can	cup	127	12.3	13	3.19	12	0.96	1.44
Soup-onion-can-water	cup	57.8	3.75	8.17	1.74	0	0.265	-
Soup-pea-green-can-water	cup	165	8.6	26.5	2.94	0	1.4	-
Soup-tomato rice-can-water	cup	119	2.11	21.9	2.72	2.47	0.519	1.7
Soup-turkey-chunky-can	cup	135	10.2	14.1	4.41	9.44	1.23	2.5
Soup-turkey noodle-can	cup	68.3	3.9	8.63	1.99	4.88	0.561	0.7
Soup-turkey vegetable-can	cup	72.3	3.09	8.63	3.04	2.41	0.892	0.964

FOOD COMPOSITION TABLE—cont'd

Food Name	Serving	KCAL Kc	PROT Gm	CARB Gm	FAT Gm	CHOL Mg	SAFA Gm	FIBD Gm
SUGARS/SWEETS								
Nuts-coconut-dri-flake-can	cup	341	2.58	31.5	24.4	0	21.6	4.4
Icing-cake-white-boiled	cup	295	1	75	0	0	0	0
Icing-cake-white/coco-boil	cup	605	3	124	13	0	11	-
Icing-cake-choc-mix/prep	cup	1035	9	185	38	0	23.4	-
Icing-cake-fudge-mix/water	cup	830	7	183	16	0	5.1	-
Icing-cake-white-uncooked	cup	1200	2	260	231	0	12.7	0
Candy-caramels-plain/choc	ounce	115	1	22	3	0	1.6	0.784
Candy-milk chocolate-plain	ounce	145	2	16	9	0	5.5	-
Candy-chocolate-semisweet	cup	860	7	97	61	0	36.2	-
Candy-choc coated peanuts	ounce	160	5	11	12	0	4	-
Candy-fondant-uncoated	ounce	105	0	25	1	0	0.1	0
Candy-fudge-choc-plain	ounce	115	1	21	3	0	1.3	-
Candy-gum drops	ounce	00	0	25	0	0	0	0
Candy-hard	ounce	110	0	28	0	0	0	0
Marshmallows	ounce	90	1	23	0	0	0	0
Honey-strained/extracted	tbsp	65	0	17	0	0	0	0.06
Jams/preserves-regular	tbsp	55	0	14	0	0	0	0.2
Molasses-can-light	tbsp	50	0	13	-	0	-	0
Molasses-cane-blackstrap	tbsp	45	0	11	-	0	-	0
Sugar-brown-pressed down	cup	820	0	212	0	0	0	0
Sugar-white-granulated	tbsp	45	0	12	0	0	0	0
Sugar-white-powder-sifted	cup	385	0	100	0	0	0	0
Nuts-coconut-dried-shred	cup	466	2.68	44.3	33	0	29.3	3.9
Nuts-coconut-cream-raw	cup	792	8.7	16	83.2	0	73.8	1.6
Candy-milk choc/peanuts	ounce	154	4	12.6	10.8	-	5.22	-
Candy-milk choc/almonds	ounce	151	2.6	14.5	10.1	-	4.06	-
Sugar-Sweet & Low-packet	item	4	-	0.9	-	0	-	-
Sugar-Equal-packet	item	4	0	1	0	0	0	-
Candy-Life Savers	item	7.8	0	1.94	0.02	0	0	0
Candy-M & M's package	item	220	3	31	10	-	-	-
Candy-Snickers bar	item	270	6	33	13	-	4.73	-
Candy-Milky Way bar	item	260	3	43	9	-	5.05	-
Candy-Kit Kat bar	item	210	3	25	11	-	5.6	-
Candy-Bit O Honey	ounce	121	0.9	21.2	3.6	-	1.65	-
Candy-Almond Joy	ounce	151	1.7	18.5	7.8	-	1.74	-
Candy-jelly beans	item	6.6	0	2.64	0	0	0	0
Candy-peanut brittle	ounce	123	2.4	20.4	4.4	-	1.85	-
Candy-peanut butter cup	piece	92	2.2	8.7	5.35	2.5	2.8	-
Candy-lollipop	item	108	0	28	0	0	0	0
VEGETABLES								
V-8 veg juice-low sodium	cup	51	0	9.72	0	0	0	2.7
Tomato juice-low sodium	cup	41.5	1.85	10.3	0.146	0	0.02	2.8
Beans-garbanzo-can	serving	27.8	1.31	4.66	0.511	0	0.07	1.4
Beans-navy pea-dry cooked	cup	225	15	40	1	0	-	9.31
Beans-red kidney-can	cup	230	15	42	1	0	-	12.5
Peas-split-dry-cooked	cup	230	16	42	1	0	-	10.5
Asparagus-froz-boil-spears	cup	50.4	5.31	8.77	0.756	0	0.171	2.16
Beans-lima-froz-boil-drain	cup	170	10.3	32	0.578	0	0.131	8.33
Beans-snap-green-raw-boil	cup	43.8	2.36	9.86	0.35	0	0.08	2.25
Beans-green-froz-French	cup	35.1	1.84	8.26	0.189	0	0.41	2.16

FOOD COMPOSITION TABLE—cont'd

Food Name	Serving	KCAL Kc	PROT Gm	CARB Gm	FAT Gm	CHOL Mg	SAFA Gm	FIBD Gm
Beans-snap-green-can-cuts	cup	27	1.55	6.08	0.135	0	0.03	1.76
Beans-snap-wax-raw-boil	cup	43.8	2.36	9.86	0.35	0	0.08	2.25
Beans-snap-yellow/wax-can	cup	27.2	1.56	6.12	0.136	0	0.03	1.77
Beans-mung-sprouted-boil	cup	26.3	2.54	5.24	0.113	0	0.031	2.7
Beets-can-sliced-drain	cup	52.7	1.55	12.2	0.238	0	0.039	2.89
Cowpeas-blackeye-raw-boil	cup	160	5.23	33.5	0.627	0	0.158	11
Cowpeas-blackeye-froz-boil	cup	224	14.4	40.4	1.12	0	0.298	9.8
Broccoli-raw	cup	24.6	2.62	4.61	0.308	0	0.048	2.46
Broccoli-raw-boil-drain	cup	43.4	4.62	7.84	0.543	0	0.084	4.03
Cabbage-white mustard-raw	cup	9.1	1.05	1.53	0.14	0	0.018	0.7
Broccoli-froz-boil-drain	cup	51.8	5.74	9.85	0.21	0	0.033	7.3
Cabbage-common-raw-shred	cup	21.6	1.09	4.83	0.162	0	0.021	1.8
Cabbage-common-boil-drain	cup	30.5	1.39	6.92	0.363	0	0.046	4
Cabbage-red-raw-shredded	cup	18.9	0.973	4.28	0.182	0	0.024	1.4
Cabbage-celery-raw	cup	12.2	0.912	2.45	0.152	0	0.033	0.76
Cabbage-white mustard-boil	cup	20.4	2.65	3.03	0.272	0	0.036	2.72
Carrot-raw-whole-scraped	item	31	0.74	7.3	0.137	0	0.022	2.3
Carrot-raw-shred-scraped	cup	47.3	1.13	11.2	0.209	0	0.033	3.52
Carrots-boil-drain-sliced	cup	70.2	1.7	16.3	0.28	0	0.053	5.77
Carrots-can-sliced-drain	cup	33.6	0.934	8.08	0.277	0	0.052	2.19
Cauliflower-raw-chopped	cup	24	1.99	4.92	0.18	0	0.027	2.4
Cauliflower-raw-boil-drain	cup	30	2.32	5.74	0.22	0	0.046	27.3
Cauliflower-froz-boil	cup	34.2	2.9	6.75	0.396	0	0.059	3.24
Celery-Pascal-raw-stalk	item	6.4	0.3	1.46	0.056	0	0.015	0.64
Celery-Pascal-raw-diced	cup	19.2	0.9	4.38	0.168	0	0.044	1.92
Collards-raw-boil-drain	cup	34.6	1.73	7.85	0.243	0	-	2.1
Collards-frozen-boil-drain	cup	61.2	5.05	12.1	0.697	0	-	5.2
Corn-kernels from 1 ear	item	83.2	2.56	19.3	0.986	0	0.152	2.85
Corn-kernels & cob-froz-boil	item	117	3.92	28.1	0.932	0	0.144	2.65
Corn-froz-boil-kernels	cup	134	4.98	33.9	0.116	0	0.018	3.47
Corn-sweet-cream style-can	cup	184	4.45	46.4	1.08	0	0.166	3.07
Corn-sweet-can-drained	cup	134	4.32	30.7	1.65	0	0.254	2.31
Cucumber-raw-sliced	cup	13.5	0.562	3.03	0.135	0	0.034	1.04
Endive-raw-chopped	cup	8.5	0.625	1.68	0.1	0	0.024	-
Lettuce-butterhead-leaves	slice	1.95	0.194	0.348	0.03	0	0.004	0.15
Lettuce-iceberg-raw-leaves	piece	2.61	0.202	0.418	0.038	0	0.005	0.2
Lettuce-iceberg-raw-chop	cup	7.15	0.556	1.15	0.105	0	0.014	0.55
Lettuce-looseleaf-raw	cup	9.9	0.715	1.93	0.165	0	0.022	0.76
Mushrooms-raw-chopped	cup	17.5	1.46	3.26	0.294	0	0.039	0.91
Onions-mature-raw-chopped	cup	60.8	1.86	13.8	0.256	0	0.042	2.56
Carrots-frozen-boil-drain	cup	52.6	1.74	12	0.161	0	0.031	5.4
Onions-mature-boil-drain	cup	92.4	2.86	21.3	0.399	0	0.065	1.68
Onions-young green	item	1.25	0.087	0.278	0.007	0	0.001	0.12
Parsley-raw-chopped	tbsp	1.32	0.088	0.276	0.03	0	0.005	0.176
Peas-green-can-drained	cup	117	7.51	21.4	0.595	0	0.105	5.78
Peas-green-froz-boil-drain	cup	125	8.24	22.8	0.432	0	0.078	6.08
Peppers-hot-red-dried	tsp	5	0	1	0	0	0	0.685
Potato-French fried-raw	item	13.5	0.2	1.8	0.7	0	0.17	0.16
Potato-French fried-froz	item	11.1	0.173	1.7	0.438	0	0.208	0.16
Potato-hashed brown-froz	cup	340	4.93	43.8	17.9	0	7.01	1.5

FOOD COMPOSITION TABLE—cont'd

Food Name	Serving	KCAL Kc	PROT Gm	CARB Gm	FAT Gm	CHOL Mg	SAFA Gm	FIBD Gm
Potato-mashed-milk/butter	cup	223	3.95	35.1	8.88	4.2	2.17	3.15
Potato-mashed-dehy-prep	cup	166	4.2	27.5	4.62	4	1.43	1.2
Potato chips-salt added	item	10.5	0.128	1.04	0.708	0	0.181	0.029
Radishes-raw	item	0.765	0.027	0.162	0.024	0	0.001	0.1
Sauerkraut-canned	cup	44.8	2.15	10.1	0.33	0	0.083	6.06
Spinach-raw-chopped	cup	12.3	1.6	1.96	0.196	cup	0.032	1.46
Spinach-raw-boil-drain	cup	41.4	5.35	6.75	0.468	0	0.076	3.96
Spinach-froz-boil-chopped	cup	57.4	6.44	10.9	0.431	0	0.068	4.51
Squash-summer-boil-sliced	cup	36	1.64	7.76	0.558	0	0.115	2.52
Squash-winter-bake-mash	cup	80	1.82	17.9	1.29	0	0.267	5.74
Sweet potato-bake-peel	item	117	1.96	27.7	0.125	0	0.027	3.42
Sweet potato-boil-mashed	cup	344	5.41	79.6	0.984	0	0.21	9.84
Sweet potato-candied	piece	144	0.914	29.3	3.41	0	1.42	1.1
Sweet potato-can-mashed	cup	258	5.05	59.2	0.51	0	0.11	4.59
Tomato-raw-red-ripe	item	25.8	1.05	5.71	0.406	0	0.056	1.6
Tomato-red-can-whole	cup	48	2.23	10.3	0.576	0	0.084	1.93
Tomato juice-can	cup	41.5	1.85	10.3	0.146	0	0.02	2.9
Tomato powder	ounce	85.8	3.67	21.2	0.125	0	0.018	-
Alfalfa seeds-sprouted-raw	cup	9.57	1.32	1.25	0.228	0	0.023	0.726
Artichokes-boil-drain	item	60	4.18	13.4	0.192	0	0.044	4
Beans-lima-can	cup	186	11.3	34.4	0.744	0	0.168	10.4
Beans-pinto-froz-boil	ounce	46	2.64	8.77	0.136	0	0.016	1.39
Beans-shelled-can	cup	73.5	4.31	15.2	0.466	0	0.056	12
Chives-raw-chopped	tbsp	0.75	0.084	0.114	0.018	0	0.003	0.096
Eggplant-boiled-drained	cup	26.9	0.8	6.37	0.221	0	0.042	2.69
Garlic-raw-cloves	item	4.47	0.191	0.992	0.015	0	0.003	-
Leeks-boil-drain	item	38.4	1.01	9.45	0.248	0	0.033	3.97
Mushrooms-boil-drain	item	3.24	0.26	0.617	0.056	0	0.007	0.264
Mushrooms-can-drain	item	2.88	0.224	0.595	0.035	0	0.005	0.216
Onion rings-froz-prep-heat	item	40.7	0.534	3.82	2.67	0	0.858	0.382
Peppers-jalapeno-can-chop	cup	32.6	1.09	0.664	0.816	0	0.084	-
Potato-skin-baked	item	115	2.49	26.7	0.058	0	0.015	3.02
Potato-au gratin-home rec	cup	323	12.4	27.6	18.6	56.4	11.6	4.41
Potato-hash brown-prep-raw	cup	239	3.77	11.6	21.7	-	8.48	3.12
Potato-scallop-home rec	cup	211	7.03	26.4	9.02	29.4	5.52	4.41
Potato-scallop-mix-prep	ounce	26.4	0.602	3.63	1.22	-	0.748	0.54
Potato pancakes-home rec	item	495	4.63	26.4	12.6	93.5	3.42	-
Pumpkin pie mix-can	cup	281	2.94	71.3	0.351	0	0.176	-
Rutabagas-boil-drain	cup	57.8	1.87	13.2	0.323	0	0.042	2.5
Seaweed-wakame-raw	ounce	12.8	0.861	2.6	0.182	0	0.037	1.2
Squash-zucchini-raw-sliced	cup	18.2	1.51	3.77	0.182	0	0.038	2
Squash-zucchini-raw-boil	cup	28.8	1.15	7.07	0.09	0	0.018	2.3
Squash-zucchini-froz-boil	cup	37.9	2.56	7.94	0.29	0	0.06	3.23
Squash-zucchini-italia-can	cup	65.8	2.34	15.5	0.25	0	0.052	7.02
Succotash-boil-drain	cup	221	9.73	46.8	1.54	0	0.284	14
Tomato-red-raw-boil	cup	64.8	2.57	14	0.984	0	0.137	2.1
Tomato-stew-cook-home rec	cup	79.8	1.98	13.2	2.71	0	0.526	1.04
Tomato-red-can-stewed	cup	66.3	2.37	16.5	0.357	0	0.051	2.04
Tomato-paste-can-low sod	cup	220	9.9	49.3	2.33	0	0.333	11.3
Tomato puree-can-low sod	cup	103	4.18	25.1	0.3	0	0.04	5.75

FOOD COMPOSITION TABLE—cont'd

Food Name	Serving	KCAL Kc	PROT Gm	CARB Gm	FAT Gm	CHOL Mg	SAFA Gm	FIBD Gm
Vegetable juice-can	cup	46	1.52	11	0.218	0	0.032	2.7
Nuts-chestnuts-roasted	ounce	67.9	1.27	14.9	0.34	0	0.05	2.19
Squash-hubbard-boil-mash	cup	70.8	3.49	15.2	0.873	0	0.179	4.2
Squash-butternut-baked	cup	82	1.84	21.5	0.185	0	0.039	3.5
Squash-acorn-baked	cup	115	2.29	29.9	0.287	0	0.059	4.3
Lettuce-romaine-raw-shred	cup	8.96	0.9	1.33	0.112	0	0.014	0.952
Soybean-dry-cooked	cup	234	19.8	19.4	10.3	0	-	-
Tofu-soybean curd	piece	86	9.4	2.9	5	0	-	1.44
Tomato-can-low sodium diet	cup	48	2.23	10.3	0.576	0	0.084	1.69
Spinach-can-solids/liquids	cup	44.5	4.94	6.83	0.866	0	0.14	5.08
Tomato paste-can-salt add	cup	220	9.9	49.3	2.33	0	0.332	11.3
Tomato puree-can-salt add	cup	103	4.18	25.1	0.3	0	0.04	5.75
Miso-fermented soybeans	cup	567	32.5	76.9	16.7	0	2.41	9.9
Beans-baked beans-canned	cup	236	12.2	52.1	1.14	0	0.295	19.6
Beans-refried beans	cup	271	15.8	46.8	2.7	0	10.4	11.6

INDEX